METHODS IN MOLECULAR BIOLOGY™

Series Editor
John M. Walker
School of Life Sciences
University of Hertfordshire
Hatfield, Hertfordshire, AL10 9AB, UK

For other titles published in this series, go to
www.springer.com/series/7651

MicroRNAs and the Immune System

Methods and Protocols

Edited by

Silvia Monticelli

Institute for Research in Biomedicine, Bellinzona, Switzerland

Humana Press

Editor
Silvia Monticelli
Institute for Research in Biomedicine
Bellinzona
Switzerland
silvia.monticelli@irb.unisi.ch

ISSN 1064-3745 e-ISSN 1940-6029
ISBN 978-1-4939-6150-4 ISBN 978-1-60761-811-9 (eBook)
DOI 10.1007/978-1-60761-811-9

Cover Illustration: Image courtesy of Lorenzo Deho'

Printed on acid-free paper

Humana Press is part of Springer Science+Business Media (www.springer.com)

Preface

The hematopoietic system is a paradigm for the differentiation of distinct cell lineages from multipotent progenitors. Differentiation is modulated by an intricate network of growth and transcription factors that simultaneously regulate the commitment, proliferation, apoptosis, and maturation of hematopoietic stem and progenitor cells. MicroRNAs (miRNAs) are endogenous small noncoding RNAs that regulate gene expression by binding to target messenger RNAs and inducing translational repression, cleavage, or destabilization of the target. Each miRNA can potentially regulate expression of a distinct set of genes and therefore miRNAs appear ideally suited to rapidly adjusting protein concentrations in cells, as would be expected to be required during cell differentiation. In fact, certain miRNAs are differentially expressed, both spatially and temporally, in many types of immune cells. Moreover, consistent with the discovery that miRNAs modulate gene expression, altered miRNA expression has been associated with various types of diseases, including cancer.

The overall importance of miRNAs during hematopoiesis has been investigated by specific disruption of steps in miRNA biogenesis, indicating a critical function for miRNAs in the biology of cells that constitute the immune system. In this volume of Methods in Molecular Biology, various methods to study miRNA expression in cells of the immune system are described, such as splinted ligation and qRT-PCR assays, as well as high-throughput profiling through cloning, deep sequencing and microarrays. A complementary approach to expression profiling is the use of miRNA reporter vectors for assaying miRNA activity. Moreover, a method to visualize miRNAs in situ in bone marrow cells is described. Besides providing an overview for the most up-to-date techniques to study miRNA expression, this book encompasses methods to study miRNA functions in various cell types of the immune system, using loss- and gain-of-function techniques, both at a single cell-type level and in entire model organisms, as well as for studies of miRNAs in the context of viruses and the immune response.

One of the most elusive areas in the miRNA field is target recognition. As a result, different computational approaches have been developed to predict miRNA target sites throughout the transcriptome. Here, tools are also provided to help understanding and navigating these bioinformatics databases. Besides the analysis of miRNA expression and function, a major challenge is represented by the precise understanding of miRNA function at a molecular level. We therefore, provide protocols for the emerging field of miRNAs posttranscriptional modifications (i.e., RNA editing), as well as for NMR structures of miRNA:mRNA complexes.

This volume of Methods will be of interest to immunologists approaching the study of miRNAs in cells of the immune system, biochemists and molecular biologists interested in the exploration of the posttranscriptional modifications and mechanisms of action of miRNAs, as well as to virologists and bioinformaticians.

Dr. Silvia Monticelli

Acknowledgments

I would like to especially thank Dr. Luisa Granziero for the invaluable help and support throughout the preparation of this volume.

Contents

Contributors

K. MARK ANSEL • *Department of Microbiology & Immunology, Strategic Asthma Basic Research Center, University of California San Francisco, San Francisco CA, USA*

ALESSIA BACCARINI • *Department of Genetics and Genomic Sciences, Mount Sinai School of Medicine, New York NY, USA*

BRIAN D. BROWN • *Department of Genetics and Genomic Sciences, Mount Sinai School of Medicine, New York NY, USA*

GEORGE CALIN • *Department of Experimental Therapeutics and Department of Cancer Genetics, University of Texas M.D. Anderson Cancer Center, Houston TX, USA*

STEFANO CASOLA • *IFOM, The FIRC Institute of Molecular Oncology Foundation, Milan, Italy*

MIRKO CEVEC • *Slovenian NMR Centre, National Institute of Chemistry, Ljubljana, Slovenia*

SANGPEN CHAMNONGPOL • *Affymetrix, Inc, Cleveland, OH, USA*

JEN-TSAN CHI • *Department of Molecular Genetics and Microbiology, The Institute for Genome Sciences and Policy, Duke University School of Medicine, Durham NC, USA*

CHAD J. CREIGHTON • *Dan Duncan Cancer Center, Baylor College of Medicine, Houston TX, USA*

VIRGINIA G. DE YÉBENES • *DNA Hypermutation and Cancer Group, Spanish National Cancer Research Center (CNIO), Madrid, Spain*

SILVANA DEBERNARDI • *Medical Oncology Centre, Barts & The London School of Medicine and Dentistry, Institute of Cancer, Queen Mary University of London, London, UK*

AMANDA DIXON-MCIVER • *Medical Oncology Centre, Barts & The London School of Medicine and Dentistry, Institute of Cancer, Queen Mary University of London, London, UK*

DYLAN E. DUPUIS • *Department of Biological Sciences, Lehigh University, Bethlehem PA, USA*

MATTHIAS EDER • *Medizinische Hochschule Hannover, Department of Hematology, Hemostasis, Oncology and Stem Cell Transplantation, Hannover, Germany*

MULLER FABBRI • *Department of Molecular Virology, Immunology and Medical Genetics, the Ohio State University, Columbus, OH, USA*

LAURA FONTANA • *Department of Hematology, Oncology and Molecular Medicine, Istituto Superiore di Sanità, Rome, Italy*

PREETHI H. GUNARATNE • *Department of Biology & Biochemistry, University of Houston, HoustonTX, USA Department of Pathology, University of Houston, Houston TX, USA Human Genome Sequencing Center, University of Houston, Houston TX, USA*

VIGO HEISSMEYER • *Helmholtz Center Munich, Institute of Molecular Immunology, Munich, Germany*

KAI P. HOEFIG • *Helmholtz Center Munich, Institute of Molecular Immunology, Munich, Germany*
DONG-YAN JIN • *Department of Biochemistry, The University of Hong Kong, Pokfulam, Hong Kong*
KIN-HANG KOK • *Department of Biochemistry, The University of Hong Kong, Pokfulam, Hong Kong*
GREGORY LAMONTE • *Department of Molecular Genetics and Microbiology, The Institute for Genome Sciences and Policy, Duke University School of Medicine, Durham, NC, USA*
GARY J. LATHAM • *Asuragen, Inc, AustinTX, USA*
ULRICH LEHMANN • *Institute of Pathology, Medizinische Hochschule Hannover, Hannover, Germany*
TING LEI • *Department of Biochemistry, The University of Hong Kong, Pokfulam, Hong Kong*
IZIDORE S. LOSSOS • *Division of Hematology-Oncology and Molecular and Cellular Pharmacology, Department of Medicine, Sylvester Comprehensive Cancer Center, University of Miami, Miami FL, USA*
STEFAN MAAS • *Department of Biological Sciences, Lehigh University, Bethlehem PA, USA*
RAQUEL MALUMBRES • *Department of Oncology, Center for Applied Medical Research, PamplonaNavarra, Spain*
N. MANJUNATH • *Department of Biomedical Sciences, Center of Excellence in Infectious Disease Research, Paul L. Foster School of Medicine, Texas Tech University Health Sciences Center, El PasoTX, USA*
PATRICIA A. MARONEY • *Center for RNA Molecular Biology and Department of Biochemistry, Case Western Reserve University, ClevelandOH, USA*
RAMON J. MAYORAL • *Institute for Research in Biomedicine, Bellinzona, Switzerland*
SILVIA MONTICELLI • *Institute for Research in Biomedicine, Bellinzona, Switzerland*
JOEL NEILSON • *Department of Molecular Physiology and Biophysics, Baylor College of Medicine, Houston TX, USA*
TIMOTHY W. NIELSEN • *Center for RNA Molecular Biology and Department of Biochemistry, Case Western Reserve University, Cleveland OH, USA*
CESARE PESCHLE • *IRCCS Multimedica, Milan, Italy*
JANEZ PLAVEC • *Slovenian NMR Centre, National Institute of Chemistry, Ljubljana, Slovenia*
ALMUDENA R. RAMIRO • *DNA Hypermutation and Cancer Group, Spanish National Cancer Research Center (CNIO), Madrid, Spain*
CAROLYN SANGOKOYA • *Department of Molecular Genetics and Microbiology, The Institute for Genome Sciences and Policy, Duke University School of Medicine, DurhamNC, USA*
MICHAELA SCHERR • *Medizinische Hochschule Hannover, Department of Hematology, Hemostasis, Oncology and Stem Cell Transplantation, Hannover, Germany*
ANTONIO SORRENTINO • *Department of Hematology, Oncology and Molecular Medicine, Istituto Superiore di Sanità, Rome, Italy*
RICCARDO SPIZZO • *Department of Experimental Therapeutics and Department of Cancer Genetics, The University of Texas M.D. Anderson Cancer Center, Houston TX, USA*

EWA SURDZIEL • *Department of Hematology, Hemostasis, Oncology and Stem Cell Transplantation, Medizinische Hochschule Hannover, Hannover, Germany*
JAYANTHA B. TENNAKOON • *Department of Biology & Biochemistry, University of Houston, Houston TX, USA*
MOLLY F. THOMAS • *Department of Microbiology & Immunology, Strategic Asthma Basic Research Center, University of California San Francisco, San Francisco CA, USA*
XIAOWEI WANG • *Department of Radiation Oncology, Washington University School of Medicine, St. Louis MO, USA*
MICHAEL WATSON • *Bioinformatics Group, Institute for Animal Health, Compton, UK*
HAOQUAN WU • *Department of Biomedical Sciences, Center of Excellence in Infectious Disease Research, Paul L. Foster School of Medicine, Texas Tech University Health Sciences Center, El Paso TX, USA*

Part I

Analysis of miRNA Expression: Classic Methods Revisited

Chapter 1

A Rapid, Quantitative Assay for Direct Detection of MicroRNAs and Other Small RNAs Using Splinted Ligation

Sangpen Chamnongpol, Patricia A. Maroney, and Timothy W. Nilsen

Abstract

This protocol describes a method that uses splinted ligation for in-solution, direct labeling of small RNAs from total RNA. The liquid phase hybridization method makes it possible to achieve sensitive, specific, and quantitative detection while eliminating a number of time-consuming and labor-intensive steps required for the standard Northern blot assay. The assay uses a small RNA-specific bridge oligonucleotide to form base pairs with the small RNA and a 5′ end radiolabeled ligation oligonucleotide. The captured small RNA is internally labeled by ligation. Detection of the labeled small RNAs is performed by denaturing gel electrophoresis and autoradiography or phosphorimaging. This protocol has been successfully used to study expression of various classes of biological small RNAs from nanogram to microgram amounts of total RNA without an amplification step and is significantly more simple and more sensitive than Northern blotting or ribonuclease protection assays. Once the oligonucleotides have been synthesized and total RNA has been extracted, the procedure can be completed in 6 h.

1. Introduction

The recent discovery and characterization of small non-protein-coding regulatory RNAs, such as microRNAs (miRNAs), PIWI-associated RNAs (piRNAs and rasiRNAs), short-interfering RNAs (siRNAs), *trans*-acting siRNAs (ta-siRNAs), and other families of short RNAs has led to a rapid expansion of research directed at elucidating their expression patterns and regulatory functions (1–3). Currently, Northern blotting is the standard method for the detection of small RNAs, because it allows direct comparison of the quantity of small RNA between different samples. However, major drawbacks of Northern blotting are the time-consuming procedures and poor sensitivity, especially when monitoring expression of short nucleotide sequences. Despite the improvements in detection sensitivity provided by locked nucleic acid (LNA)

Silvia Monticelli (ed.), *MicroRNAs and the Immune System: Methods and Protocols*, Methods in Molecular Biology, vol. 667,
DOI 10.1007/978-1-60761-811-9_1, © Springer Science+Business Media, LLC 2010

substituted probes (4), Northern blotting requires relatively large amounts of starting material and involves multiple handling steps (Table 1).

Another approach for small RNA detection is based on the ribonuclease protection assay (RPA) (5), which takes advantage of liquid hybridization kinetics to improve detection sensitivity (Table 1). Both Northern blotting and RPA determine the amount of small RNA by measuring the amount of the labeled probes that are noncovalently hybridized to the small RNA, providing a relative quantification of the small RNA levels. In addition, the critical procedures that determine the assay efficiency, which are the hybridization and wash steps in the Northern Blot assay and the hybridization and ribonuclease treatment in RPA, usually require optimization because insufficient treatment may lead to nonspecific detection while excess treatment may compromise the detection sensitivity.

The detection of individual small RNAs can be performed without the use of radioactivity. However, nonisotopic detection does not have sufficient sensitivity to allow direct detection. To achieve the sensitivity for detection of small RNAs from biological samples, an amplification reaction or expensive specialized equipment is often required (6–9). Moreover due to the short length of small RNAs, these assays typically involve a procedure for labeling and detection that has inherent biases to the method such as the ligation of RNA adapters, Poly(A) tailing, T7 RNA polymerase transcription, and RT-PCR amplification.

Here we describe a protocol for the direct labeling and quantitative detection of small RNAs by splinted ligation (10). This assay retains the simplicity of Northern blotting but eliminates its disadvantages. The described assay takes advantage of liquid hybridization kinetics and avoids a procedure that requires optimization such as transfer, prehybridization, and washing steps required for Northern blotting. Comparison of the two techniques reveals that the splinted-ligation assay is approximately 50 times more sensitive than Northern blotting using DNA probes (11). Similar to Northern blotting, this protocol does not require specialized equipment or any amplification step, and thus allows direct and accurate measurement of specific small RNAs (11–13).

The splinted-ligation technique (Fig. 1) is a nucleic acid hybridization assay that uses a bridge oligonucleotide with perfect Watson–Crick complementarity to a target small RNA and a 5′ end radiolabeled ligation oligonucleotide. Simultaneous base-pairing between both the small RNA and ligation oligonucleotide to the bridge oligonucleotide yields a double-stranded structure with a nick on one strand, which can be ligated with T4 DNA Ligase, thus labeling the target small RNA. In addition, because the labeled phosphate provided by the ligation oligonucleotide is

Table 1
Comparison of the amplification-independent assays for small RNA detection

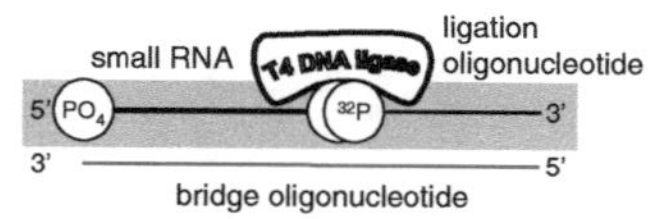

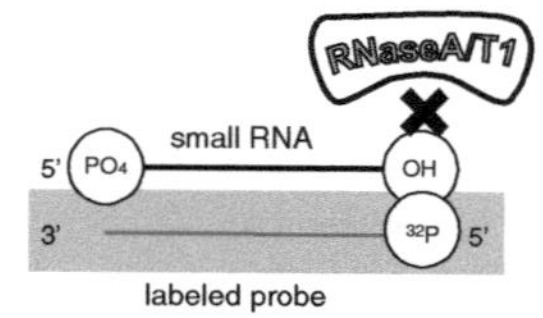

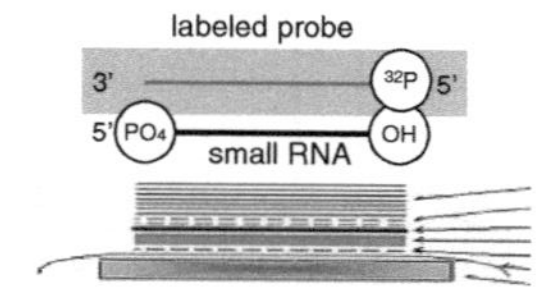

	Splinted ligation	Ribonuclease protection assay	Northern blot
Assay principle	Direct labeling and detection of ligated small RNAs	Indirect detection of the labeled probes protected by small RNAs from ribonuclease digestion	Indirect detection of the labeled probes hybridized to small RNAs
Hybridization	In-solution hybridization	In-solution hybridization	Membrane hybridization
Probe labeling	End-labeled with radioactivity	End-labeled with radioactivity	End-labeled with radioactivity
Starting materials	Nano to microgram quantities of total RNA	Nano to microgram quantities of total RNA	Microgram quantities of total RNA
Assay protocol	Add-and-incubate	Ribonuclease treatment and RNA precipitation	Membrane transfer, hybridization, and wash
Sample separation	Denaturing PAGE	Denaturing PAGE	Denaturing PAGE
Detection	X-ray film or phosphorimager	X-ray film or phosphorimager	X-ray film or phosphorimager
Time from start to finish	6 h–1 day	1–2 days	2–3 days

PAGE polyacrylamide gel electrophoresis

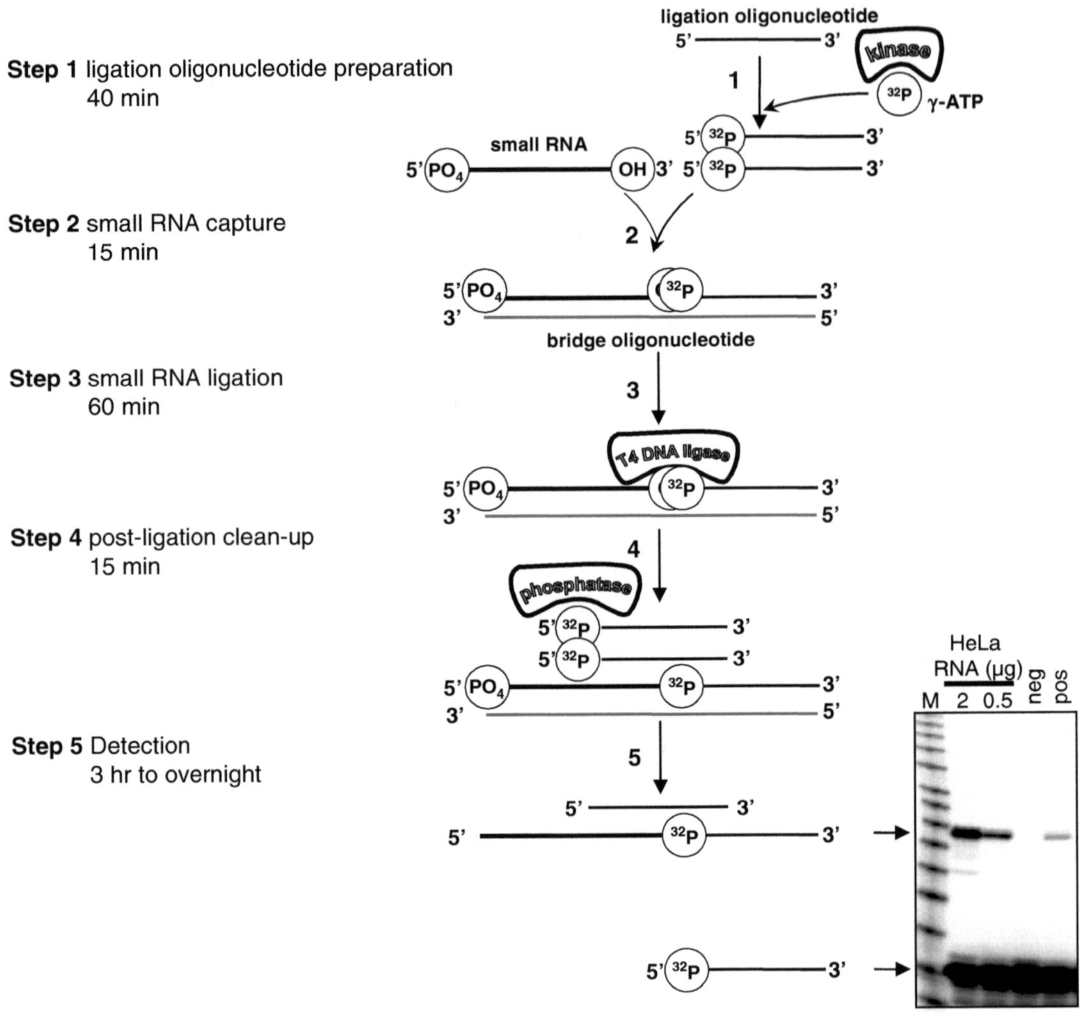

Fig. 1. Flowchart depicting each step of the small RNA detection using splinted-ligation method. The protocol is divided into five steps: step 1, labeling of the ligation oligonucleotide; step 2, capturing of the ligation oligonucleotide and small RNA on a bridge oligonucleotide, and linking of the ligation oligonucleotide to the small RNA using T4 DNA ligase; step 4, partial removal of labeled phosphate from the unligated oligonucleotide; and step 5, fractionation on a denaturing gel and detection by a phosphorimager. The gel image shows detection of *miR-21* by splinted ligation. Assay reactions were performed with the indicated amounts of HeLa cell total RNA. *Lanes* designated "neg" is a no RNA negative control and "pos" is a synthetic *miR-21* positive control. These controls were complete reactions in which the RNA samples were replaced by water and 2.5 femtomoles synthetic *miR-21* RNA, respectively. *Lane M* is 5′ end-labeled oligodeoxynucleotides markers. The *top arrow* indicates the position of *miR-21* ligated to the ligation oligonucleotide. The *bottom arrow* indicates residual radiolabeled 14 nt ligation oligonucleotide that is present due to incomplete removal of the 5′ end-^{32}P.

rendered insensitive to phosphatase activity, the label present on the unligated oligonucleotide can be removed by incubation with phosphatase after the ligation step. Following the splinted-ligation reaction, labeled small RNAs carrying nucleotide extension and any residual labeled ligation oligonucleotides can then be separated by denaturing gel electrophoresis and visualized by autoradiography or phosphorimaging.

This method is based on nucleic acid hybridization technology and therefore is designed to characterize small RNAs of known sequence. In addition, the small RNAs must have a 3′ hydroxyl group to create a covalent phosphodiester linkage between the small RNA and the 5′ phosphate group of the ligation oligonucleotide. Although this method is not a high-throughput assay, the assay setup is simple and thus allows easy processing of multiple samples.

This method has been successfully used to detect different classes of small RNAs in unfractionated RNA samples and was shown to validate tissue-specific microRNA expression in animals and plants, the expression of viral microRNAs in infected fibroblasts, the testis-specific expression of piRNAs, and the expression of low abundance *ta*-siRNAs and other small RNAs in *Arabidopsis* (11). This method was also used to determine *miR-21* distribution on polyribosomes after hypertonic stress (14).

2. Materials

2.1. Reagents (see Note 1)

1. Ligation oligonucleotide (5′-CGCTTATGACATTC/dideoxy-C/-3′, see Note 2).
2. Small RNA-specific bridge oligonucleotide (Fig. 2, see Notes 3 and 4).
3. Synthetic RNA positive control (synthetic RNA oligonucleotide corresponding to the sequence of a known small RNA, see Note 5).
4. Bridge oligonucleotide for synthetic RNA positive control (see Note 3 and 4).
5. Low molecular weight marker, 10–100 nt (e.g., USB, see Note 6).

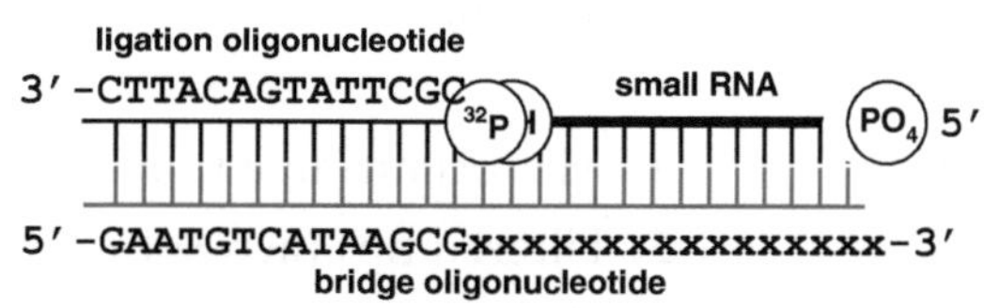

Fig. 2. Schematic representation and example of bridge oligonucleotide sequence design described in this protocol. The 22 base *miR-21* miRNA sequence is 5′-uagcuuaucagacugauguuga-3′. The 14 base ligation oligonucleotide sequence is 5′-CGCTTATGACATTC-3′. The combined *miR-21* miRNA sequence and ligation oligonucleotide sequence is 5′-uagcuuaucagacugauguugaCGCTTATGACATTC-3′. The reverse-complement DNA sequence is 5′- GAATGTCATAAGCGtcaacatcagtctgataagcta-3′. The sequence of *miR-21* miRNA-specific bridge oligonucleotide is 5′-/modification/-GAATGTCATAAGCGtcaacatcagtctgataagcta-/modification/-3′. Note that the modification is optional.

6. [γ-^{32}P]-ATP (6,000 Ci/mmol, 150 mCi/ml) (see Note 7).
7. OptiKinase™ (10 units/μl) with 10× Reaction buffer: 0.5 M Tris–HCI, pH 7.5, 100 mM $MgCl_2$, 50 mM DTT.
8. 10× Capture buffer: 100 mM Tris–HCl, pH 7.5, 750 mM KCl.
9. PrepEase® Sequencing Dye Clean-Up Kit (USB, or other gel matrix spin columns for nucleic acid clean-up and purification).
10. Ligate-IT™ Rapid Ligation Kit (USB). Other commercially available T4 DNA Ligase can be used, but the ligation efficiency may be affected by the difference in buffer and enzyme compositions.
11. RNase inhibitor (Human Placenta).
12. Shrimp alkaline phosphatase.
13. 2× Formamide loading dye: 95% formamide, 20 mM EDTA, 0.025% bromophenol blue, 0.025% xylene cyanol.
14. 40% Liquid acrylamide stock solution (19:1) (see Note 8 for UREA-PAGE gel preparation).
15. Urea (see Note 8).
16. Glycerol tolerant gel (GTG) buffer, 20× Solution: 1.78 M Tris, 0.57 M taurine, 0.01 M EDTA (see Note 8).
17. Tris–Borate–EDTA buffer (TBE), 5× Solution: 0.445 M Tris, 0.445 M boric acid, 0.01 M EDTA (see Note 8).
18. Ammonium persulfate (APS) (see Note 8).
19. N,N,N′,N′-Tetramethyl ethylenediamine (TEMED) (see Note 8).
20. Water, RNase-free.
21. TE buffer, 1× Solution: 10 mM Tris–HCl, pH 8.0, 1 mM EDTA.
22. TRIzol® Reagent.
23. Phenol:chloroform.
24. Glycogen.

2.2. Equipment

1. Microcentrifuge tubes, RNase-free.
2. Filtered tips (aerosol-resistant pipette tips, RNase-free).
3. Vortex mixer.
4. Microcentrifuge.
5. Thermalcycler PCR machine or waterbath.
6. Vertical gel-electrophoresis apparatus. Most commercially available vertical gel electrophoresis systems for SDS-polyacrylamide gel electrophoresis (PAGE) or DNA-sequencing applications are suitable.

7. Electrophoresis power supply. Most commercial power supplies sold for SDS-PAGE or DNA-sequencing applications are suitable.
8. Autoradiography film cassette and Kodak BioMax MR film (Kodak) or cassette and storage phosphor screen. Access to a darkroom equipped with film developer is needed for film autoradiography. Access to a phosphorimager instrument is needed for storage phosphor screen phosphorimaging.

3. Methods

3.1. General Recommendation to Prevent RNase Contamination When Working with RNA

1. Wear gloves at all times while handling reagents, materials, and equipment to prevent RNase contamination from hands. Change gloves after touching non-RNase-free surfaces.
2. Avoid using equipment and work areas that have been exposed to RNases. Clean the equipment and work surfaces with ethanol or commercially available RNase decontamination solutions.
3. Clean the interior and exterior of micropipette shafts with ethanol or commercially available RNase decontamination solutions and use barrier tips.
4. Use RNase-free plasticware and RNase-free buffers and reagents.

3.2. Total RNA Preparation

Prepare total RNA using guanidine isothiocyanate such as TRIzol® Reagent and phenol:chloroform according to standard total RNA isolation protocols (15) with the exception that an inert carrier such as glycogen or linear polyacrylamide is added to each sample. We recommend adding 20 µg of glycogen per 1 ml during alcohol precipitation to increase the recovery of small RNAs. Samples can also be prepared by commercially available column-based methods for small RNA isolation. Dilute RNA sample with TE buffer or RNase-free water. The purified RNA should be kept at −80°C. Avoid leaving the RNA at room temperature or 4°C and avoid multiple freeze–thaw cycles after isolation.

The amount of total RNA required per assay depends on the abundance of the small RNA of interest. This assay has a linear detection range from 0.2–20 fmol based on assaying a synthetic 22 nt RNA. The recommended protocol allows up to 8 µl of total RNA or RNA enriched for small RNAs per assay reaction. A typical reaction uses 0.5–4 µg of RNA diluted in TE buffer or RNase-free water.

3.3. Timing

After total RNA preparation, the entire procedure can be completed in a single day. The small RNA-labeling reaction (see subheading 3.7, steps 1 and 2) can be done in less than

3 h. The time required for step 3 varies depending on the gel electrophoresis system and the sensitivity of the image processing system (Fig. 1).

3.4. General Guidelines for Assay Setup

1. Thaw reagents on ice, mix thoroughly before use, and immediately return unused materials to –20°C.
2. When preparing working reagents, measure components accurately, mix thoroughly, spin briefly, and keep on ice.
3. Assemble reactions on ice or at indicated temperature throughout the procedure.

3.5. General Guidelines for Assay Control Setup

1. Prepare a "positive control" to assess assay components and procedure by substituting the RNA sample with a synthetic RNA positive control. The positive control is a premix of a 20–30 nt synthetic RNA oligonucleotide and a bridge oligonucleotide for capturing the synthetic RNA.
2. Prepare a "no RNA negative control" to assess sample background signal by substituting the RNA sample with RNase-free water.
3. For use as an "internal/loading control," we suggest that it is possible to detect small RNAs known to be constitutively expressed in the test samples by substituting the target-specific bridge oligonucleotide with a control-specific bridge oligonucleotide. Alternatively, stain gels for detecting tRNA with ethidium bromide or other single-stranded nucleic acid staining dyes.

3.6. Anticipated Results

For an example of typical results, see Fig. 1. The expected size of the ligated small RNA is the size of the small RNA plus 14 nucleotides of the labeled ligation oligonucleotide. The size may be compared to a radiolabeled low molecular weight marker. The synthetic RNA positive control shown in Fig. 1 contains a 22 nt synthetic *miR-21* which in combination with the 14 nt ligation oligonucleotide generates a 36 nt ligated fragment after separation and detection. The "neg-no RNA control" lane should have no signal.

This assay is also a quantitative technique. In order to determine the amount of a small RNA in a sample, a dilution series of a synthetic oligoribonucleotide of known concentration is analyzed in parallel with the sample. A linear standard curve can be generated from which the concentration of small RNA in the sample can be calculated.

3.7. Protocol

Step 1: Ligation oligonucleotide preparation. Timing – 40 min.

The first step is to 5′ end-label the ligation oligonucleotide with [γ-^{32}P]-ATP and remove the unincorporated isotope.

Table 2
Composition of 5′ end-labeling reaction

Components	Volume (μl)
10 μM ligation oligonucleotide[a]	2
RNase-free water	12
10× OptiKinase™ Reaction buffer	2
[γ-^{32}P]-ATP (6,000 Ci/mmol, 150 mCi/ml)	2
OptiKinase™	2
Total volume	20 μl

[a]Replace ligation oligonucleotide with marker such as low molecular weight marker when preparing radiolabeled markers

1. Thaw frozen reagents for **step 2** on ice, mix thoroughly followed by a spin at maximum speed in a microcentrifuge for 10 s at room temperature and then place on ice.
2. Prepare [^{32}P]-labeled ligation oligonucleotide by combining the following components at room temperature (25°C) (Table 2).
3. Mix thoroughly followed by a spin at maximum speed in a microcentrifuge for 10 s at room temperature. Incubate for 30–60 min at 37°C.
4. While the reactions are incubating, prepare the PrepEase® Sequencing Dye Clean-Up Kit for removing the unincorporated [γ-^{32}P]-ATP. Centrifuge the column at 750×*g* for 30 s at room temperature to collect the dry resin at the bottom of the column.
5. Hydrate the resin by adding 600 μl of RNase-free water and vortex. Remove air bubbles by vortexing or tapping the column. Incubate at least 30 min at room temperature.

The column can be hydrated overnight at 4°C.

6. Resuspend the settled resin by inverting the column several times. Ensure that no air bubbles are visible. Remove the bottom plug and place in a 2 ml collection tube.
7. Centrifuge at 750×*g* for 2 min at room temperature to remove the remaining water. Discard the flow-through.
8. After 30–60 min of incubation, dilute the labeling reactions (from step 3) to 100 μl by adding 80 μl of RNase-free water.
9. Place the column from step 7 in a clean 1.5 ml microcentrifuge tube. Without disturbing the gel bed, carefully apply

the diluted sample (from step 8) directly onto the top of the gel bed.

10. After loading the sample, centrifuge the column at 750 × *g* for 4 min at room temperature. Discard the used column in a radioactive waste container. The concentration of the labeled detection oligonucleotide should be 100 nM (0.1 pmol/μl).

    Store at −20°C if not required immediately. Keep on ice when in use.

Steps 2–4: Small RNA capture, ligation, and post-ligation clean-up. Timing – 90 min.

11. Thaw frozen reagents for step 12 on ice, mix thoroughly followed by a spin at maximum speed in a microcentrifuge for 10 s at room temperature, and then place on ice.
12. Assemble the capture reaction on ice by making a master mix of 1 μl of bridge oligonucleotide in 10× Capture buffer plus 1 μl of radiolabeled ligation oligonucleotide per sample. Add 2 μl of this master mix to each test sample, which had been diluted to 8 μl with RNase-free water (Table 3).
13. Mix thoroughly followed by a spin at maximum speed in a microcentrifuge for 10 s at room temperature. Incubate the mixture at 94°C for 1 min, 65°C for 2 min, and 37°C for 10 min.
14. It is highly recommended to incubate the reaction in this step in a Thermalcycler PCR machine.
15. Make a Ligase master mix by combining 3 μl of 5× Ligate-IT™ buffer, 1 μl of Ligate-IT™ enzyme and 1 μl of RNase-free

Table 3
Composition of capture reaction

Components	Positive control (μl)	No RNA control (μl)	Sample (μl)
RNA sample	0	0	Up to 8 μl
Synthetic RNA positive control	1	0	0
Adjust to 8 μl with RNase-free water			
0.1 pmole/μl Bridge oligonucleotide in 10× Capture buffer	1	1	1
Radiolabeled ligation oligonucleotide	1	1	1
Total volume	10	10	10

water, per sample. Add 5 μl of the Ligase master mix to each sample.

16. Mix thoroughly followed by a spin at maximum speed in a microcentrifuge for 10 s at room temperature. Incubate for 1 h at 30°C.

    It is highly recommended to incubate the reaction in this step in a Thermalcycler PCR machine.

    If not proceeding to the next step immediately, inactivate the reaction by incubation for 10 min at 75°C and store at −20°C for later use.

17. Add 1 μl of Shrimp Alkaline Phosphatase to each reaction.
18. Mix thoroughly followed by a spin at maximum speed in a microcentrifuge for 10 s at room temperature. Incubate for 15 min at 37°C.

    It is highly recommended to incubate the reaction in this step in a Thermalcycler PCR machine.

    If not proceeding to the next step immediately, inactivate the reaction by incubation for 10 min at 75°C and store at −20°C for later use.

Step 5: Electrophoretic analysis and detection. Timing – 2 h to overnight.

19. Prepare a 12% or 15% UREA-polyacrylamide gel with 1× running buffer (see Note 8).
20. Pre-run to warm the gel for 20–30 min.
21. Transfer an aliquot (up to 15 μl) of the reaction (from step 17) to a new tube. Add an equal volume of 2× formamide loading dye.
22. Transfer an aliquot (up to 15 μl) of the [^{32}P]-labeled low molecular weight marker to a new tube. Add an equal volume of formamide loading dye.

    We suggest using 5–10 μl of a 1:50 dilution of [^{32}P]-labeled low molecular weight marker per lane for detection after 2–4 h exposure using an intensifying screen. The radiolabeled markers can be stored at −20°C and used up to 2 months, although it is necessary to adjust the volume of markers needed per lane due to decay of the radioisotope.

23. Mix the tubes from steps 21 and 22 thoroughly followed by a brief spin in a microcentrifuge and incubate for 3 min at 95°C to denature the samples. Immediately cool on ice.
24. Thoroughly flush wells of the gel to remove acrylamide debris, urea, and air bubbles.
25. Load 2–15 μl of samples and the [^{32}P]-labeled markers (from step 22) onto the gel.

26. Run the gel at 20–30 mA for a small gel (13 cm × 15 cm), or at 60 mA for a large gel (36 cm × 43 cm) and stop when the bromophenol blue dye front has migrated to the bottom, or middle of the gel for these gel sizes, respectively.
27. At the end of the electrophoretic separation, detection of RNA can be completed using either a phosphorimager [option (a)] or X-ray film [option (b)].
    (a) Detection of RNA using phosphorimaging
        - Transfer the gel onto a sheet of paper, dry in a gel dryer, wrap with saran wrap and expose to a phosphorimager screen.
        - Process the phosphorimager screen according to the manufacturer's instructions.
    (b) Detection of RNA using X-ray film
        - Transfer the gel onto a sheet of nondiffusible support material, such as processed film, wrap with saran wrap and expose to X-ray film.
        - Expose the gel to X-ray film with an intensifying screen. Store for 2 h to overnight at −80°C. The gel can be reexposed several times if required.

4. Notes

1. All glassware and reagents must be RNase-free.
2. Prepare ligation oligonucleotide by resuspending with TE buffer or RNase-free water to 100 μM and store at −20°C. Dilute the stock solution to 10 μM with TE buffer or RNase-free water for the 5′ end-labeling reaction.
3. The bridge oligonucleotide is a DNA oligonucleotide complementary to both the ligation oligonucleotide and a specific small RNA at its 5′ and 3′ ends, respectively (Fig. 2). The bridge oligonucleotide sequence should be complementary to the entire length of small RNA of interest. Therefore, every bridge oligonucleotide should have the same 14 nt sequence at the 5′ end, which allows a single labeling reaction of the ligation oligonucleotide for detection of any small RNA of interest. In general, while addition of unligatable-modifications to the ends of the bridge oligonucleotide is not always necessary, in some cases it is desirable to block the 3′ end or both the 5′ and 3′ ends of the bridge oligonucleotide by incorporating modification(s) such as C3 spacer, amino-modifier,

inverted dT, or dideoxy-C. This ensures that unwanted side ligation reactions do not take place. We recommend use of an unmodified bridge oligonucleotide as the first option for the assay. The bridge oligonucleotide requires a standard desalting purification after synthesis. Further purification by HPLC or denatured PAGE is usually unnecessary.

4. Prepare bridge oligonucleotide by resuspending the bridge oligonucleotide with TE buffer or RNase-free water to 100 μM and store at −20°C. Dilute the stock solution to 100 nM (0.1 pmol/μl) with 10× Capture buffer and use 1 μl in a 10 μl assay reaction. The bridge oligonucleotides may be prediluted to 1 μM with RNase-free water before preparing the 100 nM stock solution in 10× Capture buffer. The concentration of the bridge oligonucleotide could affect the output signal independent of the RNA amount in the test sample. For quantitative measurement, the concentration of the bridge oligonucleotide should be carefully measured to yield 0.1 pmol per reaction.
5. Prepare synthetic RNA positive control preparation by resuspending the synthetic RNA positive control oligonucleotide with TE buffer or RNase-free water to 100 μM and store at −80°C. Dilute the stock solution to 0.2–20 nM (0.2–20 fmol/μl) with TE buffer or RNase-free water for standard and positive control reactions.
6. The low molecular weight marker suitable for this assay should be single-stranded DNA or RNA with an OH group at the 3′ end.
7. [γ-^{32}P]-ATP with lower specific activity can be used in this protocol. However longer exposure time may be required. Exposure to β-radiation and secondary X-radiation from ^{32}P is hazardous. Most research institutions specify procedures for the safe handling of this isotope, which should be followed stringently.
8. UREA-polyacrylamide gel preparation.

   A 13 cm × 15 cm × 0.75 mm mini-gel system requires 15 ml of gel solution and a 36 cm × 43 cm × 0.8 mm sequencing gel system requires 120 ml of gel solution (see Tables 4 and 5 for composition of gels).

   Due to the high glycerol content of the assay components, we recommend using glycerol tolerant gel (GTG) buffer in place of TBE buffer when loading more than half of the reaction volume on a gel. The GTG buffer is specially formulated to resolve the problem of gel distortion associated with samples that contain high amounts of glycerol.

Table 4
Composition of TBE gel polymerization mixtures

%Total volume Components	12% 15 ml Amount	15% 15 ml Amount	12% 120 ml Amount	15% 120 ml Amount
Urea (7 M)	6.3 g	6.3 g	50.4 g	50.4 g
40% Acrylamide/Bis solution (19:1)	4.5 ml	5.6 ml	36.0 ml	44.8 ml
5× TBE buffer	3 ml	3 ml	24 ml	24 ml
Stir and warm solution at 40–50°C to dissolve urea				
Cool the mixture to room temperature				
Adjust to the final volume with nuclease-free water				
Add the following reagents immediately before pouring the gel				
TEMED	7.5 μl	7.5 μl	60 μl	60 μl
10% APS in nuclease-free water	75 μl	75 μl	600 μl	600 μl
Allow to polymerize at room temperature for at least 30 min to 1 h				
Run in 1× TBE running buffer (diluted with deionized water)				

Table 5
Composition of GTG gel polymerization mixtures

%Total volume Components	12% 15 ml Amount	15% 15 ml Amount	12% 120 ml Amount	15% 120 ml Amount
Urea (7 M)	6.3 g	6.3 g	50.4 g	50.4 g
40% Acrylamide/Bis solution (19:1)	4.5 ml	5.6 ml	36.0 ml	44.8 ml
10× GTG buffer	1.5 ml	1.5 ml	12 ml	12 ml
Stir and warm solution at 40–50°C to dissolve urea				
Cool the mixture to room temperature				
Adjust to the final volume with nuclease-free water				
Add the following reagents immediately before pouring the gel				
TEMED	7.5 μl	7.5 μl	60 μl	60 μl
10% APS in nuclease-free water	75 μl	75 μl	600 μl	600 μl
Allow to polymerize at room temperature for at least 30 min to 1 h				
Run in 1× GTG running buffer (diluted with deionized water)				

References

1. Lagos-Quintana, M., Rauhut, R., Lendeckel, W., and Tuschl, T. (2001) Identification of novel genes coding for small expressed RNAs. *Science* **294**, 853–58.
2. Bartel, D. P. (2004). MicroRNAs: genomics, biogenesis, mechanism, and function. *Cell* **116** (2) 81–97.
3. Pillai, R. S. (2005) MicroRNA function: multiple mechanisms for a tiny RNA? *RNA* **11**, 1753–61.
4. Valoczi, A., Hornyik, C., Varga, N., Burgyan, J., Kauppinen, S., and Havelda, Z. (2004) Sensitive and specific detection of microRNAs by northern blot analysis using LNA-modified oligonucleotide probes. *Nucleic Acids Res.* **32**, e175.
5. Shingara, J., Keiger, K., Shelton, J., Laosinchai-Wolf, W., Powers, P., Conrad, R., Brown, D., and Labourier, E. (2005) An optimized isolation and labeling platform for accurate microRNA expression profiling. *RNA* **11**, 1461–70.
6. Hüttenhofer, A., and Vogel, J. (2006) Experimental approaches to identify non-coding RNAs. *Nucleic Acids Res.* **34**, 635–46.
7. Chen, C., Ridzon, D. A., Broomer, A. J., Zhou, Z., Lee, D. H., Nguyen, J. T., Barbisin, M., Xu, N. L., Mahuvakar, V. R., Andersen, M. R., et al. (2005) Real-time quantification of microRNAs by stem–loop RT-PCR. *Nucleic Acids Res.* **33,** e179.
8. Jiang, J., Lee, E. J., Gusev, Y., and Schmittgen, T. D. (2005) Real-time expression profiling of microRNA precursors in human cancer cell lines. *Nucleic Acids Res.* **33,** 5394–03.
9. Jonstrup, S. P., Koch, J., and Kjems, J. (2006) A microRNA detection system based on padlock probes and rolling circle amplification. *RNA* **12:** 1747–52.
10. Moore, M. J., and Query, C. C. (2000) Joining of RNAs by splinted ligation. *Methods Enzymol.* **317**, 109–23.
11. Maroney, P. A., Chamnongpol, S., Souret, F., and Nilsen, T. W. (2007) A rapid, quantitative assay for direct detection of microRNAs and other small RNAs using splinted ligation. *RNA* **13**, 930–6.
12. Maroney, P. A., Chamnongpol, S., Souret, F., and Nilsen, T. W. (2008) Direct detection of small RNAs using splinted ligation. *Nat. Protoc.* **3**, 279–87.
13. Chamnongpol, S., and Souret, F. (2008) miRtect-IT: a novel method for small RNA detection. *Biotechniques* **44**, 129–31.
14. Maroney, P. A., Yang, Y., Fisher, J., and Nilsen, T. W. (2006) Evidence that microRNAs are associated with translating messenger RNAs in human cells. *Nat. Struct. Mol. Biol.* **13**, 1102–7.
15. Sambrook, J., and Russell, D. W. (2001) "Molecular Cloning: A Laboratory Manual," Cold Spring Harbor Laboratory Press, 7.4.

Chapter 2

Normalization of MicroRNA Quantitative RT-PCR Data in Reduced Scale Experimental Designs

Gary J. Latham

Abstract

Proper normalization of quantitative RT-PCR (qRT-PCR) data is a crucial component of gene expression analysis. Although arbitrarily selected housekeeping genes have been used to normalize many published mRNA RT-PCR datasets, there is a growing awareness that such normalizers should be first validated empirically. The use of stable reference genes is particularly needed for qRT-PCR of microRNA (miRNA), which represent a novel class of biological regulators whose aberrant expression is associated with a range of disorders. Changes in miRNA levels can be modest, and yet have profound cellular consequences. As a result, precise measurements of miRNA expression are critically important. This chapter describes a detailed workflow for the selection of endogenous normalizers using the NormFinder algorithm, resulting in more accurate miRNA expression profiling results. This approach is particularly well suited to smaller scale miRNA qRT-PCR experimental designs.

1. Introduction

The choice of a data normalization approach is a critical consideration for successful gene expression profiling experiments. This is particularly true for experiments that aim to quantify differences in the expression of gene targets, such as miRNA, between normal and diseased samples. The actual differential expression that is measured can reflect sources of variation that are distinct from the molecular pathways associated with a particular pathology. For example, sources of technical variation may include sample collection and stabilization, RNA isolation, and efficiency of target quantification. Importantly, differences in measured miRNA expression can be relatively small (e.g., less than twofold), but still

Silvia Monticelli (ed.), *MicroRNAs and the Immune System: Methods and Protocols*, Methods in Molecular Biology, vol. 667,
DOI 10.1007/978-1-60761-811-9_2, © Springer Science+Business Media, LLC 2010

biologically meaningful (1, 2). As a result, accurate differential expression measurements of miRNA are of paramount importance to correctly define disease mechanisms and identify possible diagnostic and therapeutic interventions. In addition, miRNA represent additional challenges for normalization compared to mRNA. The miRNA population comprises a minute, yet variable, fraction of total RNA, and miRNA isolation requires a higher stringency than the methods used for conventional RNA extraction (3, 4). Thus, the selection of a normalizer should reflect such considerations. Early qRT-PCR studies of miRNA, however, relied primarily on normalization to total RNA (e.g., fixed mass input per reaction) or randomly selected RNAs, such as 18S rRNA or other non-miRNA controls, without prior validation of their utility. The pitfalls of such a haphazard normalizer selection have been described (1).

Several workflows for the normalization of miRNA qRT-PCR data are possible, depending on the goals of the study, availability of related miRNA expression data, and sample and resource limitations of the qRT-PCR experiment itself. The ideal workflow is to first confirm the quality and suitability of the sample RNA for qRT-PCR, then interrogate each sample group with a large number (e.g., hundreds) of representative miRNA targets, and finally apply a global normalization strategy. Such a strategy uses expression information from all of the targets in the experiment, rather than a select group, and is well established as the method of choice for, e.g., microarray analysis. As a result, variability in a small set of targets that may not reflect the population as a whole is removed. However, such large-scale experiments are costly in terms of materials, labor, and sample consumption, and thus may be impractical for many researchers. An alternative approach is to screen a smaller group of targets (but still as many as is practically possible) using the same samples intended for differential expression analysis and identify the most stable reference RNAs (preferably more than one) that can be used as normalizers for subsequent experiments (1). The least desirable option is to arbitrarily pick a normalizer without first obtaining data to support the specific experimental design and workflow planned for expression analysis. The point cannot be made firmly enough that there is no such thing as a universal reference gene for either miRNA or mRNA gene expression experiments, and there is no substitute for empirical validation of normalization that is appropriate to the particular experimental design and goals.

In this methods chapter, we will describe in detail one approach for the identification of miRNA reference genes that can be used to more accurately quantify miRNA targets for expression comparisons between sample groups.

2. Materials

2.1. Reagents for Small RNA Recovery

There are a number of RNA isolation methods that preserve the small RNA population, based both on organic extraction (TRIzol®, phenol/chloroform) as well as, or even in combination with, isolation by a silica column. The most important consideration is to match the isolation technology with the sample type (see Note 1); for example, FFPE samples require a different extraction approach than fresh or frozen solid tissue. Isolation products that we have extensively tested with satisfactory results are given below:

1. Frozen tissue or cultured cells – mirVana miRNA Isolation Kit (Ambion).
2. FFPE tissue – RecoverAll Total Nucleic Acid Isolation Kit (Ambion) (see Note 2).

2.2. Small RNA Quality Control

Some form of quality metric is necessary to help to ensure quantity and integrity of the RNA sample. For example, although miRNA is restricted in size by definition, the assurance that the sample contains intact RNA, such as mRNA, provides increased confidence that the isolate more accurately mirrors the expression profile of the sample at the time of extraction. The nature and extent of small RNA quality control (QC) assays that may be performed is dependent on the type and availability of purified RNA. For RNA extracted from solid tissue or cultured cells, we routinely perform QC procedures that require the following reagents and equipment:

1. NanoDrop ND-3300 Spectrophotometer (Thermo Scientific).
2. 2100 Bioanalyzer and RNA Nano 6000 kit (Agilent Technologies).
3. GeneAmp® 9700 PCR System (Applied Biosystems).
4. 7900HT Real-time PCR System (Applied Biosystems).
5. TaqMan® Reverse Transcription Kit (Applied Biosystems).
6. TaqMan® MicroRNA Assay (Applied Biosystems) for ubiquitous miRNA targets representing a range of expression in the samples of interest (see Note 3).

2.3. miRNA qRT-PCR

Although a number of qRT-PCR methodologies have been described (see Note 4), many of which can be suitable for quantitative miRNA expression profiling, the scope of this chapter is restricted to the TaqMan® microRNA assays that are available through Applied Biosystems (Life Technologies). These assays are among the most highly cited and most carefully vetted technologies for PCR-based miRNA gene expression measurements.

The primary equipment and reagents necessary to perform these assays are as follows:

1. GeneAmp® 9700 PCR System (Applied Biosystems).
2. 7900HT Real-time PCR System (Applied Biosystems).
3. TaqMan® Reverse Transcription Kit (Applied Biosystems).
4. TaqMan® MicroRNA Assays for the targets of interest (Applied Biosystems).

2.4. Software Tools for Normalizer Gene Selection

Multiple algorithms have been devised to process qRT-PCR Ct (or Cq, cycle of quantification (5)) data (see Note 5). However, the capability of the NormFinder algorithm (6) to estimate both intragroup and intergroup variance, identify even a single reference gene as the most stable normalizer, and provide a simple interface though the versatile and free Excel Addin, establishes this method as the preferred approach described here (see Note 6).

Installation of the Addin is described in a user guide written by the authors and available at http://www.mdl.dk/publicationsnormfinder.htm. Specifics of the install may be dependent on the version of Excel that is used.

1. NormFinder Excel Addin. Available for download at http://www.mdl.dk/publicationsnormfinder.htm.

3. Methods

3.1. Isolate miRNAs from the Samples of Interest

1. The reader is advised to follow the detailed instructions provided by the manufacturer of the recommended small RNA isolation technologies that are appropriate for their sample type.

3.2. Confirm the Recovery and Functionality of miRNAs from Each Sample

1. Using a NanoDrop ND-3300 Spectrophotometer, determine the A260/280 and A260/230 ratio for the purified RNA from each sample. The generally recommended acceptability criteria are A260/280 ≥ 1.8 and A260/230 ≥ 1.8.
2. To ensure intactness of the RNA population, analyze the purified RNA on an Agilent 2100 bioanalyzer using the RNA Nano 6000 kit. RNA populations with RNA Integrity Numbers (RIN) > 7 are recommended to ensure the preservation of high-quality RNA in the purified samples, although RNA characterized by lower RIN values may be acceptable for miRNA qRT-PCR analysis, given the small size of miRNA templates.
3. It is also desirable to establish functionality of the RNA in qRT-PCR prior to consuming significant quantities of precious samples or initiating expensive large-scale experiments.

We recommend that a set of miRNAs, such miR-24, miR-191, and miR-103, be analyzed by qRT-PCR using 1–10 ng of purified total RNA. These miRNAs span an expression range of ~100-fold in many tissues and thus can provide a broad assessment of miRNA suitability in qRT-PCR.

3.3. Select a Panel of Putative Normalizers to be Analyzed

1. Several references are now available as resources for potential normalization candidates of miRNA data (1, 2, 7). Important considerations are the inclusion of an appropriate number of candidate reference genes and samples, the lack of any known differential expression among sample groups for the experimental design of interest, and ideally the selection of candidates that are functionally distinct to avoid concerns of coregulation among combinations of normalizers.
2. Although the NormFinder approach can theoretically accommodate as few as three targets and two samples per group, the developers generally recommend five to ten candidate targets and at least eight samples per group (6).

3.4. Amplify Purified miRNAs in Each Sample and Determine the Ct for Each

1. The reader is advised to follow the detailed instructions provided for the designated amplification method, such as those for the TaqMan® MicroRNA assays.
2. To simplify the experimental execution, a single, fixed input of total RNA is recommended for each sample for amplification by each target. This exact input that is used should accommodate the broad range of target abundance that is desirable to detect (see Note 7) and balance the needs for accurate quantification with the amount of RNA and number of targets and experiments that are anticipated to complete the project. Thus, proper experimental planning is critical. An additional benefit of using a constant input of RNA per sample is that the amount of total RNA input into the reaction may also be used as a normalizer, although reference miRNA(s) can be a far superior choice (1).
3. Extraction of the Ct value for each target in each sample should be achieved using standard procedures and software packages.

3.5. Convert Cycle Quantification Data into a Format Suitable for Input into the Normalization Algorithm

1. The NormFinder Excel macro processes data that are provided in a linear scale. As such, Ct values cannot be input directly but must first be converted to relative quantities (RQ).
2. If absolute standard curves for the targets of interest are available, each respective Ct value can be converted to a copy number.
3. The data may also be converted using a defined calibrator sample or commuted to RQ for each target across all samples. For example, the lowest Ct for a given target across the set of

samples can be arbitrarily set to 1.0 and the corresponding Ct for the same target in all other samples referenced relative to this value. If the PCR efficiency of the target is 100%, then this conversion can be made simply using the equation: $RQ = 1/(2^{(Ct,sample - Ct,min)})$. For example, if the lowest Ct across all samples is 20, and the Ct of the sample of interest is 22, then the RQ for the latter sample is equal to $RQ = 1/(2^{(22-20)})$, or 0.25. See Fig. 1 for an example.

4. Although our experience is that many of the single-tube ABI TaqMan microRNA assays have a PCR efficiency (E) close to 100%, empirical confirmation is always the best practice. This is particularly true since the efficiency is dependent on both the assay design as well as the sample matrix. The most common method to measure the PCR efficiency is to perform a set of serial dilutions and measure the slope of the line when the log of the RNA concentration is plotted against the cycle number. The PCR efficiency can be computed as: $E=10^{(-1/slope)}-1$. The resulting PCR efficiency can then be used to determine a more appropriate measure of the relative quantity as described above, where 1.0 = 100% efficiency, 0.9 = 90% efficiency, etc. (see Note 8).

3.6. Analyze the Candidate Normalizers Using NormFinder

1. Once sample Ct's have been converted to a linear scale, the data are suitable for input into the NormFinder Add-in.
2. Data are entered into Excel using the format shown in Fig. 1 (samples differentiated by column, candidate reference genes by row).
3. If multiple groups are represented (e.g., normal vs. tumor), they are designated by discrete integers in a separate row, e.g., normal = 1.0, tumor = 2.0.
4. Open the NormFinder macro, which is presented as a dedicated menu option in Excel once installed.
5. Click the button to the right of the "Select input data" option, and highlight the data to be analyzed. If sample names (first row) and gene names (first column) are included, then tick the corresponding boxes. If groups are identified, tick the group identifier box as well.
6. Since RQ are provided, click "log transform data."
7. Do not tick "simple output only." The simple output reports the overall variability, but not the corresponding statistics for intragroup and intergroup variation. It is important to review both groups of information if separate groups are designated.
8. Once all fields have been correctly chosen, click "Go."
9. The results will be output to a separate Excel tab labeled "Statistics."

1) Amplify at least 5-10 candidate normalizers from each sample group (at least 8 samples per group). An example dataset consisting of 9 samples in two unpaired groups (N, normal and T, tumor) with associated Ct values for 9 candidate reference targets is given below.

Candidate Normalizer	Sample Type N	N	N	N	N	N	N	N	N	T	T	T	T	T	T	T	T	T
miR-16	21.86	21.25	21.99	20.15	21.25	21.76	21.67	22.47	20.60	23.33	23.43	23.43	23.64	23.69	22.29	22.93	23.58	23.08
miR-24	24.37	24.18	24.12	23.53	23.34	23.69	23.52	24.56	24.83	24.87	25.29	25.00	26.16	25.77	23.46	24.19	24.97	24.23
miR-27a	28.00	27.37	27.77	27.47	26.60	26.85	26.89	28.57	28.24	29.15	29.64	28.64	30.19	29.24	27.32	27.58	28.70	27.50
miR-93	27.56	26.85	27.30	25.68	26.48	27.10	26.36	27.13	26.11	27.74	27.34	27.34	28.38	27.12	25.56	27.20	27.83	26.17
miR-103	28.28	28.40	27.81	27.43	27.49	27.86	27.92	28.60	27.82	28.83	29.69	28.81	29.74	29.19	27.30	28.13	28.49	28.40
miR-106a	30.00	28.89	29.68	28.25	28.97	29.27	29.19	29.57	28.37	30.66	30.17	29.40	30.78	29.11	29.08	29.98	30.03	28.91
miR-125a	25.99	26.10	26.03	25.25	25.55	26.07	25.66	25.62	27.18	27.55	28.39	26.85	27.93	27.47	26.70	26.30	26.67	26.31
miR-146a	28.03	26.53	26.15	26.39	26.56	26.18	26.50	26.39	23.43	26.44	28.26	27.70	27.31	27.10	26.15	27.15	28.31	27.69
miR-191	27.43	27.06	27.25	26.64	27.00	26.82	27.27	27.69	26.50	28.31	28.83	28.25	29.03	28.80	27.41	27.49	28.65	26.95
Group ID	**1.00**	**1.00**	**1.00**	**1.00**	**1.00**	**1.00**	**1.00**	**1.00**	**1.00**	**2.00**	**2.00**	**2.00**	**2.00**	**2.00**	**2.00**	**2.00**	**2.00**	**2.00**

2) Convert Ct's to a linear scale (relative quantities). For purposes of the example dataset below, each assay has a PCR efficiency of 100% and the data are normalized to the lowest Ct value for each target.

Candidate Normalizer	Sample Type N	N	N	N	N	N	N	N	N	T	T	T	T	T	T	T	T	T
miR-16	0.30	0.46	0.28	**1.00**	0.47	0.33	0.35	0.20	0.73	0.11	0.10	0.10	0.09	0.09	0.23	0.15	0.09	0.13
miR-24	0.49	0.56	0.58	0.87	**1.00**	0.78	0.88	0.43	0.36	0.34	0.26	0.32	0.14	0.18	0.92	0.55	0.32	0.54
miR-27a	0.38	0.59	0.45	0.55	**1.00**	0.84	0.82	0.25	0.32	0.17	0.12	0.24	0.08	0.16	0.61	0.51	0.23	0.54
miR-93	0.25	0.41	0.30	0.92	0.53	0.34	0.57	0.34	0.68	0.22	0.29	0.29	0.14	0.34	**1.00**	0.32	0.21	0.66
miR-103	0.51	0.47	0.71	0.92	0.88	0.68	0.65	0.41	0.70	0.35	0.19	0.35	0.18	0.27	**1.00**	0.56	0.44	0.47
miR-106a	0.30	0.64	0.37	**1.00**	0.61	0.50	0.52	0.40	0.92	0.19	0.27	0.45	0.17	0.55	0.56	0.30	0.29	0.64
miR-125a	0.60	0.56	0.58	**1.00**	0.82	0.57	0.76	0.78	0.26	0.20	0.11	0.33	0.16	0.22	0.37	0.49	0.38	0.48
miR-146a	0.04	0.12	0.15	0.13	0.11	0.15	0.12	0.13	**1.00**	0.12	0.03	0.05	0.07	0.08	0.15	0.08	0.03	0.05
miR-191	0.53	0.68	0.60	0.91	0.71	0.80	0.59	0.44	**1.00**	0.29	0.20	0.30	0.17	0.20	0.53	0.51	0.23	0.73
Group ID	**1.00**	**1.00**	**1.00**	**1.00**	**1.00**	**1.00**	**1.00**	**1.00**	**1.00**	**2.00**	**2.00**	**2.00**	**2.00**	**2.00**	**2.00**	**2.00**	**2.00**	**2.00**

(continued)

3) Input relative quantities into NormFinder and assess the intragroup and intergroup variation. An addition below to the standard NormFinder output is the average of the intragroup variation; this intragroup variation is graphically presented as error bars in the plot of intergroup variation by candidate miRNA. The error bars are helpful in that they provide a confidence interval for the intergroup variation.

Gene name	Stability value
miR-191	0.095
miR-103	0.143
miR-24	0.158
miR-27a	0.181
miR-125a	0.205
miR-106a	0.209
miR-93	0.257
miR-146a	0.270
miR-16	0.323

Best gene	miR-191
Stability value	0.095
Best combination of two genes	miR-103 and miR-191
Stability value for best combination of two genes	0.070

Intragroup variation

Group identifier	1	2	Average
miR-16	0.095	0.049	0.072
miR-24	0.114	0.049	0.082
miR-27a	0.190	0.096	0.143
miR-93	0.034	0.095	0.065
miR-103	0.014	0.033	0.023
miR-106a	0.026	0.158	0.092
miR-125a	0.254	0.110	0.182
miR-146a	0.666	0.304	0.485
miR-191	0.006	0.038	0.022

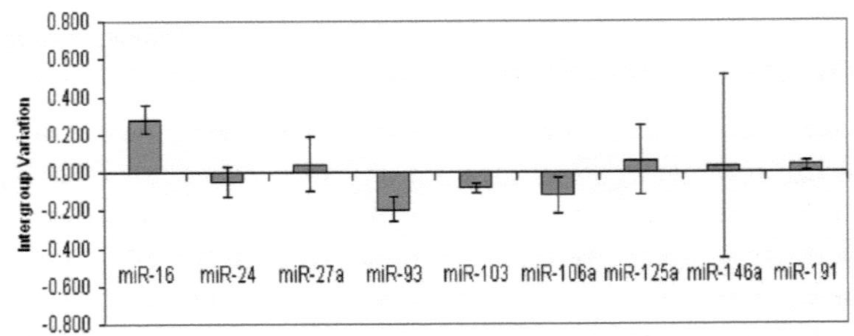

Intergroup variation

Group identifier	1	2
miR-16	0.279	-0.279
miR-24	-0.050	0.050
miR-27a	0.041	-0.041
miR-93	-0.193	0.193
miR-103	-0.083	0.083
miR-106a	-0.123	0.123
miR-125a	0.061	-0.061
miR-146a	0.032	-0.032
miR-191	0.036	-0.036

(continued)

4) Consider eliminating any candidates with large intergroup variation and re-evaluate. Here, the elimination of miR-16 shifts the best normalizer from miR-191 to miR-103 although the top two candidates remain the same.

Best gene	miR-103
Stability value	0.078
Best combination of two genes	miR-103 and miR-191
Stability value for best combination of two genes	0.044

5) Use the top candidate(s) as normalizers for all miRNA targets of interest. If multiple normalizers are advisable, compute their geometric mean for use in data normalization. In the example dataset above, the geometric mean of miR-103 and miR-191 would serve as the normalizer.

6) Determine fold change of miRNA targets of interest from the normalized data (for example, using the ddCt method).

Fig. 1. An Example Workflow for the Normalization of miRNA qRT-PCR Data using NormFinder.

3.7. Select the Most Stable Reference Targets for Normalization

1. If groups are designated, as depicted in the example in Fig. 1, then first inspect the intergroup variation statistics.
2. The extent of variation is provided for each target by group. A given target will have the same value, but a different sign, between two groups. Larger values are associated with more variation and are undesirable. The hallmark of a "good" normalizer is low intergroup variation and low intragroup variation. If all candidate normalizers manifest a relatively low intergroup variation, then the data may be used as is to select the most stable reference targets. However, if a notable outlier is present (e.g., miR-16 in Fig. 1), then it may be advisable to remove this target from the analysis and reanalyze the dataset without it. The average of the intragroup variability provides error bars for the intergroup variability and can be used to assess confidence in the intergroup difference. This filtering step can help minimize the bias that any one target has on the outcome (see Note 9). Indeed, in Fig. 1, the best single normalizer shifts from miR-191 (when miR-16 is included) to miR-103 (when miR-16 is omitted), although the best two normalizers (miR-191 and miR-103) are the same for both analyses. Note that the rank order of the remaining normalizers in this set are unchanged if miR-93, the next most variable miRNA by intergroup variation, is omitted from NormFinder analysis.
3. Typically, the top two normalizers are appropriate for normalization, and additional normalizers may not provide any additional benefit. In the example shown in Fig. 1, there is no benefit in including additional miRNA normalizers to the miR-103 and miR-191 pair.

3.8. Normalize qRT-PCR Data with miRNA Targets of Interest Using the Selected Reference Gene(s)

1. Once the reference targets have been selected through the above statistical analysis, the next step is to normalize the qRT-PCR data to the miRNA targets of interest (see Note 10).
2. The preferred approach is to calculate the geometric, rather than arithmetic, mean of the normalizers (e.g., miR-103 and miR-191 in the example present in Fig. 1). This calculation moderates the effects of outliers and differences in abundance among various targets. The geometric mean (a Ct value) can then be subtracted from the target Ct using the ddCt method (8) to reveal the fold change. For example:

   Normal sample

   Ct, target miRNA = 20
   Ct, geomean (miR-103 + miR-191) = 21

   Tumor sample

   Ct, target miRNA = 22.5
   Ct, geomean (miR-103 + miR-191) = 21.5
   ddCt = ((20 − 21) − (22.5 − 21.5)) = −(1) − (1) = −2.

Here, a ddCt = −2 corresponds to a net 2 Ct lower expression in the tumor, or approximately 25% expression relative to the normal sample.

3. The calculation above assumes that each of the targets have the same (quantitative) PCR efficiency. If this is not true, the Ct values can first be adjusted according to the difference in efficiency (see Note 8), and then compared accordingly.

4. Notes

1. Small RNA isolates should: (1) be free of protein, particularly nucleases; (2) be free of RT-PCR inhibitors (the PCR step is particularly vulnerable, and some targets may be more sensitive to inhibition than others, which can skew data comparisons); and (3) provide clear evidence of the small RNA fraction and ideally the intactness of any larger RNA species. The most important issue is to correctly match the isolation technology with the sample type (e.g., biofluid, solid tissue, or FFPE) to recover the entire miRNA population.
2. Doleshal et al. (9) have recommended procedural modifications that permit higher FFPE tissue inputs into the RecoverAll procedure. This modified protocol may be of benefit to some researchers.
3. Use of miRNAs such as let 7, miR-16, miR-24, as well as miRNAs that are typically less abundant, such as miR-191 and miR-103, can provide a rapid assessment of the compatibility of the sample for amplification of across multiple targets with a broad range of cell copy numbers. A spike-in of a defined miRNA oligonucleotide may also be used to assess general sample matrix effects, such as inhibitors.
4. The normalization selection strategy that is described is appropriate for all qRT-PCR formats, including those based on hydrolysis probes (such as TaqMan) or intercalating dyes (such as SYBR green). Results using emerging, highly multiplexed strategies, such as ABI's MegaPlex technology (10), however, should be cautiously interpreted when relative high Cts are observed (e.g., >30 Cts). Moreover, such large-scale target screens are amenable to global normalization approaches that are beyond the scope of this chapter.
5. Alternative and readily available software tools for normalization include geNorm (a free Excel add-in), BestKeeper (a free Excel spreadsheet tool), Global Pattern Recognition Data Analysis Tool (a commercial product developed by Bar Harbor Technology), as well as more comprehensive

PCR-based analysis programs such as qbasePLUS (a commercial product from Biogazelle that exploits the geNorm algorithm), and GenEx (a commercial program from MultiD Analyses with capabilities of both geNorm and NormFinder).

6. NormFinder utilizes a linear mixed effects model to estimate both intra and intergroup variation, rather than the combined variation, as with, e.g., geNorm. However, it is important to note that these estimates are usually improved by increasing the number of samples and candidate normalizers that are included in the analyses.
7. Generally, it is advisable to use normalizers whose expressions mirror the range of expression for the miRNA targets of interest.
8. An alternative data conversion is to use the known PCR efficiency for each assay to convert all Ct values to the equivalent value had the assay been performed with 100% efficiency. In this case, $\mathrm{Ct}E_{100\%} = \mathrm{Ct}E \times \log_{10}(1+E)/\log_{10}(2)$, where $0 \leq E \leq 1$ (11). For example, an assay that produces a Ct = 24 when $E = 0.9$ (90%) would be equivalent to Ct = 22.22 if $E = 1.0$ (100%). In this way, all Cts can be harmonized to common terms by a stepwise calculation that conveniently preserves the Ct unit.
9. An assumption of the NormFinder algorithm is that the collection of reference targets that are analyzed have minimal bias. In other words, bias in an individual gene can be tolerated as long as the average of all targets investigated show no systematic intergroup variation. However, estimates of variance are expected to improve by eliminating those targets with demonstrable differential expression between groups. By definition, once such targets are removed, the remaining variability should be primarily reflected in the intragroup variance.
10. The scale of the experiment may necessitate the amplification of samples and targets across multiple reaction plates. If this is the case, it is advisable to include an interplate calibrator whose resulting Ct value can be used to compensate for plate-to-plate variation.

References

1. Peltier, H. J., and Latham, G. J. (2008) Normalization of microRNA expression levels in quantitative RT-PCR assays: identification of suitable reference RNA targets in normal and cancerous human solid tissues. *RNA* **14**, 844–52.
2. Mestdagh, P., Van Vlierberghe, P., De Weer, A., Muth, D., Westermann, F., Speleman, F., and Vandesompele, J. (2009) A novel and universal method for microRNA RT-qPCR data normalization. *Genome Biol* **10**, R64.
3. Davison, T. S., Johnson, C. D., and Andruss, B. F. (2006) Analyzing micro-RNA expression using microarrays. *Methods Enzymol* **411**, 14–34.
4. Liang, Y., Ridzon, D., Wong, L., and Chen, C. (2007) Characterization of microRNA

expression profiles in normal human tissues. *BMC Genomics* **8**, 166.

5. Bustin, S. A., Benes, V., Garson, J. A., Hellemans, J., Huggett, J., Kubista, M., Mueller, R., Nolan, T., Pfaffl, M. W., Shipley, G. L., Vandesompele, J., and Wittwer, C. T. (2009) The MIQE guidelines: minimum information for publication of quantitative real-time PCR experiments. *Clin Chem* **55**, 611–22.
6. Andersen, C. L., Jensen, J. L., and Orntoft, T. F. (2004) Normalization of real-time quantitative reverse transcription-PCR data: a model-based variance estimation approach to identify genes suited for normalization, applied to bladder and colon cancer data sets. *Cancer Res* **64**, 5245–50.
7. Davoren, P. A., McNeill, R. E., Lowery, A. J., Kerin, M. J., and Miller, N. (2008) Identification of suitable endogenous control genes for microRNA gene expression anal-ysis in human breast cancer. *BMC Mol Biol* **9**, 76.
8. Livak, K. J., and Schmittgen, T. D. (2001) Analysis of relative gene expression data using real-time quantitative PCR and the 2(–delta delta C(T)) method. *Methods* **25**, 402–8.
9. Doleshal, M., Magotra, A. A., Choudhury, B., Cannon, B. D., Labourier, E., and Szafranska, A. E. (2008) Evaluation and validation of total RNA extraction methods for microRNA expression analyses in formalin-fixed, paraffin-embedded tissues. *J Mol Diagn* **10**, 203–11.
10. Mestdagh, P., Feys, T., Bernard, N., Guenther, S., Chen, C., Speleman, F., and Vandesompele, J. (2008) High-throughput stem-loop RT-qPCR miRNA expression profiling using minute amounts of input RNA. *Nucleic Acids Res* **36**, e143.
11. Kubista, M., and Sindelka, R. (2007) The Prime technique: real-time PCR data analysis. *G.I.T. Lab J* **9–10**, 33–5.

Chapter 3

MicroRNA Detection in Bone Marrow Cells by LNA-FISH

Silvana Debernardi and Amanda Dixon-McIver

Abstract

The protocol reported in this chapter describes a method for the detection and spatial localisation of microRNAs (miRNAs) in cryopreserved primary leukaemic suspension cells using digoxigenin (DIG)-labelled, Locked Nucleic Acid (LNA)-modified probes, and fluorescence in situ hybridisation (FISH). The LNA probe hybridisation yields highly accurate signals able to discrimin.ate between single nucleotide differences and hence between closely related miRNA family members. DIG-labelled LNA probes for mature miRNAs are detected using an anti-DIG fluorescein isothiocyanate (FITC) conjugated antibody and the fluorescent signals visualised with a confocal microscope, which permits the spatial localisation of the miRNAs.

Using LNA-FISH, we visualised the spatial localisation of two mature miRNAs, *miR-127* and *miR-154*, in primary acute myeloid leukaemia (AML) suspension cells, and thus, we confirmed their expression in a specific leukaemic subtype as measured by real-time PCR.

1. Introduction

MicroRNAs (miRNAs) are highly conserved small non-coding (snc) RNAs (1) that play key roles in regulatory functions, including modulation of haematopoiesis (2) and cell differentiation in mammals. MiRNAs modulate gene expression through complementarity-mediated binding to the 3′ untranslated region (UTR) of target messenger (m)RNAs (3, 4).

Examples of an association between disrupted expression of miRNAs and cancer have been shown in a variety of tissues (5, 6), and a number of miRNAs have been characterised as tumor suppressors (7, 8) or oncogenes (9). Acute myeloid leukaemia (AML) is a heterogeneous group of diseases that arises from the accumulation of myeloid precursor cells arrested at various stages of differentiation. An association between miRNA levels and

Silvia Monticelli (ed.), *MicroRNAs and the Immune System: Methods and Protocols*, Methods in Molecular Biology, vol. 667,
DOI 10.1007/978-1-60761-811-9_3, © Springer Science+Business Media, LLC 2010

AML cytogenetic subtypes has been established in our laboratory (10, 11) and by other groups (12, 13).

Locked nucleic acids (LNAs) are synthetic nucleic acid analogues that increase the thermostability of nucleic acid duplexes when incorporated into oligonucleotides (14). LNA probes provide an alternative to standard DNA probes with improved sensitivity and specificity. They are able to discriminate between single nucleotide differences and, hence, they are particularly suited for miRNA detection and analysis in cancer diagnostics (15–18).

In situ hybridisation using DIG-labelled, LNA-modified probes (LNA-ISH), and a colorimetric detection method have been used successfully for the visualisation of mature miRNAs in tissue sections (16, 17, 19). However, in haematopoietic tissue, the colorimetric method is unable to yield cellular details and thus to spatially localise the miRNAs of interest.

We further developed this methodology and successfully used a fluorescent antibody to detect the spatial localisation of miRNAs in cryopreserved primary AML suspension cells. We combined LNA-ISH with the use of a confocal microscope to visualise the signal generated by an anti-DIG fluorescein isothiocyanate (FITC) conjugated antibody. Using this adaptation [LNA Fluorescent In Situ Hybridisation (LNA-FISH)], we validated the expression of two miRNAs, previously measured by real-time PCR, in the cytoplasm of leukaemic patient cells (11). Compared to other techniques such as northern blots, LNA-FISH offers the possibility to detect miRNAs in a sparse population of cells, also providing an alternative or integrative diagnostic tool.

2. Materials

2.1. Mononuclear Cell Extraction and Cryopreservation

1. Upon informed consent, leukaemia samples used in this study were obtained from bone marrow (BM) of patients in St. Bartholomew's Hospital, London, UK.
2. Lymphoprep™ (Axis-Shield, Norway).
3. Washing solution: RPMI-1640 medium supplemented with 5% foetal calf serum (FCS) (Gibco).
4. Freezing solution: 10% dimethyl sulphoxide (DMSO) in FCS (see Note 1).

2.2. Thawing of Cryopreserved Cells

1. RPMI medium: 10% FCS in RPMI 1640; 10 mL is needed per vial to be thawed.
2. 1× Phosphate-Buffered Saline (PBS), pH 7.5: 8 g NaCl, 0.2 g KCl, 1.44 g Na_2HPO_4, 0.27 g KH_2HPO_4 are dissolved

in 800 mL ddH$_2$O. The pH is adjusted to 7.5 with HCl or NaOH; ddH$_2$O is added to 1 L. The solution is sterilised by autoclaving and stored at room temperature.

3. Trypan Blue Solution (freshly prepared): 0.1% Trypan Blue in 1× PBS.

2.3. Cytospin Preparation for Suspension Cells

1. Poly-L-lysine solution: Poly-L-lysine (Sigma-Aldrich) 0.1% (w/v) in ddH$_2$O. The solution can be stored at 4°C.
2. Shandon Cytospin® 3 cytocentrifuge (Thermo Scientific).
3. Formalin (10% Neutral Buffered): 100 mL formalin (40% aqueous solution formaldehyde), 4 g NaH$_2$PO$_4$ · H$_2$O, 6.5 g Na$_2$HPO$_4$, 850 mL ddH$_2$O. The pH is adjusted to 7.0; ddH$_2$O is added to 1 L. The solution is stored at room temperature.
4. Slide box containing silica gel (see Note 2).

2.4. Locked Nucleic Acid™-Probe Preparation

2.4.1. Labelling of miRCURY-LNA Detection Probes

1. LNA-modified probes (miRCURY-LNA Detection probe, Exiqon, Denmark) were purchased unlabelled for the studied miRNAs, positive (*U6*) and negative controls (scrambled oligonucleotide) at a stock concentration of 25 pmol/μL (see Note 3).
2. Diethylpyrocarbonate (DEPC)-treated water (Sigma-Aldrich) to dilute the LNA probes.
3. 10 M Sodium hydroxide (NaOH): 400 g NaOH are dissolved in 450 mL ddH$_2$O; ddH$_2$O is then added to 1 L.
4. 0.5 M Ethylenediaminetetraacetic acid (EDTA): 186.1 g Na$_2$EDTA · H$_2$O is dissolved in 700 mL ddH$_2$O; pH is adjusted to 8.0 with 10 M NaOH (~50 mL); ddH$_2$O is added to 1 L.
5. 1 M Tris–HCl: 121 g Tris base is dissolved in 800 mL ddH$_2$O. The pH is adjusted as desired with concentrated HCl; ddH$_2$O is added to 1 L.
6. Digoxigenin (DIG)-3′-oligonucleotide Tailing Kit (Roche Applied Science). Labelling is performed according to manufacturer's instructions.
7. Labelling master mix, to be prepared on ice (the total volume for the labelling reaction is 11 μL): 4 μL reaction buffer (1 M potassium cacodylate, 0.125 M Tris–HCl, 1.25 mg/mL bovine serum albumin (BSA), pH 6.6), 4 μL COCl$_2$ solution (25 mM COCl$_2$), 1 μL DIG-dUTP solution (1 mM DIG-11-dUTP), 1 μL dATP solution (10 mM dATP), 1 μL 400 U terminal transferase (400 U/μL terminal transferase, 60 mM K-phosphate (pH 7.2 at 4°C) 150 mM KCl, 1 mM 2-mercaptoethanol, 0.5% Triton X-100, 50% glycerol) (see Notes 4 and 5).

2.4.2. Purification of the DIG-Labelled Probe

1. Sephadex G25 column (Amersham Bioscience).

2.4.3. Labelling Efficiency and Concentration Assessment by Dot-Blot

1. DIG-dUTP/dATP tailed oligonucleotide, 2.5 pmol/μL (Roche Applied Science).
2. GE Nitrocellulose Pure Transfer Membrane.
3. 1% BSA in 1× PBS solution.
4. Blocking reagent (Roche Applied Science) (see Note 6).
5. 10× Blocking stock solution: 1% Blocking reagent (w/v) in maleic acid buffer (100 mM maleic acid, 150 mM NaCl, pH 7.5, adjusted with concentrated or solid NaOH). The blocking reagent (powder form) is dissolved in maleic acid to a final concentration of 10% (w/v) by shaking and gentle heating on a heating block. This stock solution is autoclaved and stored at 4°C (see Note 7).
6. 1× Blocking solution: the 10× Blocking stock solution is diluted with 1× maleic acid buffer to a 1× concentrated solution (always to be freshly prepared).
7. Sheep anti-DIG-alkaline phosphatase (AP) conjugated antibody, Fab fragmens, 150 U (Roche Applied Science).
8. Nitro blue tetrazolium chloride (NBT)/5-bromo-4-chloro-3-indolyl phosphate, toluidine salt (BCIP) developer (Perbio Science UK Ltd).
9. 10× TE: 100 mM Tris–HCl, pH 7.5, 10 mM EDTA, pH 8.0.

2.5. LNA Fluorescent In Situ Hybridisation

1. Sheep anti-DIG-FITC conjugated antibody, Fab fragments, 200 μg (Roche Applied Science). The lyophilised antibody is resuspended in 1 mL of ddH_2O. The stock solution is then diluted to a final concentration of 0.5 μg/mL in blocking solution briefly before use (See item 11 below for blocking solution recipe and Note 8).
2. 50× Denhardt's solution (Sigma-Aldrich).
3. Yeast tRNA (Invitrogen).
4. Hybridisation buffer: 50% deionised formamide, 0.3 M NaCl, 20 mM Tris–HCl, pH 8.0, 5 mM EDTA, 10 mM phosphate buffer, pH 8.0, 10% dextran sulfate, 1× Denhardt's solution, and 0.5 mg/mL yeast tRNA. The buffer can be stored in aliquots at −80°C.
5. RNase-free coverslip (H18200, Invitrogen).
6. Humidified HYBrite™ slide incubation chamber (Abbott Laboratories Ltd).
7. 20× Standard Saline Citrate (SSC), pH 7.5: 3 M NaCl, 0.3 M sodium citrate, the pH is adjusted to 7.5 with 1 M

HCl. The solution is autoclaved and can be stored at room temperature for up to 6 months.

8. 2× SSC/1% paraformaldehyde: SSC is diluted in ddH_2O (Fixative solution to be used in the case described in Note 9).
9. 50% Formamide/2× SSC: SSC is diluted in ddH_2O and can be stored at 4°C for up to 1 week.
10. 1× PBS/0.1% Tween 20 solution, freshly prepared.
11. 1× Blocking solution: 0.5% blocking reagent (Roche), 10% heat-inactivated sheep serum (Invitrogen), 0.1% Tween-20, and 1× PBS.
12. 1× Tris-buffered saline Tween-20 (TBST): 150 mM NaCl, 2.7 mM KCl, 25 mM Tris base, 0.1% Tween-20. Adjusted at pH 7.4 and autoclaved.
13. 4′-6′Diamidino-2-phenylindole (DAPI) (Molecular Probes) stock solution for nuclear staining: 100 μM DAPI in 1× PBS (see Note 10). DAPI staining solution: 300 nM in 1× PBS.
14. Mounting solution: ProLong® Gold antifade reagent (Invitrogen), ready to use. The antifade reagent should be stored at −20°C (see Note 11).

2.6. Microscopy and Image Analysis

1. Zeiss 510 Meta-confocal microscope equipped with a Plan-Apochromat 63×/1.4 Oil DIC lens, fitted with a motorised stage (Carl Zeiss).
2. Image stacks of cells are captured and analysed using programs LSM510, version 3.2SP2 and Image J, version 1.39d (http://rsb.info.nih.gov/ij/index.html).

3. Methods

The LNA-FISH protocol can be completed within 2 days. This includes approximately an hour's work for cytospin preparation of suspension cells and hybridisation set-up on day 1 and approximately 3 hours for washes and incubation with fluorescent antibody on day 2. Labelling of the probe with DIG and assessment of reaction efficiency can be performed in 3.5 hours. A stock of labelled probe could be prepared for future experiments.

3.1. Mononuclear Cell Extraction and Cryopreservation

1. Mononuclear cells are purified from white blood cells using the Lymphoprep™ separation kit following manufacturer's instructions.
2. Mononuclear cells are washed once in 5% FCS RPMI medium at 1,200 rpm for 10 min at 4°C. Supernatant is

discarded and cell pellet agitated or vortexed into solution. Approximately 15 million cells are aliquoted in 2 mL of freezing solution per vial. Samples are then cryopreserved in liquid nitrogen.

3.2. Thawing of Cryopreserved Cells

1. The sample vials are removed from liquid nitrogen, immediately thawed in 37°C water bath, and emptied into sterile 10-mL tubes.
2. One drop of medium is added every 10–15 s for 2 min, followed by two drops every 10–15 s for 2 min, and then gradually the number of drops is increased to 5-mL level.
3. Tubes are topped up to 10 mL and then centrifuged at 1,200 rpm for 5 min.
4. The pellets are then washed twice with 10 mL of 1× PBS.
5. Before spinning, 10 μL of cells are kept apart for cell counting and viability assessment after dilution in 10 μL of Trypan Blue Solution.
6. Cells are resuspended at a concentration of 0.5 million cells/mL in 1× PBS.

3.3. Cytospin Preparation for Suspension Cells

1. A 100-μL aliquot of suspended cells is pipetted into a cytospin column and spun at 300 rpm for 5 min on poly-l-lysine coated glass slides (see Note 12) using a Shandon Cytospin® 3 cytocentrifuge.
2. The slides are air-dried and then fixed for 10 min in neutral buffered formalin.
3. The slides are air-dried again, before proceeding to the hybridisation step (see Notes 2 and 13).

3.4. Locked Nucleic Acid™-Probe Preparation

100 pmol of LNA detection probes are labelled with DIG at the 3′ end in a final volume of 20 μL.

3.4.1. Labelling of miRCURY LNA Detection Probes with DIG

1. 100 pmol of LNA detection probes are mixed with DEPC-treated water to a volume of 9 μL and kept in ice.
2. 11 μL of labelling master mix are added to the probe, briefly vortexed, and then spun.
3. The reaction mix is incubated at 37°C for 30 min in a water bath and then placed immediately on ice.
4. The reaction is stopped by the addition of 5 μL of 0.1 M EDTA (pH 8.0).

3.4.2. Purification of the DIG-Labelled Probe

1. Before use, the Sephadex G25 column is first resuspended by inversion and centrifuged for 1 min at 720 × *g* in a 1.5-mL tube. The buffer is then discarded.

2. The probe mixture (21 μL) is added to the column. The column is centrifuged in a new 1.5-mL tube for 2 min at 720×*g*. The column is discarded and the labelled probe retained. The concentration is approximately 30 ng/μL.
3. The labelled probe can be stored at −20°C for up to 2 years (see Note 14).

3.4.3. Labelling Efficiency and Concentration Assessment by Dot-Blot

Labelling reaction efficiency and approximate concentration are determined by dot blot on nitrocellulose membrane and colorimetric detection of DIG-labelled probe performed with two colourless substrates, NBT and BCIP, which form a redox system.

1. A serial dilution of the labelled LNA oligonucleotide (approximate concentration of 30 ng/μL) as well as a DIG-dUTP/dATP-tailed oligonucleotide control is performed in DEPC-treated water. The serial dilution is as follows: 1:10, 5:50, and 5:50.
2. A 1 μL of the undiluted probes followed by a 1 μL of each dilution is spotted on a nitrocellulose membrane. The membrane is air-dried and then placed under ultraviolet light (on both sides) for 2 min (see Note 15).
3. The membrane is placed in 1× PBS for 3 min and then blocked with 1% BSA in 1× PBS for 30 min at room temperature.
4. The membrane is then incubated in 1× Blocking solution containing 1:100 anti-DIG-AP conjugated antibody for 30 min at room temperature.
5. The membrane is washed twice with 1× PBS for 10 min.
6. The membrane is covered with a thin layer of NBT/BCIP developer and incubated for 15–30 min at room temperature (dependent on the time required for the colour to become visible).
7. The reaction is stopped by replacing the developer with 1× TE buffer and the membrane examined. Concentrations and labelling efficiency are determined by eye determination of the strength of colour of the labelled probe compared to the DIG-dUTP/dATP-tailed oligonucleotide control of known concentration.

3.5. LNA Fluorescent In Situ Hybridisation

1. Slides from cytospin preparations are dehydrated in a series of ethanol rinses (70, 85, and 100%) of 2 min each at room temperature (see Note 9).
2. A 2-μL aliquot of probe is mixed with 200 μL of hybridisation buffer.
3. The mixture is incubated at 65°C for 5 min to linearise the probes and then chilled on ice.

4. A volume of 50–100 μL of hybridisation mixture is then added to slides. A RNase-free coverslip is applied and slides are incubated overnight, at a temperature 21°C below the melting temperature (Tm) of the probe, in a humidified chamber.
5. Following overnight hybridisation, the coverslips are removed (see Note 16) and slides are washed once for 5 min in 50% formamide/2× SSC at a temperature 4–6°C higher than that of hybridisation.
6. A second wash is performed at room temperature with 1× PBS/0.1% Tween 20 for 5 min.
7. Slides are incubated for 1 hour at room temperature in blocking solution.
8. Anti-DIG-FITC conjugated antibody (diluted 1:400 in blocking solution, see Note 8) is then applied to the slides and incubation is performed in a humidified chamber, for 1 hour at 37°C.
9. Following incubation, slides are washed three times in 1× TBST for 5 min each on a shaker, drained, and air-dried.
10. DAPI counter-staining and slide mounting.
    (a) Samples are washed three times in 1× PBS and the excess solution drained from slides (see Note 17).
    (b) Approximately 300 μL of dilute DAPI solution are added to the slides and incubated for 5 min at room temperature in the dark.
    (c) Slides are rinsed several times with 1× PBS. Excess buffer is drained before mounting.
    (d) A drop of ProLong® Gold antifade reagent is applied to the slides, and coverslips are then carefully lowered on the sections.

The slides can be stored at 4°C for up to 6 months without losing their signals (see Notes 18 and 19, and Table 1).

3.6. Microscopy and Image Analysis

1. Fluorescent LNA signals are visualised on a confocal microscope.
2. A minimum of 100 cells should be examined for each probe.
3. A positive signal is the presence of fluorescent green coloration and a negative signal is the absence of green coloration. An example is shown in Fig. 1.

Table 1
Troubleshooting advice

Problem	Possible explanation	Solution
No/weak signal	No probe added	Repeat the experiment ensuring addition of probe
	Inefficient labelling	Confirm labelling efficiency by dot blot (Subheading 3.4.3)
	Inadequate probe concentration	Increase the amount of probe added to hybridisation buffer (Subheading 3.5, step 2)
	Hybridisation temperature too high	Lower the hybridisation temperature (Subheading 3.5, step 4)
	Wash solutions too stringent	Decrease wash temperature and increase salt concentration (Subheading 3.5, step 5)
	Inaccessibility of probe to target	Include proteinase K or pepsin treatment prior to probe application
	Antibody concentration too low	Check antibody concentration by titration assay
High background	Cellular debris in sample preparation	Wash cell suspension in Carnoy's fixative (3:1 Methanol:Acetic Acid) prior to slide making
	High probe concentration	Lower probe concentration (Subheading 3.5, step 2)
	Post-hybridisation washes not stringent enough	Increase temperature and number/length of washes (Subheading 3.5, steps 5 and 6)
	Inadequate blocking	Change concentration and/or composition of blocking solution (Subheading 2.5, item 11)
	Contaminated blocking buffer	Check blocking buffer for possible contamination
	Antibody incubation time too long	Decrease antibody incubation time (Subheading 3.5, step 8)
	Antibody concentration too high	Decrease concentration (Subheading 2.5, item 1 and Note 8)
Partial hybridisation	Air bubbles during hybridisation	Ensure that there are no air bubbles present when applying coverslips (Subheading 3.5, step 4)

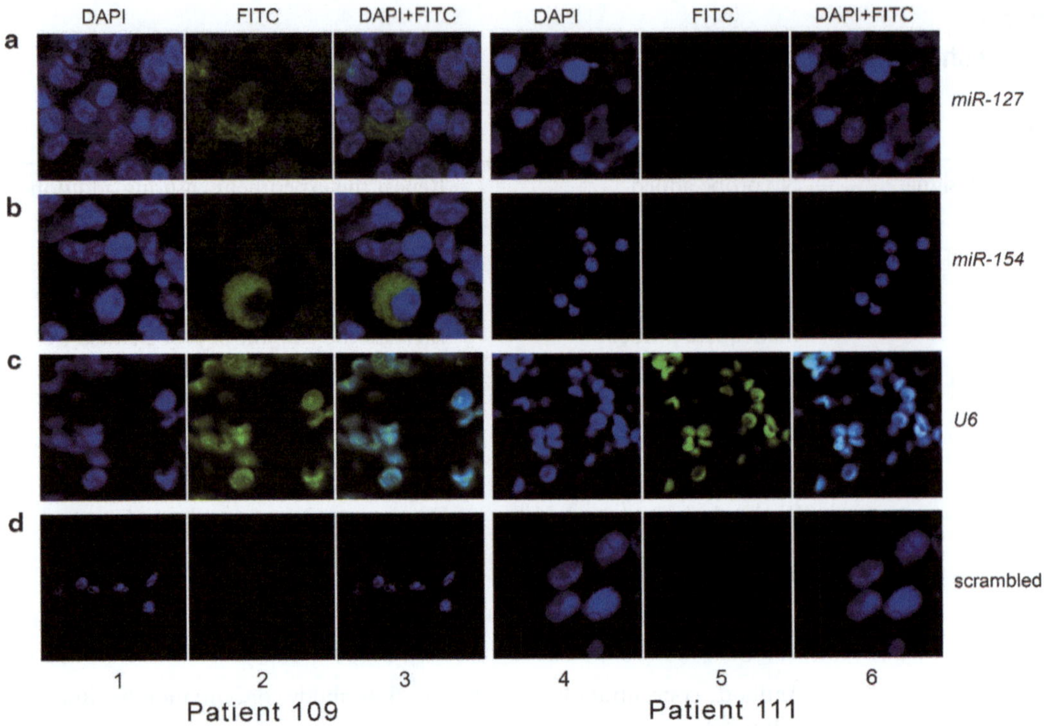

Fig. 1. MiRNA detection in cryopreserved bone marrow cells by LNA-FISH. An example of positive and negative miRNA detection is shown in two AML patients (n. 109, *lanes 1–3*, and n. 111, *lanes 4–6*, respectively). All images were obtained with the confocal microscope as described in the method (Subheading 3.6). The DAPI nuclear staining (*blue*), the fluorescent in situ hybridisation signals obtained with FITC conjugated antibody (*green*), and the combined images are indicated. The *A* and *B panels* show the detection of *miR-127* and *miR-154*, respectively. Both miRNAs are detected in the cytoplasm of cells (*lanes 2 and 3*) of sample n. 109, but not in sample n. 111 (*lanes 5 and 6*). The *C panel* shows the nuclear expression of U6, the small RNA used as positive control, in both samples (*lanes 2 and 5*). No signal is detected when cells are hybridised with a scrambled oligonucleotide (negative control), as shows in *lanes 2 and 5* of the *D panel.*

4. Notes

1. DMSO may cause eye damage and skin and respiratory tract irritation. It can also penetrate skin and carry other dissolved chemicals into the body. Therefore, it is recommended to work under the fume hood and to wear eye protection and rubber rather than nitrile gloves (as the latter can dissolve when exposed to DMSO).
2. If not immediately used, slides should be stored at –20°C in a slide box sealed with tape and containing silica gel desiccant to prevent frost building up on the slides.
3. LNA detection probes could be purchased already labelled. The LNA-FISH protocol described in this chapter has been optimised for the detection of two human miRNAs (*miR-127* and *miR-154*). The probe sequences, including

positive and negative controls, were (5′–3′): *miR-127*, AGCC AAGCTCAGACGGATCCGA; *miR-154*, CGAAGGCAACA CGGATAACCTA; *U6*, CACGAATTTGCGTGTCATCCTT; scrambled oligonucleotide, TTCACAATGCGTTATCG GATGT.

4. Wear personal protective equipment when handling potassium cacodylate. It is toxic if swallowed. It may be absorbed through the skin in harmful amounts, and it may cause eye irritation. Potassium cacodylate may cause nephrotoxicity, hepatotoxicity, and may produce abnormalities of the haematopoietic system.
5. $COCl_2$-solution, or phosgene, is a liquefied gas. It is very toxic by inhalation, corrosive to eyes, respiratory system and skin.
6. The Blocking reagent is used to decrease the background in non-radioactive hybridisation and detection of nucleic acids hybrids.
7. The blocking solution prepared with maleic acid buffer is for filter hybridisation only (Subheading 3.4.3).
8. The sheep anti-DIG-FITC conjugated antibody can be diluted also in 1× PBS/0.5% BSA (w/v), pH 7.4. However, dilution in blocking solution is preferred when a reduction of unspecific binding is necessary (Subheading 3.5, step 8).
9. Poor morphology of the cells after hybridisation is an indication of inadequate fixation (Subheading 3.5, step 1). The slides should be pre-treated with fresh fixative as follows:
   (a) Fix cells by the immersion of slides in 2× SSC/1% paraformaldehyde for 1 min.
   (b) Rinse the slides by several immersions in ddH_2O.
   (c) Dehydrate the slides through a series of 1-min EtOH rinses (70, 85, and 100%).
   (d) Air-dry the slides and continue with probe application.
10. DAPI is supplied in a unit size of 10 mg that should be stored at room temperature protected from light. The stock solution should be stored at 4°C and it will remain stable for about 6 months. DAPI is a known mutagen and should be handled with care.
11. Before use, allow the ProLong® Gold antifade reagent (Invitrogen) to equilibrate to room temperature.
12. Glass slides are washed in 70% ethanol and coated with poly-l-lysine solution for 15 min at room temperature. They are then rinsed in distilled water and air-dried.
13. To avoid cell loss, ensure that the slides are coated with poly-l-lysine prior to application (see Note 11) and do not agitate the slides too harshly during washing steps.

14. Before storing at −20°C, multiple aliquots of the probe should be prepared to avoid freezing/thawing.
15. Cross-linking of the probes, by ultraviolet light, prevents loss during the wash steps.
16. Soak coverslips off between stages in 2× SSC to prevent cell damage (Subheading 3.5, step 5).
17. Washes with 1× PBS are necessary to equilibrate the pH of the cells and increase the specificity of DAPI counter-staining.
18. A weak counter-stained signal could be observed when DAPI reagent is too old or exposed to light for extended periods. Oil droplets in the counterstain could also cause a weak signal. In this case proceed as follows:
    (a) Remove coverslip.
    (b) Immerse slides for 5 min in 2× SSC/0.1% Tween 20 at room temperature.
    (c) Dehydrate slides through a series of 1-min EtOH rinses (70, 85, and 100%).
    (d) Air-dry and re-apply counterstain.
19. Weak or absent signal, high background, and partial hybridisation could be due to a number of causes whose possible solutions are indicated in Table 1.

Acknowledgments

This work was supported by funds from Barts & The London, Research Advisory Board Studentship (ONA100P).

References

1. Bartel, D. P. (2004) MicroRNAs: genomics, biogenesis, mechanism, and function. *Cell* **116**, 281–97.
2. Chen, C. Z., Li, L., Lodish, H. F., Bartel, D. P. (2004) MicroRNAs modulate hematopoietic lineage differentiation. *Science* **303**, 83–6.
3. Doench, J. G., Sharp, P. A. (2004) Specificity of microRNA target selection in translational repression. *Genes Dev* **18**, 504–11.
4. Yekta, S., Shih, I. H., Bartel, D. P. (2004) MicroRNA-directed cleavage of HOXB8 mRNA. *Science* **304**, 594–6.
5. Lu, J., Getz, G., Miska, E. A., Alvarez-Saavedra, E., Lamb, J., Peck, D., et al. (2005) MicroRNA expression profiles classify human cancers. *Nature* **435**, 834–8.
6. Volinia, S., Calin, G. A., Liu, C. G., Ambs, S., Cimmino, A., Petrocca, F., et al. (2006) A microRNA expression signature of human solid tumors defines cancer gene targets. *Proc Natl Acad Sci U S A* **103**, 2257–61.
7. Calin, G. A., Dumitru, C. D., Shimizu, M., Bichi, R., Zupo, S., Noch, E., et al. (2002) Frequent deletions and down-regulation of micro-RNA genes miR15 and miR16 at 13q14 in chronic lymphocytic leukemia. *Proc Natl Acad Sci U S A* **99**, 15524–9.
8. Takamizawa, J., Konishi, H., Yanagisawa, K., Tomida, S., Osada, H., Endoh, H., et al. (2004) Reduced expression of the let-7 microRNAs in human lung cancers in association with shortened postoperative survival. *Cancer Res* **64**, 3753–6.

9. Metzler, M., Wilda, M., Busch, K., Viehmann, S., Borkhardt, A. (2004) High expression of precursor microRNA-155/BIC RNA in children with Burkitt lymphoma. *Genes Chromosomes Cancer* **39**, 167–9.
10. Debernardi, S., Skoulakis, S., Molloy, G., Chaplin, T., Dixon-McIver, A., Young, B. D. (2007) MicroRNA miR-181a correlates with morphological sub-class of acute myeloid leukaemia and the expression of its target genes in global genome-wide analysis. *Leukemia* **21**, 912–6.
11. Dixon-McIver, A., East, P., Mein, C. A., Cazier, J. B., Molloy, G., Chaplin, T., et al. (2008) Distinctive patterns of microRNA expression associated with karyotype in acute myeloid leukaemia. *PLoS One* **3**, e2141.
12. Garzon, R., Garofalo, M., Martelli, M. P., Briesewitz, R., Wang, L., Fernandez-Cymering, C., et al. (2008) Distinctive microRNA signature of acute myeloid leukemia bearing cytoplasmic mutated nucleophosmin. *Proc Natl Acad Sci U S A* **105**, 3945–50.
13. Jongen-Lavrencic, M., Sun, S. M., Dijkstra, M. K., Valk, P. J., Lowenberg, B. (2008) MicroRNA expression profiling in relation to the genetic heterogeneity of acute myeloid leukemia. *Blood* **111**, 5078–85.
14. Braasch, D. A., Liu, Y., Corey, D. R. (2002) Antisense inhibition of gene expression in cells by oligonucleotides incorporating locked nucleic acids: effect of mRNA target sequence and chimera design *Nucleic Acids Res* **30**, 5160–7.
15. Castoldi, M., Schmidt, S., Benes, V., Noerholm, M., Kulozik, A. E., Hentze, M. W., et al. (2006) A sensitive array for microRNA expression profiling (miChip) based on locked nucleic acids (LNA). *RNA* **12**, 913–20.
16. Kloosterman, W. P., Wienholds, E., de Bruijn, E., Kauppinen, S., Plasterk, R. H. (2006) In situ detection of miRNAs in animal embryos using LNA-modified oligonucleotide probes. *Nat Methods* **3**, 27–9.
17. Nelson, P. T., Baldwin, D. A., Kloosterman, W. P., Kauppinen, S., Plasterk, R. H., Mourelatos, Z. (2006) RAKE and LNA-ISH reveal microRNA expression and localization in archival human brain. *RNA* **12**, 187–91.
18. Stenvang, J., Silahtaroglu, A. N., Lindow, M., Elmen, J., Kauppinen, S. (2008) The utility of LNA in microRNA-based cancer diagnostics and therapeutics. *Semin Cancer Biol* **18**, 89–102.
19. Obernosterer, G., Martinez, J., Alenius, M. (2007) Locked nucleic acid-based in situ detection of microRNAs in mouse tissue sections. *Nat Protoc* **2**, 1508–14.

Chapter 4

Measuring MicroRNA Expression in Size-Limited FACS-Sorted and Microdissected Samples

Kai P. Hoefig and Vigo Heissmeyer

Abstract

MicroRNAs (miRNAs) are small noncoding RNAs of an average length of 22 nucleotides, which repress translation of a large number of target mRNAs. The particular importance of this group of small RNAs arises from the ever growing evidence that they control many biological processes, such as differentiation, proliferation, and apoptosis and that deregulation of individual miRNAs frequently results in cancer. The expression of miRNAs is spatially and temporarily fine-tuned and expression levels can reach more than 50,000 copies of one miRNA within a single cell. It is well documented that the comparison of miRNA signatures of normal and diseased tissues results in a small number of differentially expressed miRNAs, which are consequently of high diagnostic value. However, measuring miRNA expression can easily produce false-positive results, due to the high sequence similarity of the miRNAs within families and because biologically inactive pre-miRNAs as well as contaminating bystander cells may falsify the signal. The application of a quantitative PCR-based method is described here to specifically and reliably detect miRNA expression levels from as little as 50 cells. Pure cell populations were either derived from fluorescence-activated cell sorting (FACS) or laser capture microdissection (LCM). Importantly, a combination of quantitative PCR and LCM can also be applied to measure miRNA expression of cells obtained from formalin-fixed, paraffin-embedded (FFPE) tissues, thereby giving experimental access to archives with large numbers of routinely collected normal and diseased tissue samples.

1. Introduction

The biogenesis of mature microRNAs (miRNAs) is a multistep process, regulated on the transcriptional and posttranscriptional level (1). The expression of each individual miRNA is regulated during tissue differentiation, e.g., miR-181a levels strongly vary in the process of T cell development (2). Currently, there are 940 human miRNAs listed in the Sanger database; however, in most tissues, only a handful of miRNA species account for the majority of miRNA molecules (3). This results in an exceptionally high dynamic range of miRNA expression, spanning approximately

Silvia Monticelli (ed.), *MicroRNAs and the Immune System: Methods and Protocols*, Methods in Molecular Biology, vol. 667, DOI 10.1007/978-1-60761-811-9_4,

four orders of magnitude in a single cell (4). The sequences of different miRNAs often differ by just a few nucleotides (e.g., let-7 family members). From the facts presented above, one can conclude that the accurate measurement of miRNA expression levels is error-prone. It is technically challenging to reliably distinguish between pre- and mature miRNAs or between mature miRNAs that are highly similar in sequence. Additionally, due to the extreme variability of miRNA expression, meaningful miRNA measurements can only derive from well-defined and pure cell populations of the same developmental stage. Consequently, these cells may be rare and hard to obtain.

Here, we describe the use of a commercially available quantitative PCR-based miRNA assay, which meets the aforementioned technical requirements (5), in combination with two cell separation techniques, fluorescence activated cell sorting (FACS) and laser capture microdissection (LCM).

One of the two methods described here is aimed to measure miRNA expression in rare FACS-sorted cells. In recent publications, it was demonstrated that miR-155 expression is increased in activated T cells and miR-155$^{-/-}$ mice are impaired in T cell-dependent antibody responses (6, 7). Therefore, we reasoned that miR-155 expression in germinal center CD4 T cells should be increased as compared to assorted splenic CD4 T cells. We measured miR-155 expression of FACS-sorted germinal center T cells (CD4$^+$, PD1$^+$, CXCR5$^+$), derived from an immunized mouse, and compared it with mixed splenic CD4$^+$ T cells, obtained from a nonimmunized mouse. In agreement with our hypothesis, endogenous miR-155 expression was approximately six times higher in germinal center T cells than in a mixed CD4$^+$ T cell population.

In the second approach, it will be demonstrated that LCM can be used to isolate cells that cannot be accessed by FACS. As an example, the expression of tissue-specific miRNAs (miR-122/liver; miR-1/heart and muscle) was analyzed in cells derived from the respective tissues. An important application of this method would be to rid tumor samples of bystander cells and surrounding tissues to measure miRNA expression more precisely. For instance, tumor samples occasionally contain remains of epidermal layers, which can skew miRNA profiling attempts because of very high expression of epidermal-specific miRNAs, such as miR-205, miR-203, etc. (unpublished data). LCM and subsequent quantitative PCR can be applied not only on cryoconserved but also on formalin-fixed tissues. This is in agreement with several previous publications that conclusively demonstrate that formalin-fixed, paraffin embedded (FFPE) material can be used for miRNA profiling (8, 9). Hence, archived FFPE samples from diseased tissues, the common and widespread method of tissue conservation and storage in pathology departments, can be accessed to measure miRNA levels, even in small cell numbers (≥75).

The expression of cell surface markers on normal and diseased hematopoietic cells is well defined. Considering this prerequisite, the combination ofFACS sorting and miRNA measurement, as described here, should allow to address many questions of miRNA function in normal and aberrant hematopoiesis as well as in immunology. LCM expands the possibilities of obtaining pure cell samples, especially from leukemias and lymphomas with a typically low content of tumour cells in surrounding tissues, e.g., Hodgkin's lymphomas.

2. Materials

2.1. Measuring miRNA Expression

1. 96-well Multiply®-PCR Plate, half skirt, natural (Sarstedt).
2. Benchtop 96 Tube, cooling block.
3. TaqMan® MicroRNA Reverse Transcription Kit (Applied Biosystems).
4. TaqMan® MicroRNA Assays (Applied Biosystems).
5. TaqMan® Universal PCR Master Mix No Amp Erase Ung (Applied Biosystems) or LightCycler® 480 Probes Master (Roche) (both master mixes can be used).
6. LightCycler® 480 Multiwell Plate 96 (including sealing foil) (Roche).

2.2. Preparation and Staining of $CD4^+/PD1^+/CXCR5^+$ Cells for FACS-Sorting

1. Sheep blood (Oxoid GmbH).
2. PBS (phosphate buffered saline), pH 7.2:1 tablet for 500 μL of ddH_2O, autoclave.
3. Tissue culture plate, 6 well.
4. T cell medium: RPMI 1640 without L-Glutamine, 10% Fetal Bovine Serum (FBS), Pen Strep (100 U/mL Penicillin, 100 μg/mL Streptomycin), NEAA (L-Alanine 8.9 mg/L, L-Asparagine 13.2 mg/L, L-Aspartic Acid 13.3 mg/L, L-Glutamic Acid 14.7 mg/L, Glycine 7.5 mg/L, L-Proline 11.5 mg/L, and L-Serine 10.5 mg/L), Sodium Pyruvate (1 mM), MEM Eagle Vitamin Mix (D-Ca Pantothenate, 1 mg/L, Choline Chloride 1 mg/L, Folic Acid 1 mg/L, i-Inositol 2 mg/L, Nicotinamide 1 mg/L, Pyridoxine-HCL 1 mg/L Riboflavin 0.1 mg/L, and Thiamine-HCL 1 mg/L), HEPES (10 mM), β-ME-Glutamine (0.04% 2-Mercaptoethanol in 2 mM L-Glutamine).

   β-ME-Glutamine stock solution (100-fold) is produced by adding 40 μL of 2-Mercaptoethanol (0.04%) to 100 mL of a 200 mM L-Glutamine solution.

β-ME-Glutamine and MEM Eagle Vitamin Mix are kept in aliquots (100-fold concentrated) of 6 mL at −20°C. After thawing, incubate β-ME-Glutamine at 37°C until precipitates are dissolved. NEAA, Na Pyruvate, and HEPES are stored at 4°C, while Pen Strep and FBS are stored at −20°C. FBS is heat inactivated for 30 min at 57°C prior to use.

5. Cell strainer; 70 μm mesh.
6. 6 mL Syringe.
7. TAC (Tris-Ammonium-Chloride) solution for erythrocyte lysis: For 1 L TAC solution dissolve 2.06 g Tris (17 mM) in 100 mL ddH_2O and 7.47 g NH_4Cl (14 mM) in 800 mL ddH_2O. Mix both solutions, adjust pH to 7.2 using hydrochloric acid, fill up to 1 L, and autoclave.
8. CD4 (L3T4) MicroBeads, mouse (MACS/Miltenyi Biotec).
9. MACS buffer: use autoMACS running buffer (MACS/Miltenyi Biotec) or PBS pH 7.2, 0.5% BSA (bovine serum albumin) and 2 mM EDTA.
10. FACS antibodies: PE conjugated anti-mouse PD-1, clone J43 (eBioscience), rat anti-mouse CXCR5 (clone MB1 2G8-2-1/E. Kremmer, Helmholtz Center Munich), Cy™5-conjugated AffiniPure $F(ab')_2$ Fragment Goat anti-Rabbit IgG (H+L) (Jackson ImmunoResearch).
11. FACS buffer: 1× PBS, 1% FBS, 0.1% sodium azide.

2.3. Preparation of Tissue Sections from Snap-Frozen Tissues

1. Freezing medium Tissue-Tek® O.C.T. Compound.
2. C35 Type microtome blades (Feather, PMF).

2.4. Preparation of Tissue Sections from Formalin-Fixed Tissues

1. Buffered formalin pH 7.4 (1 L): Na_2HPO_4 (7.8 g/55 mM), $NaH_2PO_4 \times 2H_2O$ (1.87 g/12 mM), Formalin 36–40% (100 mL), H_2O (fill up to 1 L).
2. Embedding cassette.
3. Paraffin embedding station (TES99, Medite).
4. Paraffin.
5. Embedding mold.

2.5. Hematoxylin and Eosin Stain

1. Preparation of hematoxylin solution:

   Stock solution: 1.0 g hematoxylin, 0.2 g sodium iodate ($NaIO_3$), 91.8 g potassium alum ($KAl(SO_4)_2 \times 12\ H_2O$), 50 g chloral hydrate, and 1.0 g citric acid.

   Dissolve hematoxylin and sodium iodate in a small volume of water. In the second solution, dissolve potassium alum in 750 mL of water by heating and stirring of the solution. Combine both solutions, add citric acid and chloral hydrate, fill up to 1 L, and pass the solution through a fluted filter. The solution is now ready to use and can be stored at RT over long periods of time.

2. Preparation of eosin solution:
   Stock solution 1:298.1 mL H_2O and 1.9 mL of acetic acid (0.575% acetic acid).

   Stock solution 2: dissolve 6.15 g sodium acetate in 750 mL H_2O (0.82% sodium acetate).

   Put together 295 mL of stock solution 1.705 mL of stock solution 2, and 5 g of eosin Y. Mix well and pass through fluted filter. Precipitates may form upon prolonged storage at room temperature. The precipitates can be removed by an additional passage through a fluted filter.

2.6. Performing Laser Capture Microdissection

1. PALM® Membrane Slides, 1 mm glass, PEN membrane (Zeiss).
2. Mineral oil, light white oil.
3. 500 μL reaction tubes.

3. Methods

3.1. Preparation of Cell Lysates for miRNA First Strand Synthesis

In the Subheadings 3.1–3.3, we describe a procedure that demonstrates that miRNA expression can be measured accurately, directly after heat disruption of ≤100 cells (Fig. 1), without prior RNA isolation (see Note 1). Subsequently, the same approach

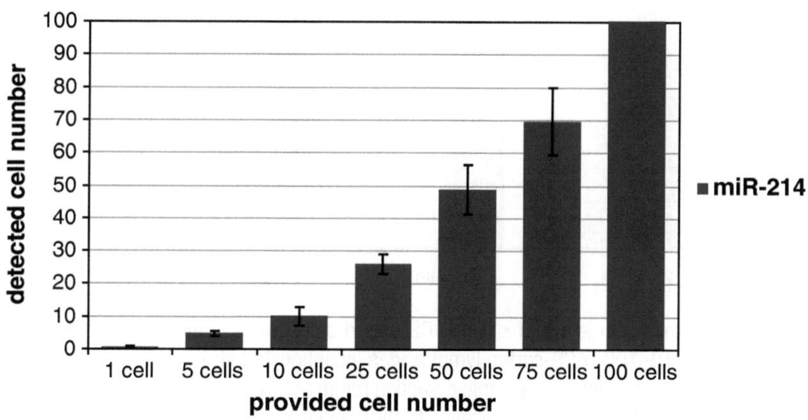

Fig. 1. Measuring the abundantly expressed miR-214 in a dilution series of MEF cells accurately reflects the performed dilution steps, without need for normalization. From each of the seven dilutions, 3× 4.58 μL were transferred into three conical wells of a microtiter plate. A RNA isolation procedure was omitted. Instead, cells were disrupted through heat treatment (5 min, 95°C) and subsequent fast cooling. miR-214 expression was measured as described in the Subheadings 3.1–3.3. The detected Cp value for 100 cells was considered to be most accurate and was used as a reference to calculate the expected Cp values for all other dilutions.

will be used in combination with cell isolation methods, such as FACS sorting (Subheadings 3.4–3.7) and LCM (Subheadings 3.8–3.10) (Figs. 2 and 3). In general, cell isolation methods are performed such that a defined number of cells (≤100) are present

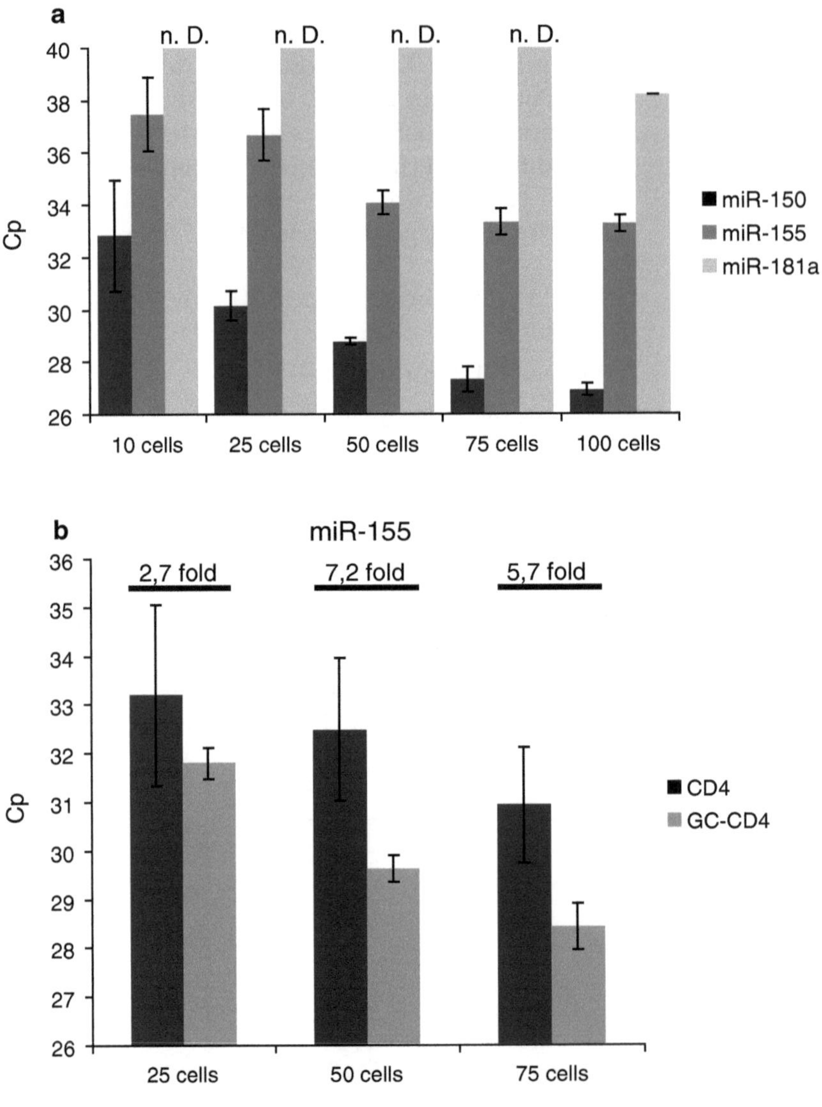

Fig. 2. Determining miRNA expression levels of ≤100 FACS-sorted cells. (**a**) Low, medium and highly abundant miRNA expression was measured on 10–100 FACS-sorted lymphocytes (lymphocyte gate). In 100 cells, the detected Cp values ranged from ~27 to ~37, thereby spanning a dynamic detection range of three orders of magnitude. This is, for instance, similar to the dynamic range of Affymetrix miRNA arrays. (**b**) Differential expression of miR-155 in FACS-sorted germinal center CD4 T cells and mixed splenic CD4 T cells. Even without normalization, it is evident that miR-155 expression is higher in germinal center than in assorted CD4 T cells. Differences in miR-155 expression can be detected from as little as ten cells, however the standard deviations suggest that reliable differential expression can be measured from ≥50 cells. However, normalization to a reference, such as U6, miR-103, or miR-191, could even reduce the minimum number of cells necessary to obtain accurate miRNA expression results. The Cp scale is logarithmic (log2), and smaller values indicate stronger expression. *n.D.* not detected.

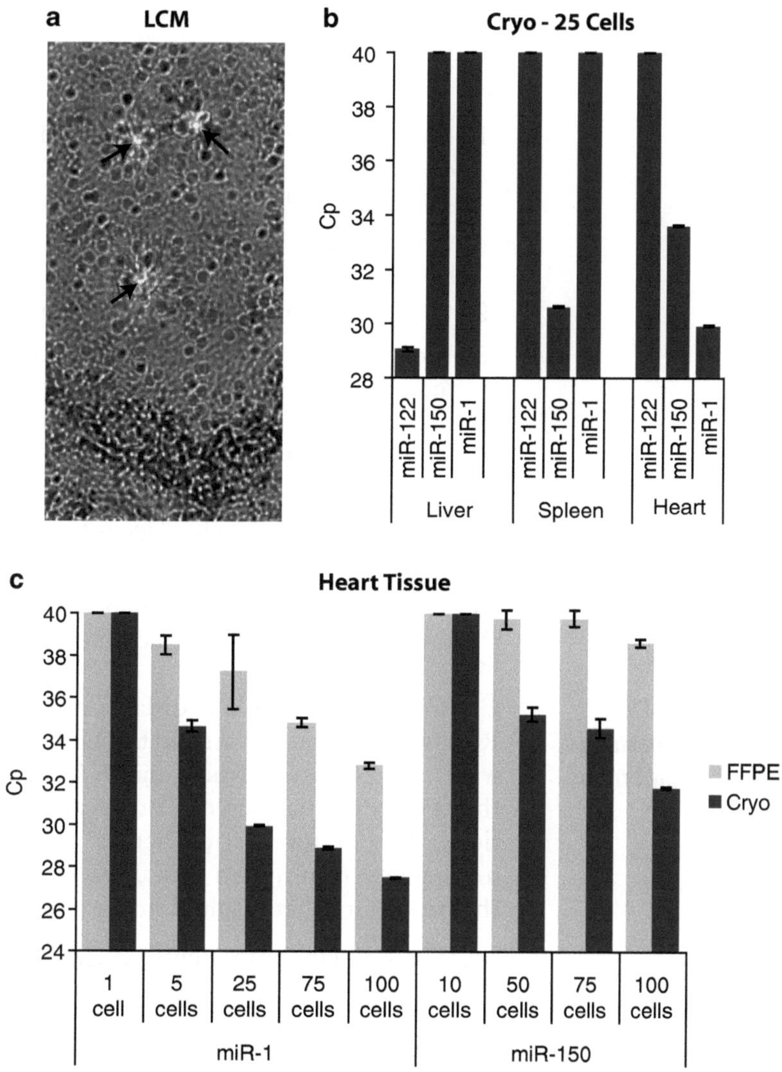

Fig. 3. Measuring miRNA expression in laser capture microdissected (LCM) samples. (**a**) To indicate the accuracy of laser-assisted dissection, this image shows an area of a germinal center from which three cells had previously been catapulted into the lid of the reaction tube (*arrows*). (**b**) Expression of three miRNA species, which are predominantly expressed in certain tissues [miR-150 (hematopoiesis), miR-122 (liver), and miR-1 (heart/muscle)], was measured in 25 microdissected cells derived from either spleen, heart, or liver tissue. As expected, miR-122 is strongly expressed in liver cells, but not in spleen or heart cells. Similarly, miR-1 is expressed in the heart, but not in liver or spleen. In good accordance with miRNA expression results obtained from human heart tissue (11), miR-1 is among the highest expressed miRNAs of the heart, but miR-150 can also be detected. (**c**) Expression of miR-1 (high abundance) and miR-150 (medium to low abundance) in a dilution series ranging from 1 to 100 microdissected cells, derived from formalin-fixed paraffin-embedded (FFPE) heart tissue and compared to samples obtained from cryoconserved heart sections. Although formalin-fixation reduces the miRNA signal, all miRNA species are affected to a similar degree (8). Therefore, miRNA expression can be measured using FFPE material. The Cp scale is logarithmic (log2), and smaller values indicate stronger expression.

in a volume of 4.58 μL of PBS or FACS buffer in a 96-well conical bottom plate. This allows continuing with Subheading 3.1, step 2 (below).

1. Mouse embryonic fibroblast (MEF) cells are diluted to yield concentrations of 1, 5, 10, 25, 50, 75, and 100 cells per 4.58 μL of PBS (see Note 2). From each dilution, 4.58 μL cell suspension is transferred into three wells to finally measure miRNA expression in triplicate (Fig. 1).
2. Centrifuge 96-well plate for 1 min at 3,000 × *g* and 4°C.
3. Program a thermal cycler to heat up to 95°C for 5 min, including lid. Start the program and wait until 95°C is reached. Swiftly open the lid, place the 96-well plate into the PCR block, and close the lid.
4. Just before the 5 min is up, open the lid, take out the 96-well plate and immediately place into a benchtop 96-tube cooling block (4°C) or alternatively onto ice.
5. The 96-well plate can now be stored at −20°C or directly be used for a miRNA-specific first strand synthesis.

3.2. Specific First Strand Synthesis to Produce cDNA from miRNAs

Commercially available TaqMan® microRNA assays, the TaqMan® Reverse Transcription kit and the LightCycler® 480 Probes Master were applied to determine miRNA expression. First strand synthesis was essentially carried out as per the manufacturer's instructions. For better cost-efficiency, we used half volumes of all ingredients, resulting in a total reaction volume of 7.5 μL. Below, the procedure that resulted in Fig. 1 is described.

1. Thaw all kit components on ice.
2. Prepare master mix according to Table 1.
3. Add 2.92 μL of master mix into each well [already containing 4.58 μL disrupted cell suspension (Subheading 3.1)].
4. Seal the plate with sealing foil.
5. Centrifuge at 3,000 × *g* for 1 min at 4°C.
6. Perform first strand synthesis by placing the 96-well plate into a thermal cycler, using the following program: 16°C, 30 min/42°C, 30 min/85°C, 5 min and 4°C, hold.
7. Continue with the quantitative PCR reaction or store at −20°C.

3.3. Quantitative PCR Reaction to Measure miRNA Expression

1. Thaw primer/probe mix on ice and prepare the master mix according to Table 2.
2. Distribute 21× 18.67 μL of master mix into a LightCycler® 480 Multiwell Plate 96. Use the same pattern as previously used for the first strand synthesis.

Table 1
Preparation of the microRNA first strand synthesis master mix

Component	1× Master mix (μL)	22× Master mix (μL)
100 mM dNTPs	0.075	1.65
MultiScribe™ Reverse Transcriptase, 50 U/μL	0.5	11
10× reverse transcription buffer	0.75	16.5
RNase inhibitor, 20 U/μL	0.095	2.09
miR-214 primer	Mix 1.5	33
Total	2.92	64.24

Table 2
Preparation of the microRNA qPCR master mix

Component	1× Master mix (μL)	22× Master mix (μL)
miR-214 PCR primer and probe	1.00	22
TaqMan 2× Universal PCR Master Mix	10.00	220
Nuclease-free water	7.67	168.74
Total volume	18.67	410.74

3. Transfer 1.33 μL of first strand from the 96-well plate into the corresponding well of the LightCycler® 480 Multiwell Plate 96 (which already contains 18.67 μL master mix).
4. Seal the plate with sealing foil.
5. Centrifuge at 3,000 × *g* for 1 min at 4°C.
6. Run the following program (Table 3) on a Light Cycler 480 device (see Note 3):
7. Use the "second derivative maximum method" (default setting) to calculate crossing points (Cp) and "absolute quantification" to analyze the results. The Cp represents the number of PCR cycles at which the growth curve enters the log-linear phase. In the experiment described here, the Cp values are compared directly (see Note 4).

3.4. Immunization of Mice

The procedures described in the following sections (Subheadings 3.4–3.7) will result in a FACS-sorted cell population of rare germinal center CD4 cells (Fig. 2). To increase the number of germinal center T cells, immunization of mice with sheep red blood cells (SRBC) is a suitable tool. Pure cell populations

Table 3
Program for microRNA qPCR

Detection format: mono color hydrolysis probe/UPL

Step	Cycles	Analysis mode
Pre-incubation	1	None
Amplification	45	Quantification
Cooling	1	None

Step	Temperature (°C)	Time (s)	Acquisition mode	Ramp rate
Pre-incubation	95	600	None	4.4
Amplification	95	15	None	4.4
	60	60	Single	2.2
Cooling	40	30	None	2.2

provide the best starting point for the measurement of miRNA expression, as described in subheadings 3.1–3.3.

One BALB/C mouse (10-week-old male) was used for immunization with 2×10^8 SRBC to induce germinal center T cell differentiation. Prior to intraperitoneal injection, SRBC were treated as follows:

1. Add 48 mL of PBS to 2 mL of sheep blood.
2. Centrifuge at 1,455 ×*g* for 10 min at 4°C.
3. Take off supernatant and resuspend pellet in 50 mL PBS.
4. Repeat steps 2 and 3 twice.
5. Before the last centrifugation step take off 10 μL cell suspension, dilute 1:50 in PBS, and count cells in a Neubauer counting chamber.
6. After the last centrifugation step, take off supernatant and use PBS to produce a cell suspension of 2×10^8 cells/200 μL.
7. Inject 200 μL of erythrocyte cell suspension into one mouse, intraperitoneally.
8. Sacrifice the mouse after 1 week, remove the spleen, and place into a cell strainer, which was previously placed into one well of a 6-well plate, containing 7 mL T cell medium. Continue with CD4 T cell isolation.

3.5. CD4 T Cell Isolation Using MACS Beads

1. Use the pistil of a 6 mL syringe and press hematopoietic cells of the spleen through the cell strainer.

2. Transfer the cell solution into a 15-mL tube, add 8 mL of T cell medium, and centrifuge at 282 ×*g* for 5 min at 4°C.
3. Remove the supernatant and vigorously flick the pellet loose.
4. Add 5 mL of ice-cold TAC buffer to lyse the erythrocytes. Quickly pipet up and down once and incubate for exactly 6 min on ice.
5. Add 10 mL of T cell medium and centrifuge at 282 ×*g* for 5 min at 4°C.
6. Remove the supernatant, flick the pellet loose and resuspend in 10 mL MACS buffer.
7. Take-off 10 μL, dilute 1:10 in PBS and count the cells in a Neubauer counting chamber.
8. Centrifuge at 282 ×*g* for 5 min at 4°C, take off the supernatant, flick the pellet loose, and resuspend in 90 μL of MACS buffer per 10^7 cells.
9. Add 10 μL of CD4 MicroBeads per 10^7 cells and mix well.
10. Incubate for 15 min in a fridge (4°C).
11. Wash cells by adding 1–2 mL of MACS buffer per 10^7 cells and centrifugation at 282 ×*g* for 5 min at 4°C.
12. Take off the supernatant, flick the pellet loose, and resuspend up to 10^8 cells in 500 μL MACS buffer. Scale the volume of MACS buffer up if the cell number exceeds 10^8. Keep a volume of 500 μL MACS buffer if the cell number is below 10^8.
13. Use autoMACSpro separator (rinsed) and a program for positive selection (Possel).
14. Place the 15-mL tube in the upper left corner of the chill1 5-block of the separator and two empty 15-mL tubes in the wells below that. Start the program.
15. Purified, positive-selected CD4 cells will be deposited in the bottommost 15-mL tube.
16. Count the cells in a Neubauer counting chamber and continue with the FACS staining procedure.

3.6. FACS Staining of PD1⁺, CXCR5⁺ Double-Positive CD4 Cells

1. Use two million CD4 cells for the double stain and, depending on the yield of CD4 cells, one to two million cells for compensation controls.
2. Antibodies for the FACS stain are used in the following end concentrations (Table 4): PD1-PE (1:100), CXCR5 (1:10), and F_{ab}-Cy5 (1:200).

Table 4
FACS labelling protocol

	First step labelling	Volume FACS buffer and antibody (μL)	Second step labelling	Volume FACS buffer and antibody (μL)
Sample to sort	PD1-PE + CXCR5	99 + 1 + 10	Cy™5- F(ab')2	99.5 + 0.5
Control 1	CXCR5	90 + 10	Cy™5-F(ab')2	99.5 + 0.5
Control 2	Untreated	100	Cy™5- F(ab')2	99.5 + 0.5
Control 3	PD1-PE	99 + 1	Cy™5- F(ab')2	99.5 + 0.5
Control 4	Untreated	100	Untreated	100

3. Transfer the appropriate volume of CD4 cells into FACS tubes. Fill up with PBS and centrifuge at 282 ×*g* for 5 min at 4°C.
4. Remove supernatant of all samples carefully, vortex vigorously, add FACS buffer and antibodies as indicated in Table 4 (first labeling step).
5. Place all five tubes for 20 min on ice. Cover with aluminum foil.
6. Wash by adding 2 mL FACS buffer, vortex vigorously, and centrifuge at 282 ×*g* for 5 min at 4°C.
7. Remove the supernatant, vortex vigorously, add 2 mL FACS buffer, vortex again, and centrifuge at 282 ×*g* for 5 min at 4°C.
8. Remove the supernatant, vortex vigorously, and add antibodies and FACS buffer as indicated in Table 4 (second labeling step).
9. Incubate 20 min on ice. Cover with aluminum foil.
10. Wash twice as described in step 7.
11. After centrifugation, take off the supernatant, vortex, and resuspend the cells in 200 μL FACS buffer. Continue with FACS sorting.

3.7. FACS Sorting of Germinal Center CD4 T Cells and Assorted CD4 T Cells

It is a current standard to consult with a FACS facility to obtain sorted cells. We used an in-house service center equipped with a MoFlo XDP cell sorter (http://www.helmholtz-muenchen.de/imi/zs/) and Summit 4.1 software. Importantly, cells were sorted directly into a 96-well conical bottom plate, which contained 4.58 μL of PBS in each well (see Note 5). After the sort, proceed immediately with cell disruption (Subheading 3.1, step 2).

3.8. Preparation of Tissue Sections from Snap-Frozen Tissues for LCM

1. A 10-week-old male mouse (C57BL/6) was sacrificed. Heart, liver, and spleen were snap-frozen in liquid nitrogen and stored at −80°C.
2. A Leica CM1950 cryostat microtome was used for sectioning the tissues. The chamber and block temperatures were set to −17°C and −20°C, respectively.
3. To prepare the tissues for sectioning, place them onto specimen holder within the cryostat chamber and completely cover in freezing medium (Tissue-Tek® O.C.T. Compound), which quickly hardens at low temperatures and attaches the tissue to the holder.
4. Start making a series of sections of a width of 12 μm.
5. Stop sectioning when slicing through the tissue part of interest and remove all sections that stick to the microtome blade.
6. Make one more section, which will stay on the microtome blade. Transfer tissue section from the blade onto a membrane-covered slide, which is suitable for LCM. Press the membrane-covered side of the slide against the section and, at the same time, place thumb on the other side of the glass. The comparably high temperature of the thumb will cause the section to stick to the slide.
7. Air-dry the slide for 30 min.
8. Tissue fixation is performed in a coplin staining jar by placing the slide into a solution of 95% ethanol (190 mL) and 5% acetic acid (10 mL) for 60 s.
9. Place the slide into empty coplin jar and rinse with tap water for 5 min.
10. Place the slide into a hematoxylin-containing coplin jar and incubate for 1 min.
11. Rinse with tap water.
12. Place the slide into an eosin-containing coplin jar and incubate for 30 s.
13. Rinse with tap water and air-dry for 10 min.
14. Use immediately for LCM or store at −20°C.

3.9. Preparation of Tissue Sections from Formalin-Fixed Tissues for LCM

1. Trim the tissue that was previously incubated in buffered formalin for ~24–48 h with a scalpel blade so that it will fit into an embedding cassette. The cassette will encase the tissue during the procedure described below, until the tissue is transferred into paraffin. Thereafter, the cassette will be used as a specimen holder to attach the paraffin-embedded tissue to it.
2. Rinse in tap water for 30 min to remove the formalin.

Table 5
Series of incubation steps performed prior to paraffin embedding of the tissue

Solution	Incubation time (h)	Temperature (°C)
Ethanol 70%	1	37
Ethanol 70%	1	37
Ethanol 80%	1	37
Ethanol 96%	2	37
Ethanol 96%	2	37
Ethanol 100%	1	37
Ethanol 100%	2	37
Ethanol 100%	2	37
Xylol	1	37
Xylol	1	37
Xylol	1	37
Paraffin	3	60
Paraffin	3	60
Paraffin	3	60

3. Place embedding cassettes into a vacuum infiltration processor to proceed through the alcohol series described in the Table 5 and eventually for transfer into paraffin.
4. Use a paraffin embedding station to fill a tissue embedding mold with 60°C warm paraffin. Take the tissue out of the embedding cassette and place it in the embedding mold. Use forceps to bring the tissue to the desired orientation and put the embedding cassette on top of the paraffin in the embedding mould.
5. Place the whole arrangement on a −20°C metal plate of paraffin embedding station for 10 min. The tissue block is now ready for sectioning.
6. Fix tissue block in the specimen holder of a microtome and start making sections of 8 μm.
7. Use a brush to transfer sections from the microtome blade to a water bath, where the sections will stretch out, due to the surface tension of the water.
8. Take a membrane-covered slide to fish a section out of the water bath.

9. Incubate at 50°C overnight to increase adhesion between tissue section and slide.
10. Perform HE-staining by first removing paraffin by the incubation of the slide for 10 min in a xylol-containing coplin jar.
11. Place the slide into a hematoxylin-containing coplin jar and incubate for 4 min.
12. Rinse with tap water until no more blue stain is released from the slide.
13. Place the slide into an eosin-containing coplin jar and incubate for 20 s.
14. Rinse with water as described above and air-dry for 10 min.
15. Use immediately for LCM or store at room temperature.

3.10. Performing Laser Capture Microdissection

In principle, LCM is easy to perform; however, it may be cumbersome to adjust the laser to the tissue section at hand (see Note 6).

1. Switch on the laser, the microscope, and the computer 10 min prior to use.
2. Place the slide carrying the cryosection onto the stage of the microscope and let it adjust to room temperature (FFPE sections are stored at room temperature and can be used directly).
3. Start the Palm@RoboV2.2 software. Set UV-Energy to 50, UV-Focus to 60, and the Selected Speed to 25. The Laser Setting is "cut" and under "Laser" in the menu bar choose "LPC".
4. Choose the 10× objective of the microscope to find the tissue area of interest. For laser capture dissection, switch to the 40-fold magnification – at the microscope and in the software (upper right corner).
5. Add 50 μL of RNAse-free light white mineral oil into the lid of a 500-μL reaction tube and immediately suck it off.
6. Place the 500-μL tube in the holder of the robotic arm, which is attached to the microscope. The lid of the tube has to point downwards while the tube is open.
7. Press the red button at the right of the pad that is used to control the robotic arm. The lid of the 500-μL tube will be moved such that it comes to rest directly over the tissue part of interest.
8. Select and mark ~10 cells at a time by using the "spot" tool on the lower task bar.
9. Start the laser (middle right). The cells will be catapulted from the tissue into the lid of the PCR tube. The mineral oil on the surface of the lid will make the cells stick.

10. After the desired number of cells has been collected, press the red button on the control pad for the robotic arm again and remove and close the reaction tube. Cells derived from cryosections should be stored on ice, which is not necessary for those dissected from FFPE material.
11. Centrifuge reaction tubes at 10,000 × g for 5 min at 4°C.
12. Add 4.58 μL PBS and transfer, mix well by pipetting up and down, and transfer the mineral oil-PBS-cell suspension into one well of a microtiter plate. Continue with section 3.1, step 2.

4. Notes

1. RNA isolation is omitted since losses during purification procedures are relatively high, especially when using small samples. The procedure described here (5) probably also results in better reproducibility.
2. Planning to measure the expression of more than one miRNA species from the exact same sample, it is recommended to increase the volume of PBS by multiples of 4.58 μL (e.g., for the measurement of three different miRNAs use 13.74 μL), then disrupt the cells as described above. Subsequently, dispense 2 × 4.58 μL into neighboring wells. Go on with first strand synthesis or freeze at −20°C.
3. The assay can also be performed and is indeed designed to run on a real-time PCR system from Applied Biosystems ("TaqMan"). The Light Cycler 480 (Roche) is our preferred system, mainly due to smaller well-to-well variations.
4. To compare the expression of one miRNA in two different samples with the highest precision, it is necessary to include at least one reference (such as U6 or miR-103 (10)) in the measurement of each sample. Analysis would be performed using relative quantification. Relative quantification was omitted here to demonstrate the accuracy of the described method, without normalization.
5. It is of crucial importance to adjust the conical 96-well microtiter plate accurately so that the cells that leave the cell sorter aim towards the center of the well. This can be tested and visualized by sealing the plate with sealing foil and ejection of FACS buffer onto the seal. Remove sealing foil before the actual sort. Most of the variance measured in the subsequent miRNA quantitative PCR is probably due to cells that do not enter the well or stick to the surface on the side of a well.
6. To adjust the laser settings, it is recommended to first choose a part of the membrane slide without tissue. Set the magnification

on the microscope (objective) and in the software (upper right corner) to 40. Pick the "line" button in the lower task bar and draw a horizontal line. Set the UV-Energy to 30 and the UV-Focus to 50. Start the laser by pressing the respective button (middle right). If the laser does not cut the membrane, gradually increase the UV-Energy. Once the laser energy is high enough to slice through the membrane, you can adjust the UV-Focus similarly to find the optimal width for your individual experiment. After optimization of the settings, chose a tissue area of interest, mark the cell(s) using the "spot" or the "circle" tool in the task bar at the bottom and set the laser (menu bar "Laser") to "LPC" or Robo LPC, respectively. Gradually, increase the UV-Energy settings as necessary.

Acknowledgments

We gratefully acknowledge the contribution of Dr. J. Ellwart, in performing FACS sorting and of the group of Dr. I. Esposito for their expertise in tissue preparation for microdissection. Furthermore, we thank Dr. A. Walch for access to the P.A.L.M laser capture mikrodissection microscop and Dr. E. Kremmer for the CXCR5 monoclonal antibody.

References

1. Hoefig KP, Heissmeyer V. MicroRNAs grow up in the immune system. Curr Opin Immunol 2008;20:281–7.
2. Li QJ, Chau J, Ebert PJ, et al. miR-181a is an intrinsic modulator of T cell sensitivity and selection. Cell 2007;129:147–61.
3. Lagos-Quintana M, Rauhut R, Yalcin A, Meyer J, Lendeckel W, Tuschl T. Identification of tissue-specific microRNAs from mouse. Curr Biol 2002;12:735–9.
4. Chang J, Nicolas E, Marks D, et al. miR-122, a mammalian liver-specific microRNA, is processed from hcr mRNA and may downregulate the high affinity cationic amino acid transporter CAT-1, RNA Biol 2004;1:106–13.
5. Chen C, Ridzon DA, Broomer AJ, et al. Real-time quantification of microRNAs by stem-loop RT-PCR. Nucleic Acids Res 2005;33:e179.
6. Rodriguez A, Vigorito E, Clare S, et al. Requirement of bic/microRNA-155 for normal immune function. Science 2007;316:608–11.
7. Thai TH, Calado DP, Casola S, et al. Regulation of the germinal center response by microRNA-155. Science 2007;316: 604–8.
8. Hoefig KP, Thorns C, Roehle A, et al. Unlocking pathology archives for microRNA-profiling. Anticancer Res 2008;28:119–23.
9. Nelson PT, Baldwin DA, Kloosterman WP, Kauppinen S, Plasterk RH, Mourelatos Z. RAKE and LNA-ISH reveal microRNA expression and localization in archival human brain. RNA 2006;12:187–91.
10. Peltier HJ, Latham GJ. Normalization of microRNA expression levels in quantitative RT-PCR assays: identification of suitable reference RNA targets in normal and cancerous human solid tissues. RNA 2008;14:844–52.
11. Liang Y, Ridzon D, Wong L, Chen C. Characterization of microRNA expression profiles in normal human tissues. BMC Genomics 2007;8:166.

Part II

High-Throughput Analysis of miRNAs

Chapter 5

MicroRNA Cloning from Cells of the Immune System

Haoquan Wu, Joel Neilson, and N. Manjunath

Abstract

MicroRNAs have emerged as – important posttranscriptional regulators of gene expression. Small RNA cloning is a powerful method to identify new microRNAs (miRNAs) and to profile miRNA expression. In addition, it reveals end heterogeneity that may be important in miRNA function. Here, we describe a protocol that is optimized to clone small RNAs from limited amounts of starting material. This is often the case for studying miRNAs in a highly purified population of immune cells or other primary cell types with limited numbers. The small RNAs cloned with this protocol will have a 5′-PO_4 and 3′-OH group, typical features of miRNAs, so majority of the cloned small RNAs will be miRNAs.

1. Introduction

Although the first microRNA (miRNA) was discovered by genetic analysis in 1993 (1), most other miRNAs have been identified only after the development of small RNA cloning method by the Ambros, Bartel, and Tuschl groups in 2001 (2–5). Small RNA cloning is not only a powerful tool to identify new miRNAs but also one of the most reliable methods to profile miRNA expression. It is hard for most other methods to distinguish miRNAs with high degree of sequence similarity as commonly occurs within miRNAs belonging to the same family. It is the only way to visualize the details of small RNA such as RNA editing and end variation. There are several protocols for cloning miRNAs, including the recently developed commercial ones. To study miRNAs in a particular population of primary cell population isolated ex vivo, the cell numbers and thus the available RNA quantity is often limited. The protocol we describe here is modified from the protocol developed by Lau et al. (3), and it is optimized for cloning miRNAs from small amount of starting material (6, 7). Essentially, the procedure consists of extraction of small RNA

Silvia Monticelli (ed.), *MicroRNAs and the Immune System: Methods and Protocols*, Methods in Molecular Biology, vol. 667,
DOI 10.1007/978-1-60761-811-9_5, © Springer Science+Business Media, LLC 2010

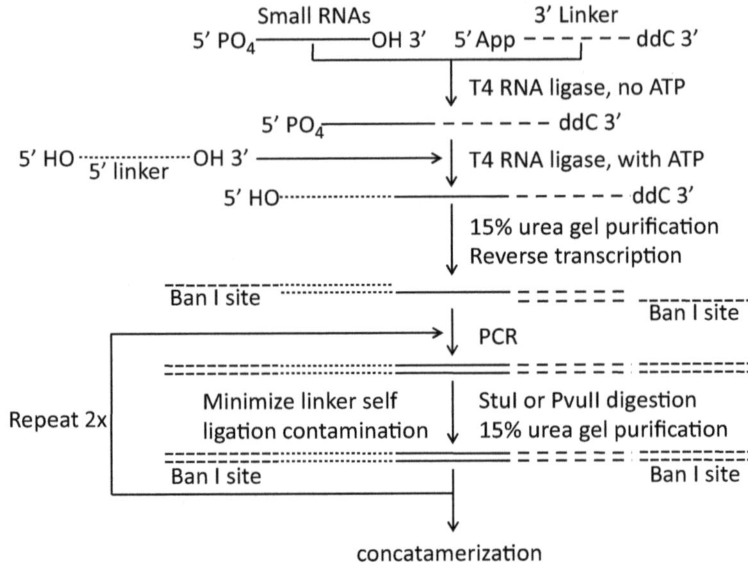

Fig. 1. **Flowchart for cloning of short RNAs**. Use of two linker sets reduces the possibility of microRNA loss in the digestion set and partially offsets the ligation bias of T4 RNA ligase.

fraction from the cells, sequential addition of 3′ and 5′ linkers, gel purification of the linker attached RNA, PCR amplification using linker-specific primers, concatemerization of the amplified products, and traditional sequencing (Fig. 1). Individual amplicons can also be sequenced using modern high-throughput sequencing methods.

Other protocols currently available for cloning miRNAs generally require three steps of denaturing gel purification, as shown in the flowchart (Fig. 1). Only one step of denaturing gel purification is used before PCR amplification in the protocol we describe. The avoidance of gel purification steps before and after addition of 3′ linker is designed to minimize the loss of material at each step. However, this modification greatly increases the chance of self-ligation between linkers. To solve this problem, a restriction enzyme digestion step is introduced to minimize the linker self-ligation. The linkers are designed to form a restriction enzyme site if the 5′ linker is joined with 3′ linker directly (half of the restriction site is at 3′ end of 5′ linker, while the other half is at 5′ end of 3′ linker). Thus, in the enzyme digestion step, after PCR amplification, the self-ligated linkers will be cut and eliminated by gel purification. The disadvantage of this strategy is that the miRNAs containing this restriction site will also be cut and thus will not be cloned. The problem can be solved by using another pair of linkers with a different restriction enzyme site. StuI and PvuII are used in this protocol.

The purpose of complicated linker ligation steps is mainly to minimize self-ligation of small RNAs. The self-ligation of small

RNAs can be minimized by either dephosphorylating small RNAs before ligating to the 3′ linker or ligating in a ligation reaction without ATP. In both cases, the 3′ end of the 3′ linker should be blocked by a dideoxycytidine (ddC) to prevent 3′ linker self-ligation. The latter approach will mostly clone small RNAs that have 5′-PO_4 and 3′-OH groups. These represent the typical structure of miRNAs and thus minimize the chance of cloning RNA degradation fragments. Without ATP, T4 RNA ligase cannot ligate the 3′-OH and 5′-PO_4 between small RNAs, thus avoiding self-ligation. However, since the 5′ end of 3′ linker is preadenylated, this enables the 3′ linker to be ligated to the 3′-OH of small RNAs in a reaction system without ATP. After 3′ linker ligation, the 5′ linker will be ligated to the 5′ end of small RNA in a ligation reaction with ATP. To prevent 5′ linker self-ligation, 5′ linker should be synthesized with free 5′-OH and 3′-OH. The small RNAs ligated with both 5′ and 3′ linkers will be gel purified and subject to reverse transcription and PCR amplification to obtain the small RNA cDNA library. The cDNA library can be sequenced directly (provided altered adaptors are used) by second generation sequencing technology that is discussed in detail in other chapters of this book. A small-scale sequencing method will be described here. Briefly, the small RNA library will be concatamerized and cloned into T vector and sequenced with the traditional sequencing methods.

2. Materials

1. 2× 3′ ligation buffer: 100 mM Tris–HCl, pH 8.0, 30 mM $MgCl_2$, 30% DMSO, 200 μg/ml BSA, 20 mM DTT, 40 μM adenylated 3′ linker (The oligo sequences are listed in Table 1.), 4 μM non-adenylated but 5′-phosphorylated 3′ linker (The oligos sequences are listed in Table 1.) (see Note 1).
2. 3× 5′ ligation buffer: 150 mM Tris–HCl, pH 8.0, 20 mM DTT, 300 μg/ml BSA, 2.6 mM ATP, 10 mM $MgCl_2$.
3. miRNeasy mini kit (Qiagen).
4. Safe Imager blue-light transilluminator (Invitrogen).
5. RNase-free water.
6. 1 M Tris–HCl, pH 7.8 (RNase free).
7. 1 M $MgCl_2$ (RNase free).
8. 10 mM ATP (RNase free).
9. 0.1 M DTT (RNase free).
10. 50 mg/ml ultrapure BSA (RNase free).
11. DMSO.

Table 1
Oligos used for small RNA cloning

5′linker Stu	ACC ACA GAG AAA CCG rArGrG
3′ linker Stu	CCT GTA TCT GTG TAT GGddC
5′ linker Pvu	ACC ACA GAG AAA CCG rCrArG
3′ linker Pvu	CTG GTA TCT GTG TAT GGddC
5′ PCR primer Stu	GAG CCA ACA GGC ACC ACA GAG AAA CCG AGG
3′ PCR primer Stu	GAC TAG CTT GGT GCC ATA CAC AGA TAC AGG
5′ PCR primer Pvu	GAG CCA ACA GGC ACC ACA GAG AAA CCG CAG
3′ PCR primer Pvu	GAC TAG CTT GGT GCC ATA CAC AGA TAC CAG
Stu RT priming	GCC ATA CAC AGA TAC AGG
Pvu RT priming	GCC ATA CAC AGA TAC CAG

12. T4 RNA ligase.
13. 2× Novex TBE Urea Sample Buffer (2×) (Invitrogen).
14. 15% TBE urea gel (Invitrogen).
15. SybrGold and SybrSafe (Invitrogen).
16. 5 mg/ml Linear acrylamide (RNase free).
17. 0.3 and 5 M NaCl (RNase-free).
18. 54 nt and 61 nt size markers.
19. DNA ligation kits, Ver. 2.1, Takara Bio.
20. Absolute ethanol.
21. Calf intestinal alkaline phosphatase (CIP).
22. 25:24:1 (v/v/v) phenol/chloroform/isoamyl alcohol.
23. Chloroform.
24. SuperScript III First-Strand Synthesis System (Invitrogen).
25. Regular agarose and agarose DNA fragment 50–1,000 bp (US Biological).
26. 10-bp DNA ladder and 100-bp DNA ladder.
27. BanI restriction enzyme.
28. Low-melting agarose gel.
29. Water-saturated phenol, pH 7.9.
30. TOPO-TA cloning kit with TOP10 competent cells (Invitrogen).
31. ExoSAP-IT (USB Corporation).

3. Methods

3.1. Ligate 3′ and 5′ Adaptors to Small RNAs

1. Prepare crudely fractionated small RNA using Qiagen miRNeasy mini kit as per the manufacturer's instructions. Roughly, 12-μl small RNA will be recovered. 4-μl small RNA will be used for small RNA cloning. The remaining small RNA can be kept in reserve.
2. Add 4 μl of small RNA into 5 μl of 2× 3′ ligation buffer containing 3′ linker for 10 μl total reaction volume (see Note 2). To control for good ATP-independent ligation, set up reaction with 1 μl of 300 μM 5′ linker as substrate.
3. Add 1 μl T4 RNA ligase. Incubate at 37°C for 1 h (see Note 3). Set aside control reaction until gel isolation.
4. Add to the reaction in following order: 2 μl of 5′ ligation buffer, 1 μl (300 μM) of 5′ linker and 1 μl T4 RNA ligase, and 2 μl of ddH_20. Incubate at 37°C for 1 h.
5. Add 0.5 μl (10 μM) of 54 and 61 nt size marker and 16-μl 2× Urea sample buffer to each reaction. Heat samples at 70°C for 3 min.
6. To purify the ligated small RNA, samples are loaded into 15% TBE urea gel. Before loading the samples, the wells should be washed thoroughly three times to remove the urea in the wells. Run the gel for 1 h at 180 V. After running, stain the gel in 1× SybrGold for 15 min. Using a blue-light transilluminator to light up the bands, cut out the gels between 54 and 61 nts (see Note 4). Note that the control ligation gives a major band at 36 nt.
7. Crush the gel slice into small pieces in a 1.5-ml tube with a regular 1 ml tip with flame-sealed end, add 400 μl of RNase-free 0.3 M NaCl, and elute at 4°C under constant agitation overnight.
8. Spin for 5 min at maximum speed (16,000 ×*g*) and take the supernatant. Add 1 μl linear acrylamide and three volumes of EtOH and keep the tube in a methanol/dry ice bath for at least 1 h to precipitate the nucleic acids.
9. Spin in a microfuge at maximum speed (16,000 ×*g*) for 10 min. The pellet that is mostly linear acrylamide should be clearly visible. Wash the pellet with 80% EtOH once. Dissolve the pellet with 8.5 μl H_2O.

3.2. Reverse Transcription of Ligated RNAs

1. To 8.5-μl ligated small RNAs, add 0.5-μl RT primer (10 μM) (see Table 1 for primer sequence) and 1-μl 10 mM dNTPs.
2. Heat at 80°C for 5 min, chill on ice for at least 1 min.

3. Make cDNA reaction mix:
   (a) 10× RT buffer, 2 μl
   (b) 25 mM $MgCl_2$, 4 μl
   (c) 0.1 M DTT, 2 μl
   (d) RNAseOUT, 1 μl
4. Mix 9 μl cDNA reaction mix with each reaction, add 0.5 μl Superscript reverse transcriptase, and incubate at 50°C for 50 min.
5. To each reaction add: 1 μl 0.1 M EDTA and 7.6 μl 1 M KOH. Heat 10 min at 90°C to hydrolyze the RNA.
6. Neutralize with 5 μl 1 M HCl and 0.5 μl 0.2 M $MgCl_2$.
7. Add 300 μl 0.3 M NaCl, adjust pH to around 8 with 1 M HCl or 1 M KOH. Add 1 μl linear acrylamide and three volumes of EtOH and keep the tube in a methanol/dry ice bath for at least 1 h. Spin at maximum speed (16,000 × *g*) for 10 min. Wash with 80% EtOH once and resuspend in 40 μl H_2O.

3.3. PCR Amplification

1. For small amounts of RNA, amplify half of cDNA in one 100 μl PCR reaction:
   (a) 100 μM Stu/Pvu Forward Primer, 1 μl
   (b) 100 μM Stu/Pvu Reverse Primer, 1 μl
   (c) 10× Hot Start buffer, 10 μl
   (d) 25 mM $MgCl_2$, 6 μl (1.5 mM final concentration)
   (e) Hot start Taq polymerase, 1 μl
   (f) 10 mM dNTP, 2 μl
   (g) H_2O, to 100 μl
2. PCR conditions:
   (a) 94°C 5 min
   (b) 94, 55, 72°C 45 s each, 3 cycles
   (c) 94, 62, 72°C 45 s each, 7 cycles
   (d) 72°C 5 min
   (e) 4°C-hold
3. Add 6 μl 5 M NaCl, 300 μl 0.3 M NaCl, 400 μl Phenol/chloroform/isoamyl alcohol extraction, followed by 400 μl chloroform extraction. Add 1-μl linear acrylamide, three volumes of EtOH to the supernatant. Keep the tube in a methanol/dry ice bath for at least 1 h.
4. Spin in a microfuge at maximum speed (16,000 × *g*) for 10 min. Wash with 80% EtOH once. Resuspend each sample in 200-μl 1×NEB buffer 4 (buffer 2 for PvuII) (see Note 5).

3.4. StuI/PvuII Digestion

1. Before adding enzymes, set aside 5 μl of all samples for gel analysis.
2. Add 100 U of StuI or PvuII accordingly and incubate for 2 h at 37°C.
3. Adjust with 5 M NaCl to final concentration 0.3 mM. Add 1-μl linear acrylamide and three volumes of EtOH and keep them in a methanol/dry ice bath for 1 h.
4. Spin at maximum speed (16,000 × *g*) for 10 min. Wash with 80% EtOH once.

3.5. Gel Isolation

1. Resuspend samples in 1× urea sampling buffer and run on 15% urea gel. Use multiple lanes of 100 ng of 10 bp ladder to mark excision points on gel. After running, stain the gel in 1× SybrSafe for 15 min. Using a blue-light transilluminator to light up the bands.
2. Cut out desired region of gel:
   (a) For small RNAs 18–24 bases long, the PCR products will be 78–84 bases long.
   (b) Cutting from 80 bases to ~88 bases will bias the population towards small RNAs of correct size.
   (c) Linker digestion products run between 40 and 60 bases.
3. Crush gel slice and add 600 μl of 0.3 M NaCl.
4. Incubate under constant agitation at 4°C overnight.
5. Spin for 5 min at maximum speed (16,000 × *g*) and take the supernatant. Add 1 μl linear acrylamide and three volumes of EtOH and keep the tube in a methonal/dry ice bath for at least 1 h. Spin at maximum speed (16,000 × *g*) for 10 min. Wash the pellet with 80% EtOH once. Dissolve the pellet with 1 mM $MgCl_2$.

Repeat step 1 of Subheading 3.3 to step 5 of Subheading 3.5 until there is a clearly visible set of bands above 80 bps at step 5 of Subheading 3.5. You should see the bands by 30 cycles of total amplification at the latest. For the first amplification round, use a Hotstart Taq. For subsequent amplification rounds, use PFU polymerase and anneal only at 62°C. The gel isolation (Subheading 3.5, step 1) can also use the 4% agarose gel (Agarose DNA fragments 50–1,000 bp) and purify the bands with a regular gel purification kit, such as QIAquick Gel Extraction kit from Qiagen.

3.6. Large-Scale PCR Amplification

1. Take half of step 5 of Subheading 3.5 DNA to prime a 500 μl PCR reaction using PFU polymerase:
   (a) 10× PFU buffer, 50 μl
   (b) PFU, 5 μl

(c) 100 μM forward primer, 5 μl

(d) 100 μM reverse primer, 5 μl

(e) 10 mM dNTPs, 10 μl

(f) H_2O, 420 μl

2. Split and dispense into five tubes (5 × 100 μl). Amplify at 94, 62, 72°C 45 s each, 6–10 cycles.
3. Collect the entire product and add 30 μl 5 M NaCl to make a final concentration of 0.3 M.
4. Extract with 500 μl phenol/chloroform/isoamyl alcohol, followed by 500 μl chloroform. Add two volumes of EtOH to the supernatant. Incubate in a methanol/dry ice bath for 10 min.
5. Spin at maximum speed (16,000 × *g*) for 10 min. Wash with 80% EtOH once. Resuspend each sample in 195 μl 1× NEB buffer 4.

3.7. Concatamerization

1. Add 10 μl of 20 U/μl Ban I and 1 μl of StuI or PvuII accordingly, incubate for 2 h at 37°C.
2. Remove 4 μl for gel analysis. Run side by side with predigestion DNA on 4% agarose gel (Agarose DNA fragment 50–1,000 bp). Digest removes 24 nt from cloned RNAs. 18–24 nt small RNAs now run at 54–60 postdigestion.
3. Add 12 μl 5 M NaCl and 300 μl 0.3 M NaCl. Extract with 500 μl phenol/chloroform/isoamyl alcohol, followed by 500 μl chloroform. Add 1.8 volume of EtOH to the supernatant. Incubate at 4°C for 2 h.
4. Spin at maximum speed (16,000 × *g*) for 10 min. Wash with 80% EtOH once. Resuspend samples in 50 μl of 1 mM $MgCl_2$ (see Note 6).
5. Take 15 μl digested DNA and add 15 μl Sol I (DNA ligation kit) and then incubate for 10 min at room temperature.
6. Incubate at 65°C for 10 min to inactivate T4 DNA ligase. Pipette vigorously for 2 min to break up loosely ligated DNAs (see Note 7).
7. Run on 0.9% GPG low-melting point agarose gel with 1× TAE buffer at 4°C.
8. Run the gel until the concatamers could be seen clearly separated from other DNAs, cut out the brightest band of concatamers that usually should appear around 800 bp. Reduce the ligation time to lower the concatamers length if the brightest band is longer than 1,500 bp.
9. Cut gel slices to weigh 150 mg or less. Add >2 volumes of TE buffer (pH 8.0, to decrease the agarose percentage to <0.4%) and incubate for 10 min at 65°C to melt gel slices.

10. Add 600 μl of 37°C saturated phenol (pH 7.9), vortex immediately for 5 s, and spin 15 min at room temperature.
11. Take the aqueous phase, extract with 500 μl Phenol/chloroform/isoamyl alcohol, followed by 500 μl chloroform extraction. Add 1 μl linear acrylamide and two volumes of EtOH to the supernatant, and keep the tube in a methanol/dry ice bath for at least 1 h.
12. Spin at maximum speed (16,000 ×*g*) for 10 min. Wash with 70% EtOH once. Resuspend each sample in 15 μl 1× Taq PCR mix:
    (a) 10× Taq buffer, 1.5 μl
    (b) 2 mM dNTP, 1.5 μl
    (c) Taq, 0.2 μl
    (d) H_2O, 11.8 μl
13. Incubate at 72°C for 10 min.

3.8. TOPO Cloning

1. To 4 μl of Taq filled-in DNA, add 1 μl salt solution and 1 μl of pCR4 vector.
2. Incubate for 10 min at room temperature. Transform TOP 10 cells with 2 μl of TOPO mix, 30 min on ice, heat shock for 30 s, and recover for 50 min.
3. Plate 50 μl, 250 μl of transformation mix/plate of LB with 25 μg/ml kanamycin at 37°C overnight. It is recommended to use kanamycin rather than ampicillin because the colony usually grows bigger in a medium with kanamycin, which will make colony picking easier.

3.9. PCR Screen

1. Pick colonies into 20 μl standard PCR mix, using M13F and M13R primers. Care should be taken to only touch the middle of the colony to avoid contamination. PCR condition:
    (a) 94°C 8 min
    (b) 94°C 20 s, 60°C 30 s, 72°C 90 s, 30 cycles
    (c) 72°C 5 min
    (d) 4°C infinity
2. Run 5 μl on 2% agarose gel using 100 bp ladder as a size marker. Most colonies should generate a band 600 bases or longer. Multichannel pipettes and a compatible gel box are recommended to avoid tandem injury, which is likely the result of loading hundreds of samples using single channel pipettes.
3. Before sending the amplicon for sequencing, the M13 primer in the PCR reaction has to be degraded. Take 5 μl PCR product and add 2 μl ExoSAP-IT. Incubate at 37°C for 15 min. Heat at 80°C for 15 min to inactivate ExoSAP-IT. The DNA is ready to be sequenced.

4. Notes

1. ATP is purposely not included in the 2× 3′ ligation buffer. Ligation to 3′ linker without ATP is critical to minimize the self-ligation of small RNAs. Adenylated 3′ linker can be ligated to small RNA 3′ end directly without ATP, while self-ligation of small RNA can not occur without ATP. However, T4 RNA ligase might be precharged with AMP that not only increases ligation efficiency but also the chance of small RNAs self-ligation. AMP is transferred from ligase adenylate to the 5′-PO_4 of small RNA to form an RNA-adenylate intermediate (AppRNA), so the adenylated small RNAs are ligated to the 3′-OH of another small RNA without ATP in the reaction buffer. Thus, if precharged T4 RNA ligase is used for the reaction, 4 μM nonadenylated but 5′-phosphorylated 3′ linker should be added to the ligation buffer to absorb the pre-charged AMP and increase the ligation efficiency. If the T4 RNA ligase is not precharged with AMP, nonadenylated but 5′-phosphorylated 3′ linker should not be added to the ligation buffer. The method of preparation of preadenylated 3′ linker can be found on the Bartel laboratory Web site: http://web.wi.mit.edu/bartel/pub/protocols/miRNAcloning.pdf. Preadenylated 3′ linker is also commercially available. If commercially available 3′ linkers are used, 5′ linker should be redesigned to create the restriction enzyme site.
2. To minimize loss of starting material, it is recommended to use low binding or siliconized tubes and tips in all the steps before PCR amplification.
3. T4 RNA ligase efficiency is often a problem for small RNA cloning. Incubation at 5–16°C overnight could significantly improve the ligation efficiency.
4. Blue-light transilluminator, rather than UV transillminator, is recommended to light up DNA and RNAs throughout the whole protocol because multiple steps of gel extraction performed in the protocol may introduce mutations if UV transilluminator is used. It is recommended to use SybrGold to visualize RNA and SybrSafe for DNA.
5. Care should be taken to avoid denaturing of DNA throughout the protocol except a few steps specified in the protocol. If the DNA is denatured and renatured, they will form bulged DNA duplex because all the small RNA cDNAs now have the same 5′ and 3′ linker sequences. They cannot be digested by restriction enzyme, thus the self-ligation contamination will not be decreased. To avoid denaturing, the DNA pellet should never be dried out, and buffer rather than water

should always be used to dissolve the DNA pellet. PCR amplification of the small RNA cDNA library should never be allowed to go out of the exponential range. Also, to purify small RNA cDNA library, most commercially available kits, such as QIAquick Gel Extraction Kit and PCR Purification Kit from Qiagen, should not be used because the kits will denature the DNA. This is the reason why any commercially available kit is not used to purify small RNA cDNAs in the protocol and also why low-melting agarose gel is used to purify the concatamerized DNA.

6. It is common to add 3 μl of 100 μM forward and reverse PCR primers to soak up digested ends to prevent religation after digestion with Ban I. However, the huge amount of PCR primers might decrease ligase efficiency. So, this step is skipped in this protocol. Instead, 1.8 volume of EtOH is used to precipitate the DNA in previous step to decrease the amount of digested ends.

7. Most ligated DNA will break down into small pieces after phenol extraction, thus most colony will generate short DNAs around 250 bp after PCR amplification. These colonies are not desirable to be sequenced because most likely they contain only one small RNA sequence. We believe that the problem is because most ligated DNAs are loosely joined together, and these loosely joined DNA will break down easily during phenol extraction. So, we pipette the ligated DNA vigorously to break these loosely ligated DNAs before loading into the low-melting agarose gel. After this simple step, most colonies will yield a band above 600 bp, thus greatly improving the sequencing efficiency.

References

1. Lee RC, Feinbaum RL, Ambros V. (1993) The C. elegans heterochronic gene lin-4 encodes small RNAs with antisense complementarity to lin-14. Cell **75**: 843–54.
2. Lagos-Quintana M, Rauhut R, Lendeckel W, Tuschl T. (2001) Identification of novel genes coding for small expressed RNAs. Science **294**:853–8.
3. Lau NC, Lim LP, Weinstein EG, Bartel DP. (2001) An abundant class of tiny RNAs with probable regulatory roles in Caenorhabditis elegans. Science **294**: 858–62.
4. Lee RC, Ambros V. (2001) An extensive class of small RNAs in Caenorhabditis elegans. Science **294**:862–4.
5. Tuschl T, Zamore PD, Lehmann R, Bartel DP, Sharp PA. (1999) Targeted mRNA degradation by double-stranded RNA in vitro. Genes Dev **13**:3191–7.
6. Neilson JR, Zheng GX, Burge CB, Sharp PA. (2007) Dynamic regulation of miRNA expression in ordered stages of cellular development. Genes Dev **21**:578–89.
7. Wu H, Neilson JR, Kumar P, et al. (2007) miRNA profiling of naive, effector and memory CD8 T cells. PLoS One **2**:e1020.

Chapter 6

High-Throughput Profiling in the Hematopoietic System

Muller Fabbri, Riccardo Spizzo, and George A. Calin

Abstract

The expression profile of microRNAs significantly varies in physiological and pathological conditions. Increasing evidence from the literature shows that abnormalities of the miRNome (defined as the full spectrum of miRNAs expressed in a genome) occur in almost all human diseases and have important pathogenetic, prognostic, and therapeutic implications. The study of the aberrancies of the miRNome has become possible by developing high-throughput profiling techniques that allow the simultaneous detection of differences in miRNA expression between normal and pathologic tissues or simply tissues at different stages of differentiation. These techniques provide the basis for further investigations focused on the miRNAs, which are most frequently and widely differentially expressed under the different investigated conditions.

1. Introduction

MicroRNAs (miRNAs) are noncoding RNAs (ncRNAs) with gene regulatory functions, involved in a variety of biological processes (1–6). Initially transcribed by RNA polymerase II as long, capped, and polyadenylated precursors (pri-miRNAs) (7, 8), miRNAs undergo a complex processing mechanism. First, a double-stranded RNA-specific ribonuclease called Drosha, in conjunction with its binding partner DGCR8 (DiGeorge syndrome critical region gene 8 or Pasha), processes pri-miRNAs into hairpin RNAs of 70–100 nucleotides (nt) known as pre-miRNAs (9). Translocated from the nucleus to the cytoplasm by means of Exportin 5, pre-miRNA is processed by a ribonuclease III (Dicer) and TRBP (HIV-1 transactivating response RNA binding protein) in an 18–24 nt duplex. Finally, the duplex interacts with a large protein complex called RNA-induced silencing complex (RISC), which includes proteins of the Argonaute family (Ago1-4 in humans). One strand of the miRNA duplex

Silvia Monticelli (ed.), *MicroRNAs and the Immune System: Methods and Protocols*, Methods in Molecular Biology, vol. 667,
DOI 10.1007/978-1-60761-811-9_6, © Springer Science+Business Media, LLC 2010

remains stably associated with RISC and becomes the mature miRNA, which guides the RISC mainly (but not exclusively) to the 3′-UTR (3′-untranslated region) of the target mRNAs. Overall, by inducing translational repression or mRNA cleavage, miRNAs silence target gene expression although recent evidences show that miRNAs are also able to directly upregulate the expression of a target gene by binding to its mRNA 5′-UTR (10).

The development of high-throughput methods to detect miRNA expression in human samples (11, 12) has provided invaluable tools to investigate the role of these ncRNAs both in physiological and pathological conditions. This chapter describes a validated array profiling approach (11), which is able to provide high-throughput miRNA expression profiling in the hematopoietic system.

2. Materials

2.1. miRNA Array Profiling

2.1.1. RNA Extraction (see Note 1)

1. TRIzol reagent: Store at +2–25°C. Warning: TRIzol is toxic if it comes in contact with skin or is swallowed. The use of TRIzol should be restricted to a chemical hood.
2. 100% chloroform: Store at room temperature (see Note 2). The use of chloroform should be restricted to a chemical hood.
3. 100% ethanol.
4. RNase- and DNase-free water (see Note 3).

2.1.2. Synthesis of Biotin-Labeled First-Strand cDNA Targets

1. Reagents:
   (a) 0.5 pM/μL 3′NNNNNNNN-$(dA)_{12}$ T (biotin) $(dA)_{12}$-biotin 5′ oligonucleotide primer.
   (b) 5× first-strand buffer.
   (c) 0.1 M dithiothreitol.
   (d) 10 mM dNTP mix.
   (e) SuperScript II RNase H^- reverse transcriptase (200 U/μL; Invitrogen).
2. Equipment and materials supplied by user:
   (a) Pipette tips (sterile, RNase free, and aerosol resistant).
   (b) Microcentrifuge tubes (sterile, RNase free, 1.7 mL).
   (c) Micropipettes (10, 20, 200, and 1,000 μL).
   (d) Nanodrop ultraviolet spectrophotometer.
   (e) Microcentrifuge (room temperature and 4°C).
   (f) Water bath (70, 65, and 37°C).

(g) Sterile, nuclease-free conical tubes (15 and 50 mL).
(h) SpeedVac concentrator.
(i) Vortex.
(j) Pipet aid and disposable pipettes.

2.1.3. Array Hybridization

1. Required reagents/kits:
   (a) 0.5% NEN blocking reagent (PerkinElmer).
   (b) Streptavidin/Alexa Fluor 647 conjugate (staining solution: a 1:500 dilution in TNB) (Molecular Probes).
   (c) Nuclease-free water.
   (d) 1× PBS, pH 7.4.
   (e) 1 M Tris–HCl, pH 7.6.
   (f) 5 M NaCl.
   (g) Tween-20.
   (h) Formamide.
   (i) 50× Denhardt's solution (Sigma).
2. Other equipment and materials:
   (a) Tecan HS 4800 hybridization station.
   (b) Axon GenePix 4000B scanner.
   (c) Computer configured for the Axon GenePix 4000B scanner.
   (d) New Brunswick Innova 4080 shaking incubator.
   (e) Sigma/Qiagen centrifuge (4–15°C) (Qiagen).
   (f) Centrifuge plate rotor: 2× 96 (Qiagen).
   (g) Pipette tips (sterile, RNase free, and aerosol resistant).
   (h) Microcentrifuge tubes (sterile, RNase free, 1.7 mL).
   (i) Micropipettes.
   (j) Powder-free gloves.
   (k) Microcentrifuge.
   (l) Microtiter plate lid, black (Corning).
   (m) Bioarray processors (GE Healthcare).
   (n) Bioarray rack (GE Healthcare).
   (o) Small reagent reservoir (GE Healthcare).
   (p) Large reagent reservoir (GE Healthcare).
   (q) Bioarray removal tool (GE Healthcare).
   (r) Bioarray position tool (GE Healthcare).

2.1.4. Posthybridization miRNA Microarray

Stock solutions for posthybridization array processing:

1. TNT buffer (20 L): 0.1 M Tris–HCl (pH 7.6), 0.15 M NaCl, and 0.05% Tween-20. Rinse a 25-L carboy with 150 mL of

isopropanol. Rinse the carboy twice with 3 L of deionized water and completely drain the carboy. Add 2 L of 1 M Tris–HCl, 600 mL of 5 M NaCl, 10 mL of Tween-20, and 17.39 L of deionized water. Mix well by swirling. Filter TNT through a 0.2-μm filter. This solution can be stored for up to 2 weeks at room temperature.

2. TNT buffer (0.75×): Add 25 mL of deionized water to 75 mL of TNT buffer (described above) per 100 mL of buffer required.
3. TNB buffer (0.5 L): 0.1 M Tris–HCl (pH 7.6), 0.15 M NaCl, and 0.5% NEN blocking reagent (PerkinElmer). Add 435 mL of nuclease-free water, 50 mL of 1 M Tris–HCl (pH 7.6), and 15 mL of 5 M NaCl. Slowly add 2.5 g of NEN blocking reagent in 0.5-g increments until all 2.5 g of the reagent are dissolved while warming in a water bath at 60°C. Filter TNB buffer through a 0.88-μm filter. Aliquot the TNB buffer into 50-ml tubes and store at −20°C. This solution can be stored for up to 12 weeks at −20°C. Thaw immediately before use.

2.1.5. Array Scanning

Equipment: Axon GenePix 4000B scanner.

2.2. Identification of Significantly Deregulated miRNAs

2.2.1. Data Normalization, Raw Data, and Statistical Analysis by Comparison of Treated and Control miRNA Signatures

Data statistical analysis requires different software programs, some of which are freely available on the Internet (open source), while others require to purchase a license. Among the most widely used methods, we mention the Significance Analysis of Microarray (SAM), the Prediction Analysis of Microarrays software programs (all of which are freely available on the Internet), and the GeneSpring software program, which requires a license purchase from Silicon Genetics, Redwood City, CA, USA.

2.3. Validation of Microarray Results

2.3.1. DNase Digestion

Required reagents/kits: TURBO DNase Kit (Ambion).

2.3.2. Gene-Specific Reverse Transcription for Mature miRNA

Required reagents/kits: TaqMan MicroRNA Reverse Transcription Kit (Applied Biosystems).

3. Methods

3.1. Sample Collection

We recommend performing these experiments at least three times for both the treatment and the control, and to hybridize the labeled RNAs on the miRNA chip (see Note 4).

Cells need to be collected as a pellet. If necessary RNA purification can be postponed. The pellet can be stored at −80°C, or snap-frozen in liquid nitrogen and then stored at −80°C (see Note 5). If the samples must be sent to another laboratory or to a core facility before the RNA extraction, the frozen pellets can be sent on dry ice, or the cells can be collected using stabilization reagents and delivered at room temperature or 2–8°C (see Note 6).

3.2. miRNA Array Profiling

3.2.1. RNA Extraction

RNA extraction should be performed by using the standard TRIzol reagent protocol (see Note 7). A total of 2.5–5.0 μg of RNA is sufficient for each replicate of each sample. Before the sample preparation for microarray hybridization, quantity and quality assessment of the RNA should be performed. Regarding the quality of RNA, as usual, higher is better (see Note 8).

3.2.2. Sample Preparation

The microarray platform for miRNA (microRNACHIP) described herein is based on the technology described by Liu et al. (11). We do not describe the procedure used for microRNACHIP printing, since Liu et al. previously described this method in detail (13). The microRNACHIP currently used at the microarray facility at The Ohio State University Comprehensive Cancer Center is version 4.0 (microRNACHIPv4) and contains 847 probes targeting 474 human miRNAs and 373 mouse miRNAs. Furthermore, the chip contains probes targeting other ncRNAs, such as ultraconserved sequences (14, 15) and human predicted miRNAs (16–18). The miRNA oligo probes that have been spotted on the chip are 40-nt long and target both the mature and precursor forms of each miRNA. This technology is based on direct reverse transcription with a biotin-labeled random octamer primer to obtain labeled target cDNA. After miRNA sample preparation, the biotin-labeled target cDNAs are hybridized with the probes on the array slides in a semiautomated manner. Finally, the biotinylated target/probe complexes are stained with a streptavidin/Alexa Fluor 647 conjugate.

3.2.3. Synthesis of Biotin-Labeled First-Strand cDNA Targets

1. Prepare each total RNA sample for manual target preparation:

   5 μg of total RNA (the optimal concentration should be determined for each source of total RNA; see Note 9).

   2 μL of 0.5 μg/μL primer.

   Add X μL nuclease-free water to a 12-μL final volume.

   12-μL total volume.

   5 μg of total RNA in 10 μL of RNase-free water.

   2 μL of an oligo primer (5′ biotin-AAA-AAA-AAA-AAA-[T-biotin]-AAA-AAA-AAA-AAA-NNN-NNN-NN 3′ [0.5 μg/μL] in which N stands for a random octamer).

2. Incubate for 10 min in a 70°C water bath and then immediately place the tube on ice.

3. Centrifuge for 5 s to collect the sample at the bottom of the tube and immediately place the tube on ice.
4. With the tube remaining on ice, add the following reagents to the 12-μL total RNA/control mRNA/primer mix.

   4 μL of 5× first-strand buffer.

   2 μL of 0.1 M dithiothreitol.

   1 μL of 10 mM dNTP mix.

   1 μL of SuperScript II RNase H^- reverse transcriptase (200 U/μL).

   20-μL final volume.
5. Incubate 90 min in a 37°C water bath.
6. Centrifuge for 5 s to collect the sample at the bottom of the tube.
7. RNA template degradation: After 90 min of incubation for the first-strand synthesis, add 3.5 μL of 0.5 M NaOH/50 mM EDTA into a 20-μL reaction mix and incubate at 65°C for 15 min to denature the DNA/RNA hybrids and degrade the RNA template. Next, neutralize the reaction with 5 μL of 1 M Tris–HCI, pH 7.6. Each labeled target should be in a 28.5-μL volume. The sample preparation will thus end, and the samples must be stored at –80°C until use.

3.2.4. Array Hybridization

1. Prime all channels of the Tecan HS 4800 hybridization stations.
2. Load a preprinted miRNA array face-up to the Tecan HS 4800 hybridization station (see Note 10). Close the hybridization chambers of HS 4800.
3. Run the hybridization program for the chip hybridization with labeled cDNA targets:
   (a) Prime the chip in the hybridization chamber at 23°C with 6× SSPE and 0.05% Tween-20 for 1 min.
   (b) Inject 150 μL of a prehybridization mix of 6× SSPE/2× Denhardt's solution/30% formamide and prehybridize the chip at 25°C for 30 min.
   (c) Inject the hybridization mix of labeled biotin-cDNA in 6× SSPE/2× Denhardt's solution/30% formamide and hybridize at 25°C for 18 h (see Note 11).
   (d) Wash in 0.75× TNT buffer at 23°C for 5 min.
   (e) Wash in 0.75× TNT buffer at 37°C for 10 min.
   (f) Rinse with water in the HS 4800 at 23°C for 30 s.
   (g) Unload the chips from the machine for posthybridization washing.

3.2.5. Posthybridization miRNA Microarray

1. Open the hybridization chamber of the HS 4800 and remove the slide chips as quickly as possible and place them in a slot of a bioarray rack placed in a large reagent reservoir containing 0.75× TNT prewarmed to 37°C. Move the slide into place using the bioarray position tool with the tooth side down. Wash the slides in 0.75× TNT prewarmed to 37°C with agitation in a New Brunswick Innova 4080 shaking incubator at 37°C for 40 min with agitation at 50 rpm.
2. Block the slide in TNB blocking buffer at room temperature for 30 min.
3. Stain the slide with a streptavidin/Alexa Fluor 647 conjugate in TNB buffer at 1:500 at room temperature for 30 min.
4. After staining, wash in 1× TNT at room temperature for 40 min with three-time buffer changes.
5. Briefly rinse the chips with distilled water and spin-dry them at 300 ×*g* for 1 min.

3.2.6. Array Scanning

Scan the slides at a resolution of 10 μm using an Axon GenePix 4000B scanner at a power setting of 100 and PMT 800 (see Note 12).

1. Open the .gal file provided by the builder of the slide.
2. Drag the file onto the features just collected to fit all of the blocks.
3. Set each block and press the F5 key for automatic alignment of the grid on the features.

The image data may be extracted using the GenePix software and saved as a .gpr file for further data analysis.

3.3. Identification of Significantly Deregulated miRNAs

Ideally, the same raw data should be analyzed by two distinct bioinformaticians using two independent methods of analyses. Two strategies have been used by us and developed in two different laboratories (19, 20).

3.3.1. Data Normalization

A first approach to data normalization has been adopted by Bloomston et al. (21) and can be summarized as follows. Mean values of the replicate spots of each miRNA are background-subtracted, normalized, and subjected to further analysis. miRNAs are retained when present in at least 20% of analyzed samples, or in at least the smallest group of comparison in the dataset, and when the miRNAs have a fold change in signal intensity of more than 1.5 from the median of all the samples. Prior to statistical analysis, a value of 22 (4.5 on the $\log_2$ scale) is assigned to miRNA probes with absent signal. This value is the mean minimum intensity level above the background detected in miRNA chip experiments. Three different data-normalization procedures are applied: global median, housekeeping, and cyclic loess.

A second approach has been described by Calin et al. (22) and consists of raw data normalization and analysis using the GeneSpring software program. Expression data are median centered using the GeneSpring normalization option or global median normalization option of the BioConductor open-source software program (http://www.bioconductor.org).

3.3.2. Raw Data and Statistical Analysis by Comparing Treated and Control miRNA Signatures

We have compared the SAM and Prediction Analysis of Microarrays (http://www-stat.stanford.edu/~tibs/PAM/index.html) tests performed for the different classes of comparison (usually, "cancer" vs. "normal" or "cancer set 1" vs. "cancer set 2") over the respective expression tables. Cyclic loess exhibited the best improvement in reducing variability of hybridization and yielded the highest number of significant miRNAs across the different tests in agreement with a recent evaluation of different normalization methods for CodeLink microarrays (23). Cyclic loess uses the MA plot and loess smoothing to estimate intensity-dependent differences in each pair of slides in the dataset and then removes these differences by centering the loess line at 0. This procedure is iterated until intensity-dependent differences between slides are removed from all of the arrays. We implemented cyclic loess using the BioConductor affy/normalization loess with miRNA nomenclature according to the miRNA database at the Wellcome Trust Sanger Institute (Hinxton, Cambridge, UK). Differentially expressed miRNAs between classes are identified using the *t*-test procedure, which is included in SAM. The SAM program calculates a score for each gene based on the change in its expression relative to the standard deviation for all measurements. The miRNA signatures are identified by applying the nearest shrunken centroids to the entire dataset. This method identifies a subgroup of genes that best characterizes two sample groups (i.e., tumor vs. normal). The prediction error is calculated using tenfold cross-validation. Using this specific approach, we were able to identify a common miRNA expression signature of human solid tumors that defines cancer gene targets (20). The Principal Component Analysis (PCA) is used for statistically exploring and making sense of datasets, different classes of tumor samples, and related miRNA expression values (Fig. 1). A more "classical" presentation of miRNA differential expression is by using "heat-maps" that use different colors to indicate up- or downregulation of miRNAs with respect to control tissues (Fig. 2).

The GeneSpring analysis of variance and support vector machine tools for cross-validation and test-set prediction identifies and confirms which miRNAs are able to best separate the groups of comparison using two different methods of raw-data normalization. All data are submitted to the ArrayExpress

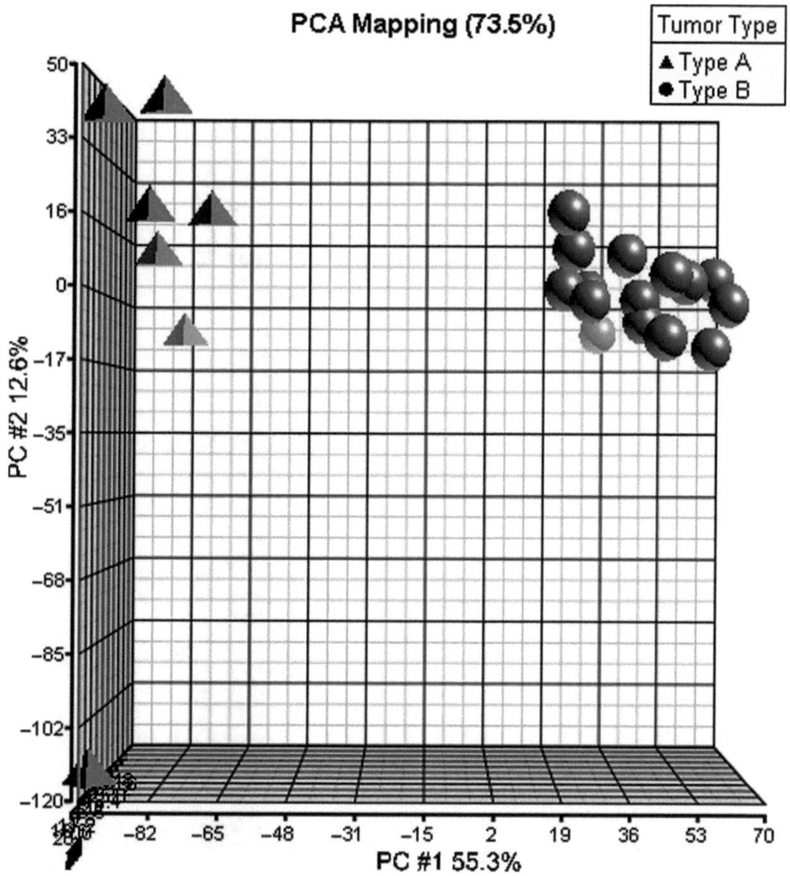

Fig. 1. Principal Component Analysis (PCA) was used for statistically exploring and making sense of datasets different classes of tumor samples and related microRNA expression values. Unsupervised PCA of normalized and filtered dataset was performed and showed perfect separation between the two classes of tumors. The most significantly differentially expressed [using Significance Analysis of Microarrays (SAM)] probes were used to build the supervised cluster of samples. We used the expression of the differentially regulated miRNAs across experiments. The tree displays their average absolute expression values after $\log_2$ transformation. The mean was computed over all samples from the same class. Genes and arrays were mean centered and normalized by using GENE CLUSTER 3.0. Single linkage clustering was performed by using Spearman correlation distance and displayed using TreeView program (http://rana.lbl.gov/EisenSoftware.htm; http://rana.lbl.gov/EisenSoftware.htm).

database (http://www.ebi.ac.uk/arrayexpress/) using MIAMExpress software program. Using this specific strategy, we were able to find a common miRNA signature for breast cancer (19) as well as for the first time, an miRNA signature of hypoxia (24).

The raw-data analysis output using this method consists of (1) dendrograms showing the clustering of multiple samples according to the transfection status and type of transfectant (e.g., miRNAs, scrambled oligos, empty vectors) and (2) gene lists containing genes differentially expressed at high statistical significance

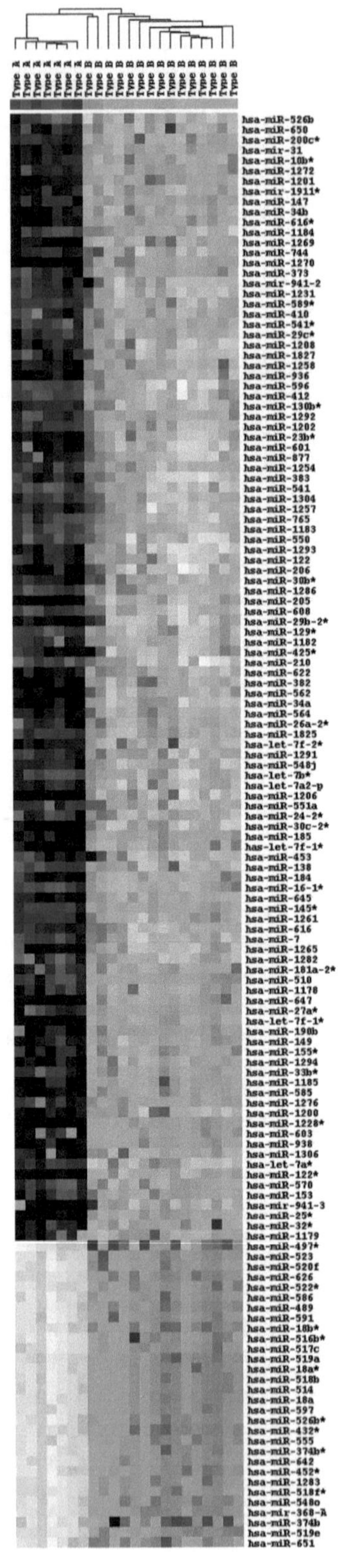

Fig. 2. Heat map showing upregulated (*darker*) and downregulated (*lighter*) miRNAs in tumors vs. normal tissues.

($P<0.05$ or, better, $P<0.01$). The level of differential expression of these genes that can be considered biologically significant is a key issue. If fold differences in gene expression of 10–20 are biologically important, then we support the view that much smaller differences (less than twofold) may also be significant. The explanation for this resides in the multiplicity of targets of specific miRNAs and the large number of altered miRNAs, meaning that two or more target protein-coding genes in the same pathway likely are consequently disturbed. An opposite view is that in some cases, the described changes in miRNA expression between normal and tumor cells may be biologically irrelevant; the main interactions of one miRNA with various targets may not accumulate but antagonize each other (e.g., repression of both proapoptotic and antiapoptotic genes) resulting in unmodified phenotype (25).

4. Notes

1. All of the solutions and plastic supplies used during cell collection must be tested using cell culture analysis, and all of the tubes and tips used to collect the samples must be RNase certified and DNase certified or autoclaved before use.
2. A few milliliters of RNase-/DNase-free water can be overlaid onto chloroform to decrease evaporation.
3. Instead of buying ready-to-use RNase-/DNase-free water, one can easily treat 18.2 MΩ-cm water overnight at room temperature with 0.1% DEPC and autoclave it the next day.
4. The other choice is to treat cell lines once and, after RNA purification, split the same sample in three replicates.
5. The first procedure is recommended, since the freezing process is quicker, and changes in the miRNome are less likely to occur.
6. Different companies, such as Qiagen and Ambion, sell these reagents. We do not have any experience with these stabilization reagents and are not sure how they may affect the miRNome. Thus, we recommend using the former procedure.
7. In the last step, "RNA wash with 75% ethanol," mixing of the sample should be avoided, because floating the RNA pellet can decrease the number of small RNA molecules such as miRNAs. When using an RNA extraction kit, carefully check the kit's protocol, as some protocols have a 200-bp RNA length cut-off value; both mature and precursor molecules would be lost during washing of the column using such protocols.

8. Using RNA column purification instead of TRIzol increases the chances of obtaining RNA samples with good quality. The cut-off size is set to 18 bp, which is very close to the miRNA size (19–24 nt), at least for Qiagen columns. This specificity is based on the ratio of water to ethanol in the samples before the transfer of the samples to the columns. For these reasons, this RNA purification technique may affect the miRNome. We have never compared the TRIzol protocol with column purification on the microarray platform that we describe here, and we do not know whether some differences between these RNA purifications exist. Thus, we strongly recommend the TRIzol purification at this point.
9. The lowest concentration allowed is 0.5 μg/μL.
10. Each slide has a code scratched on it identifying the batch. The code is located on the opposite face of the printing side.
11. Increase the volume of the sample preparation to 100 μL with prehybridization solution to ensure a more uniform hybridization.
12. The slide has to be placed face down and with the scratched code toward the operator. The direction of the slide is very important for the following superimposition of the .gal file.

References

1. Ambros, V. and Lee, R. C. (2004) Identification of microRNAs and other tiny noncoding RNAs by cDNA cloning, *Methods Mol Biol* **265**, 131–158.
2. Bartel, D. P. (2004) MicroRNAs: genomics, biogenesis, mechanism, and function, *Cell* **116**, 281–297.
3. He, L. and Hannon, G. J. (2004) MicroRNAs: small RNAs with a big role in gene regulation, *Nat Rev Genet* **5**, 522–531.
4. Plasterk, R. H. (2006) Micro RNAs in animal development, *Cell* **124**, 877–881.
5. Pasquinelli, A. E., Hunter, S., and Bracht, J. (2005) MicroRNAs: a developing story, *Curr Opin Genet Dev* **15**, 200–205.
6. Carleton, M., Cleary, M. A., and Linsley, P. S. (2007) MicroRNAs and cell cycle regulation, *Cell Cycle* **6**, 2127–2132.
7. Lee, Y., Kim, M., Han, J., Yeom, K. H., Lee, S., Baek, S. H., and Kim, V. N. (2004) MicroRNA genes are transcribed by RNA polymerase II, *EMBO J* **23**, 4051–4060.
8. Cai, X., Hagedorn, C. H., and Cullen, B. R. (2004) Human microRNAs are processed from capped, polyadenylated transcripts that can also function as mRNAs, *RNA* **10**, 1957–1966.
9. Cullen, B. R. (2004) Transcription and processing of human microRNA precursors, *Mol Cell* **16**, 861–865.
10. Vasudevan, S., Tong, Y., and Steitz, J. A. (2007) Switching from repression to activation: microRNAs can up-regulate translation, *Science* **318**, 1931–1934.
11. Liu, C. G., Calin, G. A., Meloon, B., Gamliel, N., Sevignani, C., Ferracin, M., Dumitru, C. D., Shimizu, M., Zupo, S., Dono, M., Alder, H., Bullrich, F., Negrini, M., and Croce, C. M. (2004) An oligonucleotide microchip for genome-wide microRNA profiling in human and mouse tissues, *Proc Natl Acad Sci U S A* **101**, 9740–9744.
12. Lu, J., Getz, G., Miska, E. A., Alvarez-Saavedra, E., Lamb, J., Peck, D., Sweet-Cordero, A., Ebert, B. L., Mak, R. H., Ferrando, A. A., Downing, J. R., Jacks, T., Horvitz, H. R., and Golub, T. R. (2005) MicroRNA expression profiles classify human cancers, *Nature* **435**, 834–838.
13. Liu, C. G., Spizzo, R., Calin, G. A., and Croce, C. M. (2008) Expression profiling of microRNA using oligo DNA arrays, *Methods* **44**, 22–30.

14. Bejerano, G., Pheasant, M., Makunin, I., Stephen, S., Kent, W. J., Mattick, J. S., and Haussler, D. (2004) Ultraconserved elements in the human genome, *Science* **304**, 1321–1325.
15. Calin, G. A., Liu, C. G., Ferracin, M., Hyslop, T., Spizzo, R., Sevignani, C., Fabbri, M., Cimmino, A., Lee, E. J., Wojcik, S. E., Shimizu, M., Tili, E., Rossi, S., Taccioli, C., Pichiorri, F., Liu, X., Zupo, S., Herlea, V., Gramantieri, L., Lanza, G., Alder, H., Rassenti, L., Volinia, S., Schmittgen, T. D., Kipps, T. J., Negrini, M., and Croce, C. M. (2007) Ultraconserved regions encoding ncRNAs are altered in human leukemias and carcinomas, *Cancer Cell* **12**, 215–229.
16. Altuvia, Y., Landgraf, P., Lithwick, G., Elefant, N., Pfeffer, S., Aravin, A., Brownstein, M. J., Tuschl, T., and Margalit, H. (2005) Clustering and conservation patterns of human microRNAs, *Nucleic Acids Res* **33**, 2697–2706.
17. Xie, X., Lu, J., Kulbokas, E. J., Golub, T. R., Mootha, V., Lindblad-Toh, K., Lander, E. S., and Kellis, M. (2005) Systematic discovery of regulatory motifs in human promoters and 3 UTRs by comparison of several mammals, *Nature* **434**, 338–345.
18. Berezikov, E., Guryev, V., van de Belt, J., Wienholds, E., Plasterk, R. H., and Cuppen, E. (2005) Phylogenetic shadowing and computational identification of human microRNA genes, *Cell* **120**, 21–24.
19. Iorio, M. V., Ferracin, M., Liu, C. G., Veronese, A., Spizzo, R., Sabbioni, S., Magri, E., Pedriali, M., Fabbri, M., Campiglio, M., Menard, S., Palazzo, J. P., Rosenberg, A., Musiani, P., Volinia, S., Nenci, I., Calin, G. A., Querzoli, P., Negrini, M., and Croce, C. M. (2005) MicroRNA gene expression deregulation in human breast cancer, *Cancer Res* **65**, 7065–7070.
20. Volinia, S., Calin, G. A., Liu, C. G., Ambs, S., Cimmino, A., Petrocca, F., Visone, R., Iorio, M., Roldo, C., Ferracin, M., Prueitt, R. L., Yanaihara, N., Lanza, G., Scarpa, A., Vecchione, A., Negrini, M., Harris, C. C., and Croce, C. M. (2006) A microRNA expression signature of human solid tumors defines cancer gene targets, *Proc Natl Acad Sci U S A* **103**, 2257–2261.
21. Bloomston, M., Frankel, W. L., Petrocca, F., Volinia, S., Alder, H., Hagan, J. P., Liu, C. G., Bhatt, D., Taccioli, C., and Croce, C. M. (2007) MicroRNA expression patterns to differentiate pancreatic adenocarcinoma from normal pancreas and chronic pancreatitis, *JAMA* **297**, 1901–1908.
22. Calin, G. A., Ferracin, M., Cimmino, A., Di Leva, G., Shimizu, M., Wojcik, S. E., Iorio, M. V., Visone, R., Sever, N. I., Fabbri, M., Iuliano, R., Palumbo, T., Pichiorri, F., Roldo, C., Garzon, R., Sevignani, C., Rassenti, L., Alder, H., Volinia, S., Liu, C. G., Kipps, T. J., Negrini, M., and Croce, C. M. (2005) A microRNA signature associated with prognosis and progression in chronic lymphocytic leukemia, *N Engl J Med* **353**, 1793–1801.
23. Wu, W., Dave, N., Tseng, G. C., Richards, T., Xing, E. P., and Kaminski, N. (2005) Comparison of normalization methods for CodeLink Bioarray data, *BMC Bioinformatics* **6**, 309.
24. Kulshreshtha, R., Ferracin, M., Wojcik, S. E., Garzon, R., Alder, H., Agosto-Perez, F. J., Davuluri, R., Liu, C. G., Croce, C. M., Negrini, M., Calin, G. A., and Ivan, M. (2007) A microRNA signature of hypoxia, *Mol Cell Biol* **27**, 1859–1867.
25. Calin, G. A. and Croce, C. M. (2006) MicroRNA signatures in human cancers, *Nat Rev Cancer* **6**, 857–866.

Chapter 7

Construction of Small RNA cDNA Libraries for Deep Sequencing

Molly F. Thomas and K. Mark Ansel

Abstract

Since the phenomenon of small RNA-mediated gene silencing was first described over 15 years ago (Lee et al. Cell 75:843–854, 1993; Wightman et al. Cell 75:855–862, 1993), it has become evident that a variety of endogenous small RNAs play an important role in establishing and maintaining cell lineages. MicroRNAs (miRNAs), in particular, have been shown to exert regulatory control over the development and function of the many specialized cells that comprise the mammalian immune system (Baltimore et al. Nat Immunol 9:839–845, 2008; Kanellopoulous and Monticelli Semin Cancer Biol 18:79–88, 2008; Xiao and Rajewsky Cell 136:26–36, 2009). The advent of next generation sequencers provides an important tool for profiling the small RNA transcriptome of many diverse cell types. Compared to traditional Sanger sequencing, next generation sequencing machines can process millions of sequence reads in parallel, generating megabases of data within just a few days. The generation of small RNA libraries for sequencing is relatively straightforward and involves the ligation of platform-specific adapter sequences to small RNAs, followed by reverse transcription of the ligated species and PCR amplification. While other hybridization-based techniques are available for profiling well-characterized small RNAs, high-throughput sequencing remains the most powerful method for discovering novel small RNAs and post-transcriptional editing.

1. Introduction

The identification of small RNAs and their specific expression patterns is an important component of understanding the complex gene regulatory networks that govern the immune system (1–5). Hybridization-based detection methods, such as qPCR, northern blot, and microarrays, are effective for probing the expression of known miRNAs; however, high-throughput sequencing remains the best technique for the discovery of novel small RNAs (6, 7). Furthermore, sequencing allows the possibility to assess the posttranscriptional modification of miRNAs such as

Silvia Monticelli (ed.), *MicroRNAs and the Immune System: Methods and Protocols*, Methods in Molecular Biology, vol. 667, DOI 10.1007/978-1-60761-811-9_7, © Springer Science+Business Media, LLC 2010

miR-142, which is edited by deaminases and is highly expressed in many hematopoietic lineages (8). Several different next generation sequencers are available for use, including 454 (Roche), SOLiD (ABI), and Solexa (Illumina). While platforms vary by target sequence length, accuracy, and cost (9), all give reproducibly comparable results (10, 11). The methods described here are specific for preparing cDNA libraries for Solexa sequencing, which is optimized for short sequence reads. These techniques can be easily adapted to other platforms by substituting different adapter and primer sequences from those listed in Table 1.

Small RNA cDNA library preparation for all high-throughput sequencers is based on the same set of basic steps: RNA isolation followed by 3′ and 5′ linker ligation, reverse transcription, and PCR amplification (6) (Fig. 1). The standard protocol enriches for miRNAs by size fractionating total RNA samples and demanding that all linkered products carry a 5′-monophosphate, a hallmark feature of Dicer and Drosha cleavage products. An alternate protocol for 5′-monophosphate-independent linker ligation is also described. This protocol allows broader capture of other small RNA species, including those that carry 5′-triphosphate

Table 1
Oligonucleotide sequences for the small RNA cloning protocol

18-bp RNA size marker	rGrUrArCrGrCrGrGrGrUrUrUrArArArCrGrA
30-bp RNA size marker	rUrCrArGrGrArUrGrGrCrGrCrGrCrCrGrGrUrCrUrCrArCrUrGrArArCrGrC
5′ Solexa RNA linker	rGrUrUrCrArGrArGrUrUrCrUrArCrArGrUrCrCrGrArCrGrArUrC
3′ Solexa DNA linker	Monophosphate-TCGTATGCCGTCTTCTGCTTGidT
3′ Adenylation template	ACAAGCAGAAGACGGCATACGATATAGTGAGTC
3′ Solexa RT/PCR primer	CAAGCAGAAGACGGCATACGA
5′ Solexa PCR primer	AATGATACGGCGACCACCGACAGGTTCAGAGTTCTACAGTCCGA
Solexa sequencing primer	CGACAGGTTCAGAGTTCTACAGTCCGACGATC

Bases preceded by an "r" indicate RNA nucleotides. The remainders are DNA nucleotides. The 3′ DNA linker must contain a 5′-monophosphate so that it can be charged with an adenylation group by T4 DNA ligase. idT represents a 5′-, 3′-inverted thymidine deoxynucleotide that blocks phosphodiester bond formation at the 3′ end of the oligo and thus prevents circularization of the 3′ linker upon the addition of truncated Rnl2 (1-249). All oligonucleotides can be ordered from Integrated DNA Technology (IDT) and require no further purification beyond desalting.

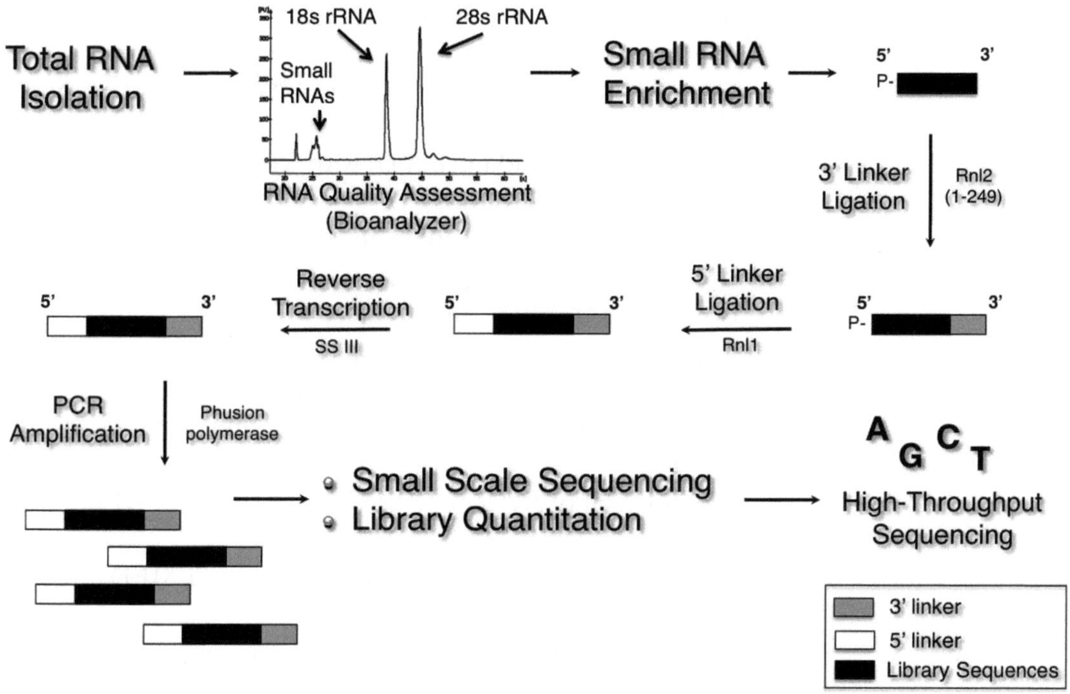

Fig. 1. Overview schematic of small RNA cloning for deep sequencing. cDNA libraries for deep sequencing are generated by ligating size-fractionated small RNAs to platform-specific linker sequences. The protocol can be easily modified for 5′-monophosphate-independent cloning by pretreating 3′-linkered RNA samples with phosphatase prior to 5′ linker ligation. Libraries are then reverse transcribed and amplified by minimal rounds of PCR to avoid library bias. The quality of the prepared libraries should be verified throughout the protocol. This includes using an electrophoretic method (i.e., Agilent Bioanalyzer) to evaluate the quality of RNA isolation, routinely visualizing linkered and PCR amplified products on acrylamide gels and carrying out small-scale sequencing of your cloned cDNAs to assess the number of known small RNAs in your final libraries.

modifications (12). As with any profiling technique, library bias can be introduced at several steps including linker ligation, reverse transcription, and PCR amplification (13, 14). Thus, sequencing results must ultimately be validated by alternative methods such as qPCR or northern blot.

2. Materials

2.1. Prepare 5′-Labeled Size Fractionation Markers

1. ATP [γ-^{32}P] – 6,000 Ci/mmol.
2. T4 Polynucleotide Kinase with 10× kinase buffer.
3. DEPC Water: Add 1 ml of diethyl pyrocarbonate to 1 l of ddH_2O and mix with a stir bar until DEPC is fully dissolved. Autoclave solution at 121°C for 30 min, which will convert the DEPC into ethanol and CO_2. Store at room temperature.
4. G25 Sephadex columns (GE Life Sciences, Pescataway, NJ).

5. 0.5 M EDTA pH 8: Dissolve 93.5 g of disodium salt dihydrate in 400 ml of DEPC H_2O. While stirring the mixture, adjust the pH to 8.0 by adding NaOH to dissolve the EDTA. Store at room temperature.
6. 2× formamide loading buffer with xylene cyanol and bromophenol blue.
7. Large format polyacrylamide gel electrophoresis apparatus.
8. RNaseZAP or similar product for cleaning RNase-contaminated equipment.
9. 5× TBE: Combine 20 ml of 0.5 M EDTA pH 8.0, 27.5 g of boric acid, 54 g of Tris base, and 800 ml of DEPC H_2O. Bring the total volume up to 1 l and store at room temperature.
10. 40% solution of acrylamide and bis-acrylamide (19:1 ratio for best results). Store at 4°C.
11. *N*,*N*,*N*′,*N*′-Tetramethylethylenediamine (TEMED). Store at 4°C.
12. 10% Ammonium persulfate (w/v). Store at 4°C for up to 1 month.
13. Phosphorimager and phosphor screens for rapidly visualizing electrophoresed radiolabeled nucleic acids.

2.2. Size Fractionate Small RNAs from Total Extracted RNA

1. 500 ml DEPC 1 M NaCl: Dissolve 29.2 g of NaCl in 500 ml of ddH_2O. Add 500 μl of DEPC and mix with a stir bar until the DEPC is full dissolved. Autoclave at 121°C for 30 min. Store at room temperature.
2. RNase-free 1.5-ml microcentrifuge safe-lock tubes (Eppendorf, Westbury, NY) and RNase-free pestles for use with 1.5-ml tubes (Kimble Chase Kontes, Vineland, NJ).
3. GlycoBlue (15 mg/ml dyed glycogen; Applied Biosystems, Austin, TX).
4. RNase-free siliconized 1.5-ml microcentrifuge tubes.

2.3. Adenylate 3′ Adapter and Ligate to Small RNAs

1. NEB Quick Ligation Kit with high concentration T4 DNA Ligase (2,000,000 U/ml) and Quick Ligation Reaction Buffer containing polyethylene glycol (PEG). Truncated T4 RNA Ligase 2 (1-249) (New England BioLabs, Ispwich, MA).
2. Molecular biology grade dimethylsulfoxide (DMSO).
3. 50% PEG (w/v).
4. 10 mg/ml ethidium bromide solution. Because ethidium bromide is a DNA intercalating agent and potential carcinogen, wear a mask to avoid inhaling powder when measuring weight. Store at room temperature protected from light.

2.4. Ligate 5′ Adapter

1. Antarctic Phosphatase, T4 DNA ligase buffer containing 10 mM ATP, and T4 RNA ligase 1 (New England BioLabs, Ispwich, MA).
2. Phenol:chloroform:isoamyl alcohol (P:C:I; 25:24:1 ratio) pH 4.5.
3. DEPC-treated 3 M NaOAc pH 5.2: Dissolve 204 g of NaOAc-$3H_2O$ in 400 ml of ddH_2O. Adjust the pH to 5.2 with glacial acetic acid and bring the volume up to 500 ml. Dissolve 0.5 ml of DEPC into the sodium acetate solution and autoclave for 30 min at 121°C. Store at room temperature.
4. TE pH 8: Make a solution of 1 M Tris–HCl pH 8 by dissolving 12.1 g of Tris base in 80 ml of ddH_2O and adjusting the pH to 8 with HCl. Bring the final volume up to 100 ml. To make TE pH 8 buffer, add 5 ml of 1 M Tris–HCl pH 8 to 100 μl of 0.5 M EDTA pH 8 and adjust the final volume to 500 ml with ddH_2O. Store at room temperature.

2.5. Reverse Transcribe and PCR Amplify Small RNA Library

1. SuperScript III First-Strand Synthesis System (containing SS III reverse transcriptase, 25 mM $MgCl_2$, 0.1 mM DTT, RNaseOUT, and 10 mM dNTPs) and 10 mM dNTP stock (Invitrogen, Carlsbad, CA).
2. Phusion high-fidelity polymerase kit (with polymerase buffers) and low molecular weight DNA ladder (New England BioLabs, Ispwich, MA).

2.6. Small-Scale Sequence Library and Determine Concentration

1. Taq DNA polymerase for addition of 3′ adenine to libraries for TOPO cloning.
2. TOPO TA cloning kit containing TOP10 chemically competent *Escherichia coli* and SOC medium (Invitrogen, Carlsbad, CA).
3. X-gal solution for blue/white colony screening: Dissolve 2 g of 5-bromo-4-chloro-3-indolyl-β-D-galactoside (X-gal) in a total volume of 50 ml of *N*,*N*′-dimethyl formamide. Aliquot the solution to 1.5-ml microcentrifuge tubes and store at −20°C protected from light.
4. SYBR Green master mix for qPCR.
5. Real-time PCR thermocycler.

3. Methods

Though there are several commercially available kits for generating small RNA libraries, it is relatively straightforward and cost effective to create libraries using standard molecular biology reagents and custom oligonucleotides listed in Table 1. The major cost of most prepackaged kits is the purchase of the preadenylated linker oligonucleotides, which can be easily synthesized through enzymatic adenylation of DNA oligos (15). Preadenylated linkers are used in the first RNA ligation step of small RNA cloning so that the reaction can be carried out under conditions that favor miRNA ligation to the linker over miRNA circularization. Once the 3′ linker has been adenylated, a truncated Rnl2 (1-249) enzyme can efficiently catalyze the formation of a phosphodiester bond between an acceptor small RNA bearing a free 3′-hydroxyl group and a donor linker adenylated at its 5′ end in the absence of ATP (7). The modified Rnl2 enzyme requires a preadenylated linker because it lacks its C-terminal domain, which is required for enzymatic charging of 5′-monophosphorylated RNA targets (including microRNAs) with adenosine monophosphate (16). While some miRNA circularization still occurs with truncated Rnl2, the reaction is much less efficient and therefore fewer ligation side products are formed with this enzyme compared to T4 Rnl1, even in ATP-depleted conditions. Furthermore, Rnl2 (1-249) allows for efficient ligation of small RNAs modified at the 3′-terminal nucleotide by 2′-O-methylation. Thus, we recommend Rnl2 (1-249) in this protocol.

This protocol can be completed in 10 days; however, the most time-intensive component of small RNA sequencing is the bioinformatics analysis and data validation. It is therefore essential that the quality of the cDNA libraries be validated prior to high-throughput sequencing. The quality of the initial sample preparation and RNA extraction should be evaluated by an electrophoresis-based method such as the Agilent Bioanalyzer. If possible, at least 10 μg of the original extracted total RNA should be set aside for later validation of sequencing results by qPCR or northern blot. Bioinformatics analysis is greatly aided by preparing cDNA libraries from multiple biological replicates, especially if RNA samples are derived from genetically heterogeneous sources (e.g., patient samples). Small-scale Sanger sequencing of cloned RNAs is recommended to verify the correct size distribution of libraries as well as enrichment for tissue or cell-specific miRNAs (e.g., miR-142 or miR-150 in hematopoietic lineages) before proceeding to high-throughput sequencing. Once sequence results are obtained, there are numerous publicly available algorithms and databases for identifying known miRNAs and predicting novel Dicer products (17, 18).

3.1. Prepare 5′-Labeled Size Fractionation Markers

1. Set up two of the following 20 μl reactions to 5′-end label 18- and 30-nt RNA size markers (see Note 1) with ATP [γ-^{32}P]: 1 μl of 1 μM size marker RNA (18- or 30-mer), 2 μl of PNK buffer, 1 μl (10 U) of PNK, 5 μl of 6,000 Ci/mmol ATP [γ-^{32}P] (1.67 μM), and 11 μl of DEPC H_2O. Incubate

the reactions for 1 h at 37°C and then heat inactivate the kinase by incubation at 65°C for 20 min.

2. Prepare G-25 columns according to the manufacturer's instructions. This involves resuspending the beads by gentle mixing and then centrifuging the column in a disposable collection tube at 735 ×*g* for 1 min to remove the packing buffer. Then place the column into a fresh RNase-free 1.5-ml microcentrifuge tube.
3. Add 30 μl of 0.1 mM RNase-free EDTA to each sample and apply this mixture to the G-25 column resin to desalt the reaction and remove unincorporated radiolabeled nucleotides. Centrifuge at 735 ×*g* for 2 min and collect the eluate.
4. Make five dilutions of each labeled marker (i.e., 1:9, 1:27, 1:81, 1:243, and 1:729) in a 10-μl total volume. Add 10 μl of 2× formamide loading dye containing xylene cyanol and bromophenol blue.
5. Run the samples on an acrylamide denaturing gel to determine the minimum amount of marker required to detect a signal. These instructions are for the Bio-Rad Protean II gel system, though they can be adapted for other electrophoresis systems. Wash the gel plates thoroughly with a rinsable detergent (e.g., Micro-90; Cole-Parmer, Vernon Hills, IL). Dry the plates and treat them with RNaseZAP to ensure that they are RNase free.
6. Prepare a 1.5-mm thick, 15% denaturing urea–TBE gel by mixing 24 g of urea with 5 ml of 5× TBE and 18.75 ml of the 40% acrylamide mix and adding water to 50 ml total. Set mixture at 37°C for 20 min to dissolve the urea, inverting occasionally to mix. Once the urea has dissolved, add 250 μl of 10% ammonium persulfate solution and 50 μl of TEMED to begin gel polymerization. Immediately pour the gel and insert well combs. The gel should set in approximately 30 min.
7. Prepare 0.5× TBE running buffer by diluting 200 ml of 5× TBE in 1,800 ml of water.
8. When the gel has set, carefully remove the well comb. Add running buffer to the chamber and carefully lower the gel apparatus into the chamber at an angle to prevent bubbles from collecting along the bottom of the gel (bubbles may disrupt the current and lead to uneven RNA migration). Use a 10-ml syringe with a 20-gauge needle to clear viscous urea solution out of the wells and prerun the gel at 400 V for 1–2 h.
9. Again use the syringe to clear urea from the wells and immediately load the gel with the ten radioactively labeled samples. Add TBE running buffer containing 1× loading dye to any

empty wells. Run the gel at 400 V for 2–4 h or until the xylene cyanol and bromophenol blue dye bands are separated by at least 2 in.

10. Remove the gel plates from the electrophoresis apparatus and gently pry them apart, leaving the gel lying flat on the inner, smaller plate. Cover the gel and plate with plastic wrap and expose to a phosphor screen for approximately 10 min before scanning the plate with a phosphorimager.
11. Determine the minimum amount of each labeled size marker that can still be detected. Minimizing the quantity of marker oligonucleotides added to each library ensures that they represent only a small fraction of the total small RNAs that will be cloned and sequenced. Using this protocol, we found that marker sequences made up less than 0.1% of our cDNA libraries.

3.2. Size Fractionate Small RNAs from Total Extracted RNA

1. Extract and purify total RNA using a technique that captures small RNAs, such as Trizol, according to the manufacturer's instructions. Note that standard protocols using column-based RNA extraction kits, such as RNeasy (Qiagen), are not recommended as they must be modified to avoid the loss of small RNAs.
2. Verify the quality of total RNA extraction either by Agilent Bioanalyzer (Fig. 1) or by running a small amount of RNA on a denaturing gel and staining with ethidium bromide (EtBr). Using these methods, you should be able to clearly detect 28S and 18S rRNAs as well as a population of smaller RNAs (mostly 5.8S and 5S rRNAs and tRNAs).
3. Quantify total RNA by UV spectroscopy. Optimally, prepare 50 μg of total starting RNA per library (as little as 10 μg can be used for 5′-dependent cloning or 20 μg if you are planning on carrying out both 5′-dependent and 5′-independent cloning – see Note 2).
4. Cast a 15% denaturing urea–TBE gel as described in Subheading 3.1, step 6. Use a 10-ml syringe with a 20-gauge needle to clear urea from wells and prerun the gel at 400 V for 1–2 h.
5. To each sample add a minimal quantity of ATP [γ-^{32}P]-labeled size markers (as determined in Subheading 3.1) and one volume of 2× formamide loading dye. Make sure to use locking or screw top microcentrifuge tubes to decrease the risk of the cap opening during heating. Denature the sample by heating for 5 min in an 80°C heat block and cool on ice for 2 min. Collect the sample by brief centrifugation.
6. Again clear urea from wells and immediately load total RNA samples with spiked size markers onto the gel, leaving at least

one empty well between libraries to prevent mixing between samples. Add TBE running buffer with 1× formamide dye to the empty wells. Run the gel at 400 V for 2–4 h or until the xylene cyanol and bromophenol blue bands are separated by at least 2 in. (see Note 3).

7. Remove the gel plates from the apparatus and gently pry them apart, leaving the gel flat on the inner, smaller plate. Underlay the plate with a grid of squares of known sizes (e.g., 2 cm per side). Dilute ATP [γ-^{32}P] 1:10,000 in 2× formamide dye. Somewhere between the top of the gel and the xylene cyanol dye, embed a small amount of the solution into the gel at approximately the intersection of several different squares, creating a grid of dots a known distance apart. Carefully cover the gel and glass plate with plastic wrap and expose them to a phosphor screen for approximately 10 min before scanning the image with a phosphorimager.
8. Print a 1:1 scale image of the scanned gel. Use a ruler to verify that the individual points making up the radioactive grid are the expected distance apart.
9. Underlay the gel plate with this printout and align the gel to the printed picture via the radioactive grid.
10. Prepare a razor blade by treating it with DEPC H_2O followed by RNaseZAP. For each library, cut out a gel slice that extends from the middle of the 18-mer signal to the middle of the 30-mer signal as shown in Fig. 2a (see Note 4).
11. Add the gel slice to a preweighed 1.5-ml microcentrifuge tube (see Note 5) and determine the weight of the gel slice. Mash the gel into small fragments using a pestle and add a volume of RNase-free 1 M NaCl that is 3/7 of the gel weight, thus bringing the final NaCl concentration to 0.3 M. Add two volumes of 0.3 M NaCl and continue to mash the gel into a fine slurry. Add three additional volumes of 0.3 M NaCl and set overnight at 4°C with rotation.
12. Spin samples at top speed in a microcentrifuge for 10 min and transfer the liquid supernatant to a fresh siliconized tube (see Note 6).
13. To precipitate RNA, add 2 μl of 15 mg/ml glycogen and three volumes of ice-cold 100% ethanol and set at −80°C for at least 2 h. Spin the samples at full speed in a microcentrifuge for 30 min and wash the RNA pellet once with 70% ice-cold EtOH. Allow the pellet to dry and resuspend it in 15 μl of DEPC H_2O. Immediately freeze 5 μl of RNA at −80°C, in case you need to return to it later, and use the remaining 10 μl for the following steps.

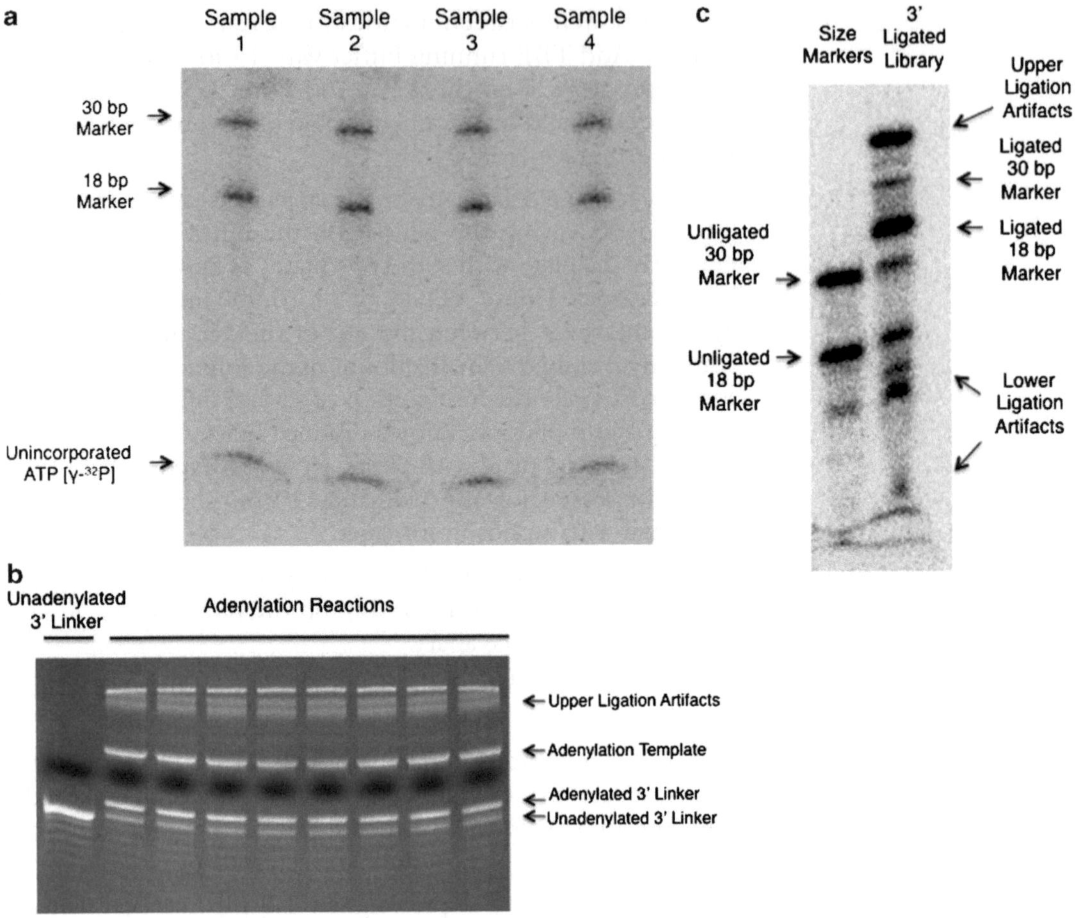

Fig. 2. 15% TBE–urea acrylamide gels for isolating oligonucleotides following small RNA size fractionation, 3′ linker adenylation, and 3′ linker ligation. (**a**) 18- and 30-nt RNA size markers were 5′-end labeled with ATP [γ-^{32}P] and run on a test gel to determine the minimal concentration of markers required for visualization on a phosphorimager (not shown). The determined concentration of markers was then spiked into four separate RNA samples to guide accurate size fractionation of libraries on a denaturing acrylamide gel. (**b**) 3′ DNA linkers were enzymatically adenylated using T4 DNA ligase. Charged adenylation products are one nucleotide longer than unadenylated linkers and can be clearly visualized on an acrylamide gel by running a unadenylated control. (**c**) 18–30 nt small RNAs were ligated to 3′ adapters, and the ligated products were selectively extracted from an acrylamide gel. Residual radiolabeled size markers from the initial RNA size fractionation serve as size references for successfully linkered products.

3.3. Adenylate the 3′ Adapter and Ligate it to Small RNAs

1. In a PCR tube, mix together 25 μl of 500 μM 3′ linker with 25 μl of 500 μM adenylation template oligo as listed in Table 1. Using a thermocycler, heat the sample to 90°C for 3 min and slowly cool to room temperature over the course of an hour to allow the oligos to anneal with each other.
2. Set up two of the following 300 μl adenylation reactions: 150 μl 2× quick ligase buffer with PEG, 18 μl of 250 μM oligo/template mixture, 30 μl (60,000 U) of high concentration T4 DNA ligase, and 102 μl of DEPC H_2O.

3. Incubate the reactions in a 37°C water bath for 5 h, flicking the tube occasionally to mix.
4. In the meantime, cast two 1.5-mm thick 20% denaturing urea–TBE gels and prerun the gels at 400 V for 1–2 h before loading samples.
5. Stop the reactions by heating to 65°C for 5 min and adding 300 μl 2× formamide loading dye. Load the samples onto the gel along with one lane containing just the 3′ adapter (as a size reference for the unadenylated oligo). Run the gel at 400 V until the bromophenol blue dye just runs off the gel – approximately 7 h.
6. Carefully pry apart the glass plates and move the gels to two separate glass dishes containing a sufficient amount of 0.5× TBE with 400 ng/ml EtBr to cover the gel. Set the gel at room temperature for 5 min with gentle rocking. Dispose of EtBr waste and incubate the gel for 5 min in 0.5× TBE with gentle rocking to wash out excess EtBr.
7. Wash a UV transilluminator box first with water, then with RNaseZAP. Carefully place the gel on the UV box and use a razor blade to cut out the adenylated 3′ linker, which should migrate slightly slower than the unadenylated linker oligo (Fig. 2b).
8. Add the gel slices to a preweighed 1.5-ml microcentrifuge tube and determine the weight of the gel slice. Mash the gel into small fragments using a pestle and add a volume of 1 M NaCl that is 3/7 of the gel weight to bring the final NaCl concentration to 0.3 M. Add two volumes of 0.3 M NaCl and continue to mash the gel into a fine slurry. Add two additional volumes of 0.3 M NaCl and set overnight at 4°C with rotation.
9. Spin samples at top speed in a desktop centrifuge for 10 min and transfer the liquid supernatant to a fresh siliconized tube. To precipitate DNA, add 2 μl of 15 mg/ml glycogen and 2.5 volumes of 100% ice-cold EtOH and set at −80°C for at least 2 h. Spin the samples at full speed for 30 min and wash the DNA pellet once with 70% ice-cold EtOH. Allow the pellet to dry and resuspend the DNA in 20 μl of DEPC H_2O.
10. Estimate the adenylated oligo concentration by UV spectroscopy or by running a small amount on a gel containing known DNA concentrations. Adjust the adenylated oligo concentration to 100 μM. You will need 200 pmol of adenylated linker per library (see Note 7).
11. Mix together 2 μl of the adenylated 100 μM linker, 2 μl of truncated Rnl2 10× buffer, 1.5 μl of DMSO, 2.5 μl of 50% PEG, and 10 μl of fractionated small RNAs containing

radiolabeled size markers. Make sure to use locking or screw top microcentrifuge tubes to decrease the risk of the cap opening during heating. Denature the samples by heating to 90°C for 30 s, then transfer to ice for 2 min to cool. Collect by brief centrifugation. Add 2 μl of truncated Rnl2 (1-249), mix, and set the reaction at room temperature for 2.5 h.

12. In the meantime, cast a 15% denaturing urea–TBE gel as described in Subheading 3.1, step 6 and prerun at 400 V for 1–2 h.
13. Stop the reaction by adding 20 μl of 2× formamide loading dye. Heat the sample for 5 min in an 80°C heat block and cool on ice for 2 min. Collect the sample by brief centrifugation. Load the samples with at least one open lane between each sample to prevent mixing. In the interdigitated lanes, load unligated size markers at half the minimal amount as determined in Subheading 3.1. These markers serve as important size references for unligated small RNAs. Run the gel until bromophenol blue and xylene cyanol dyes are separated by at least 3–4 in.
14. Disassemble the gel apparatus, leaving the gel attached to the inner glass plate. Using the methods described in Subheading 3.2, steps 7–9, scan in a phosphor screen that has been exposed to the gel and make a 1:1 scale printout of the image to underlay the glass plate. The ligated 18- and 30-nt size markers should run at 40 and 52 nt, respectively (just above the xylene cyanol dye) (Fig. 2c). Cut out a gel slice corresponding to the ligated 40–52 bp small RNAs, making sure to avoid any upper ligation artifacts.
15. Isolate the RNA from gel slices as described in Subheading 3.2, steps 10–13. Resuspend the 3′-ligated small RNAs in 24 μl DEPC H_2O. Immediately freeze down 5 μl of RNA at –80°C, in case you need to return to it later, and use the remaining 19 μl for the following steps.

3.4. Ligate to the 5′ Adapter

1. If you wish to carry out 5′-monophosphate-independent ligations in addition to 5′-monophosphate-dependent ligations, make two 8.5 μl aliquots of 3′-ligated small RNAs from each library – one for 5′-dependent ligation and one for 5′-independent ligation. Bring the total volume of the 5′-dependent aliquot up to 18 μl and set aside. If you are not planning on carrying out 5′-independent cloning, aliquot 18 μl of your 3′-ligated RNAs into an RNase-free tube and proceed directly to step 5.
2. For 5′-end processing of the 5′-independent sample, denature the 8.5-μl aliquot of 3′-ligated RNA by heating to 90°C, cool on ice for 2 min, and collect by brief centrifugation.

To remove all 5′ phosphate groups from your small RNAs, add 1 μl of 10× Antarctic Phosphatase buffer and 0.5 μl (2.5 U) of Antarctic Phosphatase. Incubate the samples at 37°C for 20 min followed by heat inactivation at 75°C for 10 min. Spin briefly in a microcentrifuge to collect the sample.

3. To add 5′-monophosphate groups to your small RNAs, add 3 μl of 10× T4 DNA ligase buffer (1 mM final ATP concentration), 16 μl of DEPC H_2O, and 1 μl (10 U) of T4 PNK. Incubate the reaction at 37°C for 30 min followed by heat inactivation at 65°C for 20 min. Add DEPC H_2O to a final volume of 200 μl.
4. Isolate PNK-treated RNA by phenol–chloroform extraction. Add 200 μl P:C:I (25:24:1, pH 4.5) (see Note 8). Vortex until thoroughly mixed and centrifuge at top speed in a microcentrifuge for 3 min. Transfer aqueous phase to a new siliconized tube and add 2 μl of glycogen (15 mg/ml), one-tenth volume of 3 M NaOAc pH 5.2, and three volumes of ice-cold 100% EtOH. Place samples at −80°C for 30 min. Centrifuge at top speed for 10 min. Remove the supernatant and wash the RNA pellet once with 70% ice-cold EtOH. Allow the pellet to dry and resuspend the 5′-independent library samples, which now all contain 5′-monophosphorylated ends, in 18 μl of DEPC H_2O.
5. Set up 30 μl 5′ adapter reactions for 5′-dependent and/or 5′-independent samples by mixing the following: 10 μl of 10× T4 RNA ligase 1 buffer, 6 μl of 100 μM 5′ linker, 3 μl (60 U) of T4 RNA ligase 1, and 18 μl of 3′-ligated small RNAs in DEPC H_2O. Incubate the reaction for 4 h at room temperature.
6. Add 120 μl of TE pH 8 to bring the reaction volume up to 150 μl total. Add 2 μl of glycogen (15 μg/ml), 15 μl of 3 M NaOAc pH 5.2, and 450 μl of ice-cold 100% EtOH to precipitate the linkered RNA. Mix by vortexing. Place the reaction tubes at −80°C for at least 2 h and then centrifuge the samples at top speed for 10 min. Aspirate the supernatant and wash the RNA pellet once with ice-cold 70% EtOH. Allow the pellet to dry and resuspend each sample in 15 μl of DEPC H_2O. Immediately freeze down 5 μl of the linkered RNA at −80°C in case you need to return to it later, and use the remaining 10 μl for the following steps.

3.5. Reverse Transcribe and PCR Amplify the Small RNA Library

1. Add 1 μl of 100 μM RT primer to 10 μl of the linkered RNA library and heat at 65°C for 3 min to denature. Cool on ice for 2 min and collect by brief centrifugation.

2. In a separate tube, combine the following in this order: 4 µl of 25 mM $MgCl_2$, 3 µl of SS III 10× buffer, 7 µl of 10 mM dNTPs, 3 µl of 0.1 M DTT, 1 µl (40 U) of RNaseOUT, and 1 µl (200 U) of SuperScript III reverse transcriptase. Heat the mixture to 48°C for 2 min and then add to the 11 µl linkered RNA sample.
3. Heat the mixed 30 µl sample at 44°C for 1 h to allow reverse transcription to proceed, then add 1 µl of RNase H, and incubate at 37°C for 30 min to digest away the RNA template. Use 10 µl of the 30 µl RT reaction for PCR and store the remainder at −80°C.
4. Set up a 50-µl PCR using the Phusion high-fidelity polymerase: 10 µl of the RT reaction, 10 µl of 5× Phusion buffer, 1 µl of 10 mM dNTPs, 0.25 µl of 100 µM 3′ PCR primer, 0.25 µl of 100 µM 5′ PCR primer, 0.5 µl (1 U) of Phusion polymerase, and 28 µl of ddH_2O (see Note 9).
5. Run the following PCR cycle:

   98°C for 30″

   15 cycles of 98°C 10″, 60°C 30″, 72°C 15″

   72°C for 10′

   4°C hold
6. In the meantime, cast a small 1.5-mm thick 6% nondenaturing TBE gel (these instructions are designed for the Bio-Rad Mini-Protean Tetra Cell, though any equivalent system can be used). Combine 1.5 ml of 40% acrylamide mix, 1 ml of 5× TBE, and 7.5 ml of ddH_2O. To begin acrylamide polymerization, add 6.5 µl of TEMED and 65 µl of 10% APS, and then immediately pour the gel between the two glass gel plates. Insert a well comb and allow the gel to polymerize for 30 min. When the gel has set, secure it in the clamping frame and insert the assembly into the electrophoresis apparatus. Fill the upper and lower gel chambers with 0.5× TBE according to the manufacturer's instructions.
7. Add 10 µl of 6× DNA loading dye to each sample and load them onto the gel, leaving at least one empty well between libraries to prevent mixing. Make sure to also load 1 µg of the NEB low molecular weight DNA ladder.
8. Electrophorese at 100 V until the bromophenol blue reaches the bottom of the gel.
9. Carefully remove the gel from the apparatus and soak for 5 min with gentle rocking in a solution of 0.5× TBE containing 400 ng/ml EtBr. Dispose of EtBr solution and rinse the gel for 2 min in 0.5× TBE to wash out excess EtBr.

10. Visualize RT-PCR products under UV light and cut out the bands corresponding to 84–96 nucleotide products as shown in Fig. 3 (see Note 10). Add gel slices to preweighed siliconized tubes and extract the DNA as described in Subheading 3.3, steps 8–9. Resuspend the DNA pellet in 50 μl 0.1 mM EDTA.

3.6. Small-Scale Sequence Library and Determine Concentration

1. Because the Phusion polymerase generates blunt DNA ends, it is necessary to add a 3′-A overhang using Taq polymerase prior to TOPO cloning. Add 5 μl of each library to 5 μl of 400 μM dATP (or 1 μl of 10 mM dNTP mix). Add 0.2 U of Taq polymerase to each reaction and set the reaction at 72°C for 15 min.
2. Add 2 μl of the Taq reaction mixture to 0.5 μl of the dilute salt solution and 0.5 μl of the TOPO vector included in the TOPO cloning kit. Set this reaction at room temperature for 20 min.
3. Add 2 μl of the TOPO reaction to one vial of Top10 chemically competent *E. coli*, mix by flicking the tube several times and incubate on ice for 30 min.
4. Heat shock the bacteria for 30 s at 42°C without shaking.

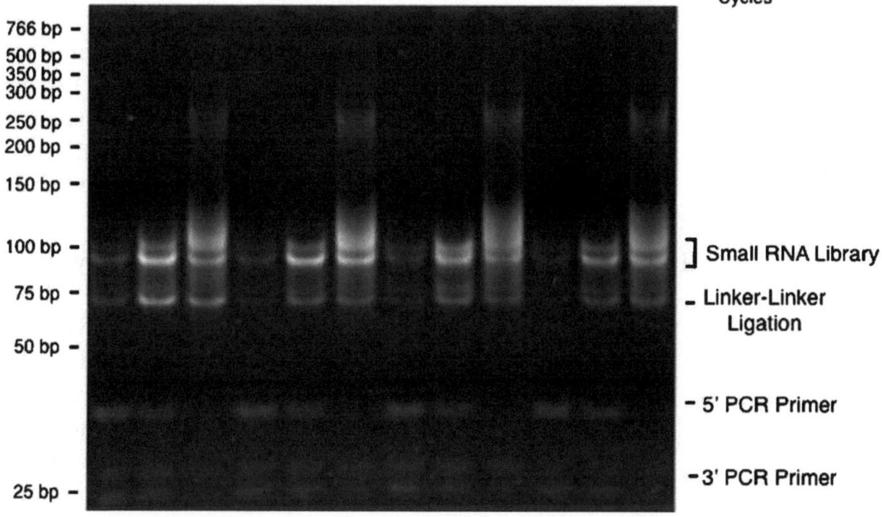

Fig. 3. PCR amplification of cDNA libraries. Linkered and reverse transcribed small RNAs were amplified by 15, 18, and 22 rounds of PCR using adapter-specific primers. Products were loaded onto a 15% TBE gel to determine the minimal number of cycles required to give products that can be easily visualized for extraction. Note that by 22 cycles of PCR most reactions are saturated, as evidenced by the depletion of PCR primers.

5. Transfer the tube to ice for 2 min and add 250 μl of SOC medium at room temperature. Cap the tube tightly and shake horizontally (200 rpm) at 37°C for 1 h.
6. In the meantime, spread 20 μl of 40 mg/ml X-gal on LB plates containing ampicillin or kanamycin (use two plates per library). Set the plates in 37°C incubator to dry. TOPO vectors that have successfully ligated cDNAs from your library will not produce β-galactosidase, an enzyme that hydrolyzes X-gal and creates an insoluble product (5-bromo-4-chloroindole) that is blue. Therefore, only uncolored bacterial colonies will contain clones of cDNA sequences from your library.
7. For each library, spread 75 μl of transformed *E. coli* onto two different LB-antibiotic plates. Place plates upside down in a 37°C incubator and grow for 20 h or until colonies are approximately 0.25 cm in diameter.
8. Pick approximately 25 white colonies per library to submit for sequencing. We have found it convenient and efficient to use rolling circle amplification for direct sequencing from transformed colonies. Use an M13R sequencing primer with the pCRII-TOPO vector.
9. BLAST your sequences using the Santa Cruz genome browser (http://genome.ucsc.edu/) or the NCBI Web site (http://blast.ncbi.nlm.nih.gov/Blast.cgi). For most cell types, a high quality 5′-monophosphate-dependent small RNA library will contain at least 50% miRNA sequences and 85% sequences that map to the genome.
10. Ideally, relative library concentrations can be determined with SYBR Green qPCR by comparing your libraries to libraries of similar size distribution that have been successfully sequenced in the past. If these are not available, you may use a standard curve to estimate your library concentration (provided that you can demonstrate 100% PCR efficiency). For qPCRs, dilute each library 1:10, 1:100, and 1:1,000 with H_2O in a 15-μl total volume.
11. Set up duplicate 20-μl PCRs for each library dilution and reference library/standard curve sample: 5 μl of library dilution or reference standard, 10 μl of 2× SYBR master mix, 0.6 μl of 10 μM forward primer, 0.6 μl of 10 μM reverse primer, and 3.8 μl of ddH_2O. Use threshold cycle (Ct) values in the linear amplification range to estimate the relative concentration of your libraries. Differences between Ct values should represent $\log_2$ differences in library concentration. Check with your sequencing core to determine at what concentration your libraries should be submitted for deep sequencing.

4. Notes

1. The 18–30 nt size markers broadly capture small RNAs including those in the piRNA size range (24–30 nt). If you wish to enrich for just miRNAs, you may use 18- and 25-nt size markers.
2. Ideally, there will be a sufficient amount of total extracted RNA such that 10–15 μg of additional RNA can be set aside for verification of sequencing results by northern blot, qPCR, etc. This allows for direct comparison of several different small RNA identification techniques. If possible, it is best to start with at least two biological replicates of each library, as this will greatly aid bioinformatics analysis of sequencing data.
3. In a 15% denaturing acrylamide gel, the bromophenol blue and xylene cyanol dyes should run at approximately 10 and 30 nt, respectively. Thus, the separation of the small RNAs can be estimated by observing loading dye migration.
4. Make sure to wash the razor blade with DEPC H_2O and RNaseZAP between cutting out different libraries to avoid library cross-contamination and RNase exposure.
5. While other combinations of pestles and microcentrifuge tubes may be used instead of those cited in Subheading 2, these brands have been selected because they fit perfectly together and allow efficient mashing of the gel into a fine slurry.
6. Siliconized microcentrifuge tubes will increase the recovery of RNA compared to polypropylene tubes, which will adsorb significant amounts of the RNA sample over time.
7. Enzymatically adenylated linkers can be a common source of RNase contamination. Therefore, you may choose to carry out a test linkering reaction with your size markers, which you can then run on a 15% denaturing gel along with unlinkered ATP [γ-^{32}P] 5′-end-labeled size markers. In addition to verifying that the linkers are RNase free, this will allow you to visualize bands corresponding to the 3′-linkered small RNAs.
8. Note that the acidic pH of the P:C:I solution is essential for extracting RNA. More basic P:C:I solutions (≈pH 8) will selectively extract DNA and you will lose most of the RNA sample.
9. You may want to test several PCRs with 10, 15, 18, 20, etc. cycles to see the minimum number of cycles needed to see a visible product on the gel (Fig. 3). The fewer number of PCR

cycles used to amplify your libraries, the less biased your libraries will be for the products that are more efficiently amplified.

10. You may see two predominant bands on your gel – the higher band (≈92 bp) corresponds to the majority of the small RNA library, while the lower band (≈65 bp) corresponds to a linker–linker ligation product (Fig. 3). Make sure to avoid cutting this lower band out of the gel.

Acknowledgments

The authors thank Josh Babiarz and Yangming Wang for helpful conversations and advice, as well as Poornima Parameswaran and Sam Gu for providing the protocol for 5′-monophosphate-independent cloning. This work was supported by the Burroughs Wellcome Fund (CABS 1006173) and the Dana Foundation.

References

1. Lee, R. C., Feinbaum, R. L., and Ambros, V. (1993) The C. Elegans Heterochronic Gene Lin-4 Encodes Small RNAs with Antisense Complementarity to Lin-14. *Cell* **75**, 843–854.
2. Wightman, B., Ha, I., and Ruvkun, G. (1993) Posttranscriptional Regulation of the Heterochronic Gene Lin-14 by Lin-4 Mediates Temporal Pattern Formation in C. Elegans. *Cell* **75**, 855–862.
3. Baltimore, D., Boldin, M. P., O'Connell, R. M., Rao, D. S., and Taganov, K. D. (2008) MicroRNAs: New Regulators of Immune Cell Development and Function. *Nat. Immunol.* **9**, 839–845.
4. Kanellopoulous, C. and Monticelli, S. (2008) A Role for microRNAs in the Development of the Immune System and in the Pathogenesis of Cancer. *Semin. Cancer Biol.* **18**, 79–88.
5. Xiao, C. and Rajewsky, K. (2009) MicroRNA Control in the Immune System: Basic Principles. *Cell* **136**, 26–36.
6. Lau, N. C., Lim, L. P., Weinstein, E. G., and Bartel, D. P. (2001) An Abundant Class of Tiny RNAs with Probable Regulatory Roles in Caenorhabditis Elegans. *Science* **294**, 858–862.
7. Hafner, M., Landgraf, P., Ludwig, J., Rice, A., Ojo, T., Lin, C., Holoch, D., Lim, C., and Tuschl, T. (2008) Identification of microRNAs and Other Small Regulatory RNAs using cDNA Library Sequencing. *Methods* **44**, 3–12.
8. Yang, W., Chendrimada, T. P., Wang, Q., Higuchi, M., Seeburg, P. H., Shiekhattar, R., and Nishikura, K. (2006) Modulation of microRNA Processing and Expression through RNA Editing by ADAR Deaminases. *Nat. Struct. Mol. Biol.* **13**, 13–21.
9. Rothberg, J. M. and Leamon, J. H. (2008) The Development and Impact of 454 Sequencing. *Nat. Biotechnol.* **26**, 1117–1124.
10. Aury, J. M., Cruaud, C., Barbe, V., Rogier, O., Mangenot, S., Samson, G., Poulain, J., Anthouard, V., Scarpelli, C., Artiguenave, F., and Wincker, P. (2008) High Quality Draft Sequences for Prokaryotic Genomes using a Mix of New Sequencing Technologies. *BMC Genomics* **9**, 603.
11. Linsen, S. E., de Wit, E., Janssens, G., Heater, S., Chapman, L., Parkin, R. K., Fritz, B., Wyman, S. K., de Bruijn, E., Voest, E. E., Kuersten, S., Tewari, M., and Cuppen, E. (2009) Limitations and Possibilities of Small RNA Digital Gene Expression Profiling. *Nat. Methods* **6**, 474–476.
12. Pak, J. and Fire, A. (2007) Distinct Populations of Primary and Secondary Effectors during RNAi in C. Elegans. *Science* **315**, 241–244.

13. Romaniuk, E., McLaughlin, L. W., Neilson, T., and Romaniuk, P. J. (1982) The Effect of Acceptor Oligoribonucleotide Sequence on the T4 RNA Ligase Reaction. *Eur. J. Biochem.* **125**, 639–643.
14. Taube, R., Loya, S., Avidan, O., Perach, M., and Hizi, A. (1998) Reverse Transcriptase of Mouse Mammary Tumour Virus: Expression in Bacteria, Purification and Biochemical Characterization. *Biochem. J.* **332**, 807–808.
15. Vigneault, F., Sismour, A. M., and Church, G. M. (2008) Efficient microRNA Capture and Bar-Coding Via Enzymatic Oligonucleotide Adenylation. *Nat. Methods* **5**, 777–779.
16. Ho, C. K., Wang, L. K., Lima, C. D., and Shuman, S. (2004) Structure and Mechanism of RNA Ligase. *Structure* **12**, 327–339.
17. Hackenberg, M., Sturm, M., Langenberger, D., Falcon-Perez, J. M., and Aransay, A. M. (2009) MiRanalyzer: A microRNA Detection and Analysis Tool for Next-Generation Sequencing Experiments. *Nucleic Acids Res.* **37**, W68–76.
18. Friedlander, M. R., Chen, W., Adamidi, C., Maaskola, J., Einspanier, R., Knespel, S., and Rajewsky, N. (2008) Discovering microRNAs from Deep Sequencing Data using miRDeep. *Nat. Biotechnol.* **26**, 407–415.

Chapter 8

MicroRNA-Profiling in Formalin-Fixed Paraffin-Embedded Specimens

Ulrich Lehmann

Abstract

The discovery of small regulatory RNA molecules during the last few years has changed our understanding of many biological and pathological processes. The most prominent and best analyzed class of these small regulatory noncoding RNAs is comprised by the microRNAs. The analysis of microRNA expression patterns is now widely used in biology and pathology employing a range of methodologies. However, many precious human tissue samples are only available as formalin-fixed paraffin-embedded (FFPE) specimen.

In this chapter, the extraction of RNA from FFPE samples and the subsequent microRNA profiling utilizing fluorescence-labeled bead technology from Luminex Inc. is described.

1. Introduction

Regulatory or noncoding (i.e. not for protein coding) RNAs emerged during the last few years as a new class of key regulators involved in development, normal physiology, and many different types of disease (1, 2). Some studies suggest that microRNA profiling is superior to mRNA profiling (e.g., ref. 3), most probably due to the pleiotropic effects of every microRNA and the inherent greater stability of the microRNA molecules in comparison with mRNA molecules.

Many DNA or RNA-based molecular studies rely on the use of fresh-frozen specimens. This is also true for most of the recently published microRNA studies. However, under many circumstances they are not available. In addition, the archives of institutes of pathology around the world contain millions of blocks with detailed documentation of histopathological diagnosis and clinical data. This represents an invaluable treasure trove for retrospective molecular studies (4). Also, in prospective trials,

Silvia Monticelli (ed.), *MicroRNAs and the Immune System: Methods and Protocols*, Methods in Molecular Biology, vol. 667, DOI 10.1007/978-1-60761-811-9_8, © Springer Science+Business Media, LLC 2010

often only FFPE material is preserved because many subtle morphological differences are only detectable in appropriately stained FFPE sections and these specimens can easily be exchanged between participating institutions. A very recent study has provided evidence that microRNA profiling of FFPE specimens outperforms mRNA expression profiling, a result, which might lead to a reevaluation of many published expression profiling studies (5).

During the last few years, many protocols for the extraction of RNA from formalin-fixed paraffin-embedded (FFPE) tissue specimens have been published. Also, several more or less comprehensive comparisons have been performed (see refs. 6–9 and references therein). Since we have already developed a protocol some time ago (10) and collected extensive data analyzing several thousands of samples following this protocol, only this protocol will be presented herein without a comprehensive discussion of alternative protocols or commercially available kits, which might also be used.

There are several options for the detection and quantification of microRNA expression levels: Northern blotting, semiquantitative in situ-hybridization, quantitative real-time PCR, fluorescence-labeled bead technology, and array hybridization (with various probe sets). Each approach has its specific advantages and shortcomings. Advantages of the fluorescence-labeled bead technology are the omission of any amplification step, which might introduce a bias of unknown extent, and the hybridization of probe and target in a homogeneous solution which avoids any boundary surface artefacts, a potential problem for every array hybridization method.

The microRNA profiling using fluorescence-labeled beads comprises the following steps (see Fig. 1):

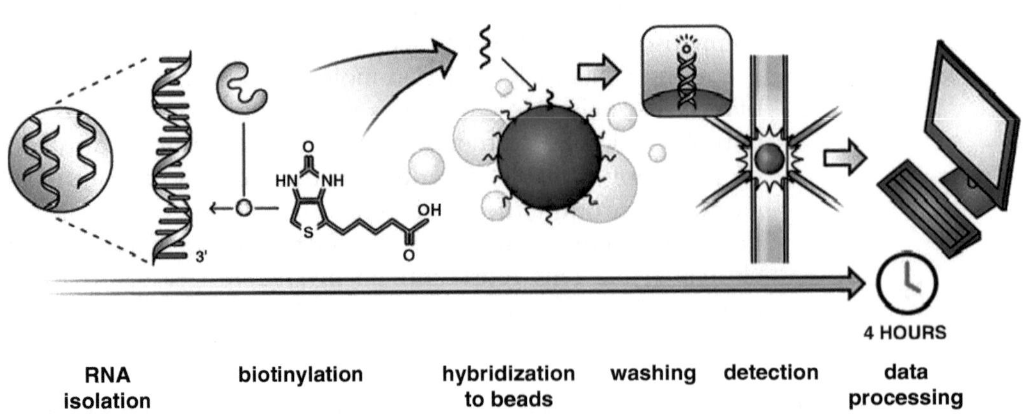

Fig. 1. Schematic overview of the workflow (with kind permission from Luminex Inc., slightly modified by the author, original in color can be found in the online version).

1. RNA isolation
2. Biotin-labeling of total RNA
3. Hybridization to fluorescence-labeled microspheres and washing
4. Detection of hybridized microRNAs
5. Data processing and evaluation

All five steps are described in detail in this chapter.

Alternative protocols and methods for microRNA profiling of FFPE specimens (based on real-time PCR or array-hybridization) have recently been published (11–17). A detailed discussion of the merits and shortcomings of these studies is beyond the scope of this chapter. It can be found in our recent publication Hasemeier et al. (18).

2. Materials

2.1. RNA Isolation

1. Digestion solution: 4.2 M guanidine-thiocyanate, 30 mM Tris–HCl, pH 7.6, 2% sodium-*N*-lauryl-sarcosine) (see Note 1).
2. Proteinase K (20 mg/ml).
3. 3 M Na-acetate, pH 5.2.
4. Chloroform.
5. Isoamylalcohol.
6. Isopropanol.
7. Glycogen (see Note 2).
8. Water-saturated phenol.
9. Xylene replacement medium (XEM 200, Vogel) (see Note 3).
10. β-Mercaptoethanol.
11. Diethylpyrocarbonate treated-water (DEPC-water) (see Note 4).
12. Spectrophotometer.
13. Thermoshaker.
14. Table-top centrifuge, refrigerated.
15. Aerosol filter tips (see Note 5).

2.2. Biotin-Labelling of Total RNA

1. FlexmiR™ MicroRNA Labeling Kit (Luminex Inc.).
2. FlexmiR™ MicroRNA Control Set (Luminex Inc.).
3. Thermocycler.
4. Table-top centrifuge, refrigerated.
5. Aerosol filter tips.

2.3. Hybridization and Washing

1. FlexmiR MicroRNA Human Panel (Luminex Inc.).
2. 96-Well filter plates (1.2 μm Millipore filter plate, Multiscreen Styrene MSBV N12XX).
3. Vacuum manifold for 96-well plates.
4. Bath sonicator.

2.4. Detection of Hybridized MicroRNAs

1. Total human brain RNA, as positive control (Ambion/Applied Biosystems).
2. Luminex 100™ or Luminex 200™ analyzer.

The flow cytometer from Luminex Inc. required for the analysis of the fluorescence labeled beads can be purchased from the following distributors:

Bio-Rad Life Science	http://www.bio-rad.com/bioplex
Invitrogen	http://www.invitrogen.com/luminex
Millipore	http://www.millipore.com
MiraiBio	http://www.miraibio.com/luminex-solutions.html
Qiagen	http://www.qiagen.com

We performed all measurements on a machine from Bio-Rad (BioPlex 200™) using the software from Luminex Inc. (Luminex IS™, version 2.3).

3. Methods

3.1. RNA Isolation

1. Three to seven 15 μm thick sections are cut from a paraffin block and collected in a safe-lock tube (see Note 6).
2. 750 μl digestion solution (see Note 1), 5.5 μl β-mercaptoethanol, and 300 μl Proteinase K are added. The mixture is thoroughly vortexed and incubated in a thermoshaker overnight at 55°C at 1,400 rpm (see Note 7).
3. Tubes are centrifuged at full speed (16,200 × *g*) in a refrigerated table-top centrifuge (4°C) for 5 min. A "paraffin cap" is formed on the top of the solution and undigested material is pelleted at the bottom of the tube.
4. 950 μl of the digested sample are transferred to a new tube without disturbing the pellet and without transferring too much of the paraffin cap.
5. 100 μl 3 M sodium acetate, pH 5.2, 630 μl acidic water-saturated phenol, and 270 μl chloroform are added and mixed thoroughly.

6. The tube are left on ice for 15 min and then centrifuged for 15 min at 4°C at 16,200 × *g*.
7. 950 μl of the aqueous supernatant are transferred to a fresh tube, and 1 μl glycogen (see Note 2) and 950 μl isopropanol are added.
8. After precipitation overnight at −20°C, the tubes are centrifuged for 20 min at 4°C at 16,200 × *g*.
9. The supernatant is removed carefully without disturbing the pellet, which might be difficult to recognize (it is transparent), and the pellet is washed with 300 μl 70% ethanol.
10. After centrifugation for 5 min at 4°C at 13,000 rpm (16,200 × *g*), the supernatant is carefully removed and the pellet is air-dried for approx. 5 min (see Note 8) and dissolved in 10–100 μl of water (depending on the amount of RNA expected to be isolated).

3.2. Biotin-Labeling of Total RNA

In contrast to other methods (see Subheading 1), the microRNA profiling approach described here does not involve an enrichment step of small RNA molecules. The labeling procedure comprises two steps: dephosphorylation using calf-intestine phosphatase (CIP) and biotinylation. If not otherwise stated, all reagents and tubes are kept on ice during pipetting.

3.2.1. Dephosphorylation

For five pools (comprising 319 microRNAs in total), 5 μg of total RNA dissolved in a volume of 5 μl is incubated with 2.5 μl CIP in a total volume of 17.5 μl. 2.5 μl CIP buffer and (optionally) 2.0 μl nonbiotinylated control are contained within this reaction mixture (see Note 9).

A negative control containing nuclease-free water instead of RNA is also set up.

The reaction mixture is incubated at 37°C for 10 min. Subsequently, it is heated at 95°C for 5 min to inactivate the CIP and then cooled on ice. It is strongly recommended to proceed to biotinylation immediately afterward.

3.2.2. Biotinylation

The inactivated and cooled CIP reaction mixture (17.5 μl) is combined with 15 μl biotinylation buffer and 7.5 μl biotinylation enzyme (see Note 10). Subsequently, the reaction is incubated at 16°C for 60 min and at 65°C for 15 min. Afterward, the reaction is cooled on ice and used immediately for hybridization (see Note 11).

3.3. Hybridization to Fluorescence-Labeled Microspheres and Washing

3.3.1. Hybridization

For hybridization of labeled RNA to the fluorescence-labeled microspheres, the following reaction mixture is set up in a 200-μl PCR tube for every bead pool (in total there exist five different pools for a comprehensive profiling comprising 319 human microRNAs (see Note 12)):

8 µl	Microsphere suspension
14 µl	Hybridization buffer
8 µl	Labeled RNA
20 µl	Nuclease-free water

The samples are incubated in a thermocycler at 95°C for 3 min followed by incubation at 60°C for 60 min.

3.3.2. Washing

1. Place filter plates on the inverted filter plate lid. This will prevent cross-contamination at the lower side of the plate.
2. Cover all unused wells with aluminium foil, add 100 µl wash solution (room temperature) to the required number of wells, and incubate at room temperature for 25 min.
3. Transfer the filter plate to the vacuum manifold and filter the wash solution. Avoid overdrying the filters and remove all liquid from the bottom of the plate by blotting the filter plate on an absorptive paper sheet.
4. Place filter plate again on the inverted filter plate lid and transfer the hybridization reaction to the filter plate (see Note 13).
5. Transfer the filter plate to the vacuum manifold and filter the hybridization reaction. Avoid overdrying the filters and remove all liquid from the bottom of the plate by blotting the filter plate on an absorptive paper sheet. Place plate again on the inverted filter plate lid.
6. Add 100 µl preheated wash solution (60°C) to each well and repeat step 5.
7. Repeat the washing step with 100 µl preheated washing solution (step 6).
8. Add 75 µl freshly prepared reporter solution (see Note 14) and 30 µl wash solution per well.
9. Mix on plate shaker at room temperature for 30 min at 600 rpm. Protect the plate from light by wrapping it in aluminium foil.
10. Proceed with detection of hybridized microRNAs.

3.4. Detection of Hybridized MicroRNAs

As described above (see Subheading 2.4), the flow cytometer required for the analysis can be purchased from different vendors. Each company also offers a software solution for data acquisition and reagents necessary for the calibration of the instrument. Luminex Inc. offers also its own software and reagents. A comprehensive discussion of the various vendors is beyond the scope of this chapter.

A major difference between different vendors is the price for the machine and the software and the service and training provided (but this might differ for different countries.). Since the actual process of calibration and measurement is very specific for the software in use, only general guidelines and hints are provided below. A detailed description of how to perform the calibration using the Luminex reagents would be totally useless for a reader performing essentially the same calibration, but using, for example, the Bio-Rad calibration kit or the software from Millipore. Also, different versions of the software which are available in parallel on the market differ in many practical details. Therefore, the situation is sometimes a bit confusing for the customer, and methodological details provided in publications are, under many circumstances, difficult to compare.

Before starting the calibration procedure, check the following points:

1. The system has to warm up at least for 30 min (see Note 15).
2. Make sure that the waste bottle is empty and the lid loosened and that the sheath bottle is full and tightly closed.
3. The system has to be free of air bubbles (by washing with 70% isopropanol) and washed with deionized water two times afterward.

The order of the calibration steps depends on the data acquisition software in use. The target values that have to be reached do not only depend on the manufacturer but they are also lot specific and may vary from lot to lot.

The specifications of proper signals are described in detail in the user manual from Luminex Inc.

For every session, a negative control (water instead of RNA) and a positive control (total human brain RNA from Ambion) are included.

3.5. Data Evaluation

In the first step, check whether basic requirements for a proper measurement are fulfilled:

- For every bead type, approximately 100 beads have to be counted. There exists no clearly defined threshold regarding how many beads have to be counted exactly. 100 beads is the target value, but 99 or 97 beads counted might also be OK.
- The negative control signals should be equal to or below the signals of loaded beads. That means all "real" signals (coming from beads loaded with labeled microRNA molecules) should be in the range of the background or above.
- For all beads, the analyzed bead population should look as shown in Fig. 2: a tight bead population within a white region. Deviations from this pattern could be caused due to several reasons: use of photobleached calibration microspheres, air bubbles in the system, lack of sheath fluid, agglutination of

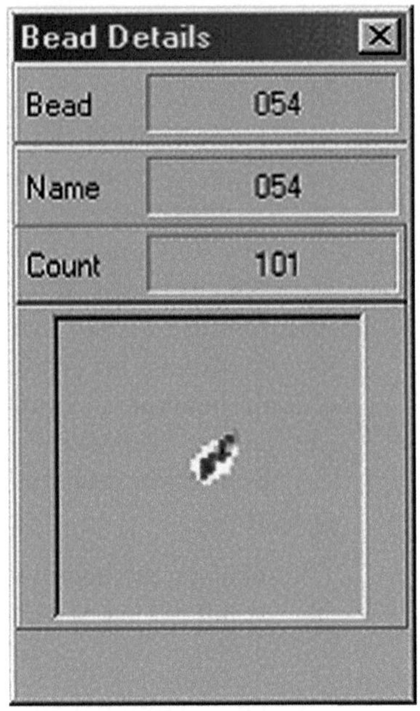

Fig. 2. Example of a proper bead population (original in color can be found in the online version): a tight bead population within a white region in the "bead map" (with kind permission from Luminex Inc.).

microspheres, incompatible solvent (details can be found in the User Manual and at the Luminex Technical Support site, http://luminexcorp.custhelp.com).

- The signal "histogram" (*Y*-axis: "Events" = counted beads, *X*-axis: Doublet Discriminator) should look as in Fig. 3: a single sharp peak. An additional peak shifted to the right is caused by microspheres sticking together. It should be as small as possible compared to the gated main peak.
- The four normalization controls included by Luminex Inc. in every bead pool should give strong signals of comparable intensity (in the range of 1,000 and more). These four normalization controls are the "housekeeping gene equivalents" snoRNA C/D box 13, C/D box U6, C/D box 2, and C/D box 6 (see Note 16).
- If five synthetic RNA oligonucleotides (provided by Luminex Inc. in the FlexmiR MicroRNA Control Set, see above Subheading 2.2) are included in the analysis, they should also give signals in the range of 2,000 and more.

It has to be mentioned that no consensus exists regarding above which signal strength a signal is "real" and without background fluctuation. But this caveat applies to many different methodologies used in experimental biology and is not a specific shortcoming of the method described in this chapter.

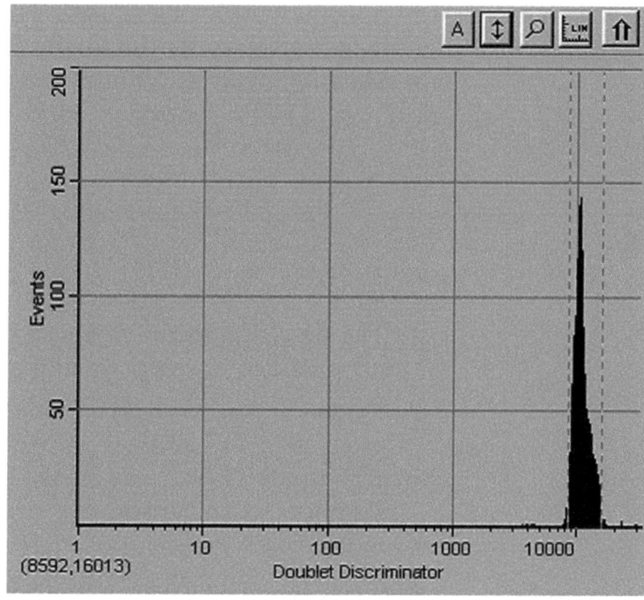

Fig. 3. Example of a good "histogram" (y-axis: "Events" = counted beads, x-axis: Doublet Discriminator). Only single sharp peak should be visible. For details see text (with kind permission from Luminex Inc.).

However, one should be aware of the fact that for many judgements and calculations performed during data processing, no strict guidelines exist. The important ones are traceability, internal consistency, and a detailed documentation of all calculations done.

The background signals (median fluorescence intensities, MFI, in the water control sample) were, in our setting, between 75 and 105 arbitrary units for the five different pools. The mean plus two times the standard deviation (95% confidence interval) were between 130 and 170. Thus, our measurements justify the "rule of thumb" given by Luminex Inc.: "Consider only signals above 200 as real". In our experience, the majority of weak "real" signals (MFI in the range of 200–300), nevertheless, showed quite a lot of variation, arguing for a more stringent threshold. Comparing two (or more) groups of samples (e.g., tumor versus normal) by dividing the background corrected fluorescence signal for every individual microRNA, one might create apparently huge differences by computing the ratio of weak signals slightly above the threshold: let us assume a signal of 240 in one sample and 210 in the corresponding control. Subtracting a background of 200 and computing the ratio might lead to the (most probably wrong!) conclusion that the expression differs by a factor of 4 (40 vs. 10). One has to decide whether high sensitivity with the risk of many false positives is desired or a more stringent threshold with the possibility of losing signals. The choice depends also on the number of differences found and the work (and costs) required for validation by an independent method (in the case of microRNA profiling of FFPE specimens: by real-time PCR).

4. Notes

1. The digestion solution has to be stored in the dark at room temperature. It can be used for approximately 3 months.
2. Originally, we used glycogen from Boehringer (now Roche, order no.: 901393) as a carrier. Alternatively, linear polyacrylamide (LPA) can be used. But we did not perform a systematic comparison of these reagents, or other carrier molecules.
3. Ordinary xylene can also be used but smells much more unpleasant and represents a health hazard.
4. DEPC represents a very toxic compound which has to be handled with appropriate care (only under a fume hood wearing protective gloves. After stirring 1 ml DEPC per 500 ml water at room temperature for several hours, it has to be destroyed by autoclaving (at least twice), because otherwise, it inactivates any enzymatic activity. Several authors now recommend to use pure 'PCR water" instead (commercially available) because of the health hazards of DEPC and the risk that it might not be inactivated completely, thereby interfering with downstream applications.
5. Aerosol filter tips are quite expensive but absolutely necessary if the RNA will be analyzed using methods involving amplification steps as well (as quantitative RT-PCR). We use filter tips from Sarstedt.
6. The actual number of sections collected for RNA isolation depends on the size and cellularity of the specimens and the total amount of RNA required for subsequent molecular studies. In order to prevent cross-contamination, the microtome blade is cleaned meticulously after every block with the xylene substitute.
7. Intensive shaking overnight is essential. It definitely supports tissue lysis and increases the RNA yield.
8. Prolonged air-drying of RNA pellets should be avoided because this might lead to an irreversible loss of solubility of the RNA (and thereby total loss of a given sample). High dilution of the RNA by dissolving in a large volume should also be avoided because this reduces the stability of the RNA.

On the other hand, complete dissolution of the RNA has to be ensured. This sometimes requires vigorous vortexing for several minutes (with intermittent cooling of the samples!).

9. If several samples are processed in parallel, the preparation of a master mix for the setup of the dephophorylation as well as the biotinylation and the hybridization reaction is strongly recommended.
10. All reagents are kept on ice during setup. The biotinylation enzyme is mixed before use by flicking the tube (don't forget a quick spin down!).The viscous biotinylation buffer has to be pipetted very slowly. The nonbiotinylated control consists of five synthetic RNA oligonucleotides, with no homology to any known RNA. These artificial small RNAs are bound to microspheres no. 83, 84, 85, 86, and 87, respectively, and serve as spike-in controls for the labeling and the hybridization procedure. The numbers of the microspheres refer to the position in the bead matrix.
11. The biotinylation reactions and the biotinylated RNA samples have to be protected from light.
12. The comprehensive and regularly updated list of all microRNA molecules detected by the FlexmiR™ Human Panel (and the distribution over the five pools) can be found on the web site of Luminex Inc. (http://www.luminexcorp.com/microrna/download.html) in the table FlexmiR Human Panel microRNA Targets. We have used version 8 of the microRNA pools.
13. Before transferring the hybridization reactions to the filter plate, homogenize by gently pipetting up and down three times. Carefully avoid any air bubbles or foaming at this step.
14. The reporter solution is prepared by diluting the reporter molecule (SA-PE) at room temperature in wash solution 1:300. This solution is light-sensitive and has to be protected from light.
15. If the system remains inactive for more than 4 h, the laser will automatically shut down. Therefore, a new warmup is necessary.
16. It is not clear whether snoRNA C/D box 13, C/D box U6, C/D box 2, and C/D box 6 are constantly expressed in all tissues of interest under all conditions one might think of (starvation, hypoxia, viral or bacterial infection, neoplastic transformation etc.). Therefore, one has to figure out, for every project, which small RNA molecules are suitable as endogenous controls. We use the software tools geNorm (19) and NormFinder (20) for this purpose; however, a steadily growing list of alternative programs is also available. Performing a

comprehensive profiling, one might identify microRNAs stably expressed in all groups, which have to be compared and might therefore serve as new endogenous controls for this project.

Acknowledgements

Indispensable help with figures and proofreading by Britta Hasemeier is acknowledged.

References

1. O'Rourke, J.R., Swanson, M.S., and Harfe, B.D. (2006) MicroRNAs in mammalian development and tumorigenesis. *Birth Defects Res C Embryo Today* **78**, 172–9.
2. Boyd, S.D. (2008) Everything you wanted to know about small RNA but were afraid to ask. *Lab Invest* **88**, 569–78.
3. Lu, J., Getz, G., Miska, E.A., Alvarez-Saavedra, E., Lamb J, Peck D, et al. (2005) MicroRNA expression profiles classify human cancers. *Nature* **435**, 834–8.
4. Lewis, F., Maughan, N.J., Smith, V., Hillan, K., and Quirke, P. (2001) Unlocking the archive – gene expression in paraffin-embedded tissue. *J Pathol* **195**, 66–71.
5. Liu, A., Tetzlaff, M.T., Vanbelle, P., Elder, D., Feldman, M., Tobias, J.W., et al. (2009) MicroRNA Expression Profiling Outperforms mRNA Expression Profiling in Formalin-fixed Paraffin-embedded Tissues. *Int J Clin Exp Pathol* **2**, 519–27.
6. Krafft, A.E., Duncan, B.W., Bijwaard, K.E., Taubenberger, J.K., and Lichy, J.H. (1997) Optimization of the Isolation and Amplification of RNA From Formalin- fixed, Paraffin-embedded Tissue: The Armed Forces Institute of Pathology Experience and Literature Review. *Mol Diagn* **2**, 217–30.
7. Lehmann, U. and Kreipe, H. (2001) Real-time PCR analysis of DNA and RNA extracted from formalin-fixed and paraffin-embedded biopsies. *Methods* **25**, 409–18.
8. Gilbert, M.T., Haselkorn, T., Bunce, M., Sanchez, J.J., Lucas, S.B., Jewell, L.D., et al. (2007) The isolation of nucleic acids from fixed, paraffin-embedded tissues-which methods are useful when? *PLoS One* **2**, e537.
9. Farragher, S.M,, Tanney, A., Kennedy, R.D., and Paul Harkin D. (2008) RNA expression analysis from formalin fixed paraffin embedded tissues. *Histochem Cell Biol* **130**, 435–45.
10. Bock, O., Kreipe, H., and Lehmann, U. (2001) One-step extraction of RNA from archival biopsies. *Anal Biochem* **295**, 116–7.
11. Nelson, P.T., Baldwin, D.A., Scearce, L.M., Oberholtzer, J.C., Tobias, J.W., and Mourelatos, Z. (2004) Microarray-based, high-throughput gene expression profiling of microRNAs. *Nat Methods* **1**, 155–61.
12. Lawrie, C.H. (2008) microRNA expression in lymphoid malignancies: new hope for diagnosis and therapy? *J Cell Mol Med* **13**, 1248–60.
13. Li, J., Smyth, P., Flavin, R., Cahill, S., Denning, K., Aherne, S., et al. (2007) Comparison of miRNA expression patterns using total RNA extracted from matched samples of formalin-fixed paraffin-embedded (FFPE) cells and snap frozen cells. *BMC Biotechnol* **7**, 36.
14. Xi, Y., Nakajima, G., Gavin, E., Morris, C.G., Kudo, K., Hayashi, K., et al. (2007) Systematic analysis of microRNA expression of RNA extracted from fresh frozen and formalin-fixed paraffin-embedded samples. *RNA* **13**, 1668–74.
15. Wang, H., Ach, R.A., and Curry, B. (2007) Direct and sensitive miRNA profiling from low-input total RNA. *RNA* **13**, 151–9.
16. Hoefig, K.P., Thorns, C., Roehle, A., Kaehler, C., Wesche, K.O., Repsilber, D., et al. (2008) Unlocking pathology archives for microRNA-profiling. *Anticancer Res* **28**, 119–23.
17. Zhang, X., Chen, J., Radcliffe, T., Lebrun, D.P., Tron, V.A., and Feilotter, H. (2008) An array-based analysis of microRNA expression comparing matched frozen and formalin-fixed paraffin-embedded human tissue samples. *J Mol Diagn* **10**, 513–9.
18. Hasemeier, B., Christgen, M., Kreipe, H., and Lehmann, U. (2008) Reliable microRNA profiling in routinely processed formalin-fixed paraffin-embedded breast cancer specimens using fluorescence labelled bead technology. *BMC Biotechnol* **8**, 90.

19. Vandesompele, J., De Preter, K., Pattyn, F., Poppe, B., Van Roy, N., De Paepe, A., et al. (2002) Accurate normalization of real-time quantitative RT-PCR data by geometric averaging of multiple internal control genes. Genome Biol **3**, RESEARCH0034.

20. Andersen, C.L., Jensen, J.L., and Orntoft, T.F. (2004) Normalization of real-time quantitative reverse transcription-PCR data: a model-based variance estimation approach to identify genes suited for normalization, applied to bladder and colon cancer data sets. *Cancer Res* **64**, 5245–50.

Part III

Functional Analysis of miRNAs in the Immune System: Gain-of-Function

Chapter 9

Expression of miRNAs in Lymphocytes: A Review

Raquel Malumbres and Izidore S. Lossos

Abstract

In this chapter, we provide a review on the functions of the most important miRNAs in lymphocytes. Most of them are involved in lymphopoiesis, immune response, and lymphoid malignancies, highlighting the importance of miRNAs in these cells.

1. Introduction

1.1. The Role of Lymphocytes in the Immune System

The immune system exerts the defense of an organism against pathogens or tumoral cells; in humans it has two main components: innate immunity and adaptive immunity. Innate immunity appeared early in evolution and is able to fight pathogens based on common features of these organisms. Adaptive immunity is a more sophisticated immune response that has evolved in vertebrates: pathogens or tumoral cells are recognized by specific protein–protein interactions carried out by specialized cells, the lymphocytes (1). The two main types of lymphocytes are B cells, which produce antibodies for the humoral response, and T cells which, depending on their subtype, are able to carry out cellular response against tumoral or virally infected cells, or to secrete cytokines that control the intensity of the immune response.

Lymphocytes and other blood cells originate from hematopoietic stem cells residing in the bone marrow. These hematopoietic cells differentiate to distinct cellular lineages in the process of hematopoiesis. Initial lymphocyte precursors are produced during lymphopoiesis in the bone marrow and undergo additional maturation steps in the secondary peripheral lymphoid organs: thymus for T cells and lymphoid follicles for B cells.

At the latter steps of bone marrow lymphopoiesis for B cells, or early maturation in the thymus for T cells, lymphocytes express

Silvia Monticelli (ed.), *MicroRNAs and the Immune System: Methods and Protocols*, Methods in Molecular Biology, vol. 667, DOI 10.1007/978-1-60761-811-9_9, © Springer Science+Business Media, LLC 2010

protein receptors on the plasmatic membrane (BCR in B cells and TCR in T cells) that are able to bind to antigens. To allow for the recognition of any possible antigen, lymphocytes have unique mechanisms that enable them to produce a large number of different receptors by genomic rearrangement of different loci; each lymphocyte will express a unique receptor that is different from receptors expressed by other lymphocytes. The main genes of the BCR and the TCR are composed by several V, D, and J subunits that are recombined differently in each lymphocyte to produce specific receptor repertoires; this process is called VDJ recombination and takes place at the Pre-B cell stage for B cells and at the Double Negative 3 stage of T cells (Fig. 1). Such variability must be controlled to avoid generating lymphocytes recognizing self antigens that might lead to autoimmune disorders. Therefore, a process of negative selection takes place in the bone marrow for B cells and in the thymus for T cells. Lymphocytes are presented with self antigens of the organism and those that are able to recognize these antigens will undergo apoptosis. T cells are also positively selected in the thymus, and only those lymphocytes able to recognize foreign antigens in the context of the major histocompatibility complex will survive and egress the thymus as mature T cells (reviewed in ref. 2).

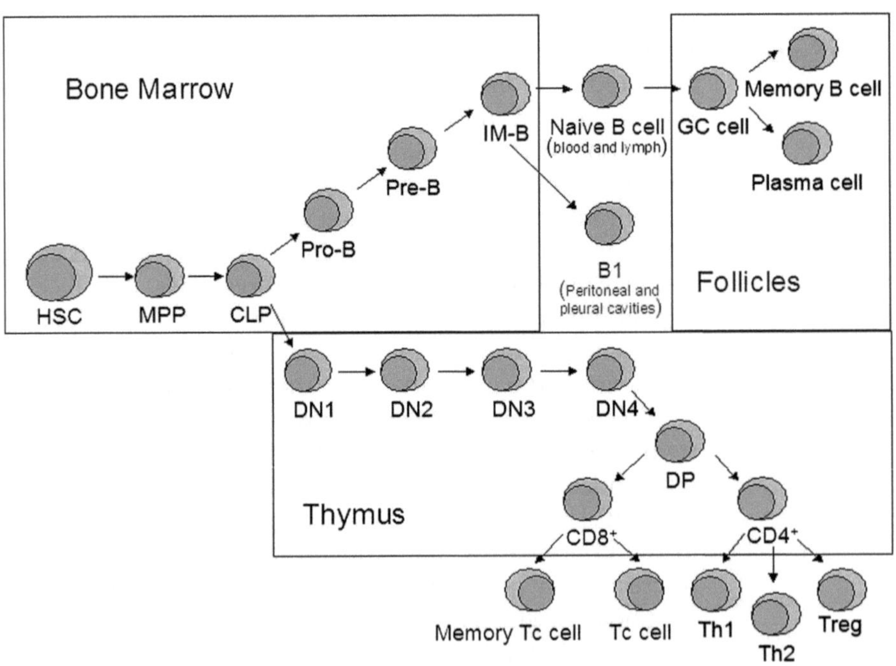

Fig. 1. Cellular stages of lymphopoiesis and peripheral maturation of B and T lymphocytes. *HSC* hematopoietic stem cell, *MPP* multipotent progenitors, *CLP* common lymphocyte progenitors, *IM-B* immature B cell, *GC cell* germinal center cell, *B1* B cell of the subtype 1, *DN* double negative stage, *DP* double positive stage CD4+ CD8+, *Treg* regulatory T cell, *Th* helper T cell, *Tc* cytotoxic T cell. CD4+ memory cells are also produced in T cell activation, but they have been excluded from the figure for simplicity.

The positive selection of B cells occurs in specialized structures of the follicles called germinal centers (reviewed in ref. 3), formed by B cells activated by antigen encounter that undergo high-rate proliferation and differentiation into germinal center cells: centroblasts and centrocytes. In the germinal centers, more variability is added to the pool of different BCRs by a process known as somatic hypermutation that further modifies the variable region of the BCR. Then, positive selection occurs: B cells harboring a BCR with high affinity for the antigen will be selected for survival and further differentiation into memory B cells or antibody-producing plasmatic cells. The rest of B cells will undergo apoptosis.

All these processes of development and maturation of lymphocytes involve several intermediate stages that are depicted in Fig. 1.

1.2. MiRNAs are Involved in the Production and Functions of Immune Cells

MiRNAs, or microRNAs, are short (21–24 nucleotides) noncoding RNA sequences that are able to bind to partially complementary sequences in the 3′ UTR of mRNAs. The multiprotein complex RISC (RNA-Induced Silencing Complex) uses miRNAs as probes to bind to these complementary sites in the mRNAs. Upon binding, RISC induces the degradation of the mRNA or the inhibition of its translation (4). This kind of post-transcriptional regulation is thought to affect up to at least one third of the human genes, probably more, as the number of confirmed targets of miRNA regulation is increasing steadily in the scientific literature.

One of the more quickly developing fields in the subject of miRNA studies has been the functions these small noncoding RNAs exert in hematopoiesis. Starting with hematopoietic stem cells, a tightly regulated program in the expression of genes and miRNAs ensures the correct production of all blood cell lineages. The particular role of some individual miRNAs has been depicted along different steps of hematopoiesis, i.e., miR-223 is a master regulator of human granulopoiesis (5), where it is involved in a regulatory loop with the transcription factors NFI-A and C/EBPalpha; furthermore, this miRNA is also involved in erythropoiesis (6) and peripheral B cell differentiation (7, 8) due to its ability to downregulate LMO2 expression. Of note, the whole miRNA expression pattern changes remarkably between the successive stages of peripheral B cell differentiation. In a recent work, we found that out of 122 miRNAs that were detected as expressed during this process by miRNA microarray hybridization, 118 showed differential expression, particularly due to the highly specific miRNA expression pattern of the germinal center cells (7). This finding agrees with the notion that the specialized and exclusive functions of the germinal center cells require the establishment of unique gene (9) and miRNA expression patterns (7, 8, 10, 11). The specificity of miRNA expression in the germinal center

Table 1
Differential expression of miRNAs during B cell peripheral differentiation

Stage	Naïve B cell	Centroblast	Memory B cell
MiRNAs	miR-223	miR-146a	miR-223
	miR-320	miR-99b	miR-320
	miR-29b	miR-125a-5p	miR-29b
	miR-101	miR-92a	miR-101
	miR-29c	miR-214	miR-29c
	miR-150	miR-125b	miR-150
	miR-151-5p	miR-191	miR-194
		miR-128b	miR-146b-5p
		miR-20b	miR-23a
		miR-18a	miR-24
		miR-130b	miR-23b
		miR-106b	miR-27b
		miR-425	miR-27a
		miR-93	miR-671-5p
		miR-28-5p	miR-146a
		miR-17	
		miR-106a	
		miR-25	
		miR-20a	
		miR-15b	
		miR-30c	
		miR-16	
		miR-181b	
		miR-151-5p	

cells allowed us to find a signature of 39 miRNAs whose expression is able to differentiate these cells from naïve and memory B cells (Table 1).

Likewise, several miRNAs are preferentially expressed at different stages of T cell differentiation. Table 2 summarizes the miRNAs that are enriched at specific stages of T cell differentiation in the thymus (12).

Table 2
Differential expression of miRNAs during T cell differentiation

Stage	DN1	DN3	DN4	DP	CD4	CD8
MiRNAs	miR-21	miR-191	miR-142-5p	miR-92	miR-669c	miR-142-3p
	miR-29b		miR-20a	miR-181a	miR-297	miR-15b
	miR-342		miR-16	miR-181b	miR-142-3p	miR-150
	miR-221		miR-128b	miR-350		miR-24
	miR-223			miR-16		miR-27a
				miR-15b		

MiRNAs regulate important processes not only during hematopoiesis and cell differentiation, but also in controlling the functions of immune cells: i.e., miR-181a is able to regulate the sensitivity and signaling strength of the TCR during T cell binding to an antigen (13).

1.3. MiRNAs and Hematological Malignancies

Interestingly, miRNAs are also commonly involved in malignant transformations. The first association of miRNAs with a malignant disease was the finding that miR-15 and miR-16, located at 13q14.3, underwent deletion in some Chronic Lymphocytic Leukemia (CLL) patients, and their expression was downregulated in most of CLL cases (14). These two miRNAs are able to downregulate the antiapoptotic factor BCL2 (15). Very frequently, miRNAs that are deregulated in lymphoid malignancies are also involved in processes that are necessary for the differentiation of normal lymphocytes: i.e., cluster miR17–92, described as “oncomiR-1” in B cell lymphomas (16), is also involved in the maturation of B cells during the germinal center response (7).

In this chapter, we will review the most important miRNAs involved in lymphoid hematopoiesis, differentiation, function, and/or malignant transformation.

2. MiR-181a

This miRNA was initially known as miR-181, but the official name has been changed to miR-181a because it is part of a family of four different sequences encompassing six different loci in the murine and human genomes: miR-181a-1, miR-181a-2, miR-181b-1, miR-181b-2, miR-181c, and miR-181d (17–20). All these sequences share the same seed region and are thought to be able to bind to the same targets, though probably not with the same affinity. In the human genome, these miRNA are included in three clusters of two miRNA each: cluster miR-181a-1-181b-1 is located at 1q31.3, cluster miR-181a-2-181b-2 at 9q33.3, and cluster miR-181c-181-d at 19p13.12.

2.1. MiR-181a in Lymphopoiesis and Lymphocyte Immune Functions

The first studies on miRNA involvement in hematopoiesis were performed in mice; miR-181a, miR-142, and miR-223 were found to be expressed in hematopoietic tissues (21). Ectopic expression of miR-181a in hematopoietic stem cells (HSCs) cultured in vitro induced an increase in the number of B cells without marked change in the number of T cells. Nevertheless, ectopic expression of miR-181a in HSCs followed by their transplant into lethally irradiated mice produced a bias in lymphopoiesis, remarkably increasing (to 80%) the proportion of B cells in peripheral blood and inducing a concomitant decrease in T cells (88%) (21). These data contrasted with the in vitro results, where miR-181a overexpression did not affect T cell production, and seemed to suggest that miR-181a impaired T cell differentiation in vivo. It appears that miR-181a is an essential regulator of T cell differentiation from DN4 to DP stage (12), inducing a decrease in the expression of three genes involved in T cell positive selection: TCRα, BCL2, and CD69. TCRα expression is necessary for the final assembly of the T Cell Receptor (TCR) that activates a signaling pathway upon antigen encounter, thus initiating the first step of the selection process. BCL2 is an antiapoptotic factor that enables the survival of positively selected T cells, and CD69 is a membrane marker that allows the mature T cells to egress the thymus. Downregulation of these three proteins by ectopic expression of miR-181a provides an explanation for the decreased number of mice peripheral blood T cells since high expression of miR-181a beyond the DP stage would decrease the egress of T cells from the thymus due to insufficient levels of CD69. In addition, the decrease of BCL2 survival stimulus in positively selected T cells would increase cell death, and the selection process itself would be compromised due to impaired TCR assembly because of the reduced expression of TCRα.

In addition to targeting TCRα, miR-181a has also a paramount role in fine-tuning the sensitivity of the TCR to antigen stimulus. Multiple phosphatases in the signaling pathway of the TCR are targets of miR-181a (PTPN22, SHP-2, DUSP5 and DUSP6). Thus, high expression of this miRNA leads to elevated steady-state levels of phosphorylated intermediates and a reduction of the T cell receptor signaling threshold (13). This regulation probably makes miR-181a expression also necessary for proper mature T cell activation and for the selection steps that take place during immature T cell stages.

2.2. MiR-181a Involvement in Lymphoid Malignancies

MiR-181 was implicated to have an antioncogenic role in CLL: miR-181 and miR-29 are involved in the downregulation of TCL1, a protein that behaves as an oncogene in T-CLL and B-CLL and is particularly overexpressed in the most aggressive subtypes of CLL (22, 23). Interestingly, miR-181a and miR-181b also act as tumor suppressors in glioblastoma (24).

3. MiR-150

MiR-150 is a miRNA preferentially expressed in thymus and spleen (25), suggesting its involvement in lymphocyte maturation. In contrast to miR-181 family, no other miRNA with the same seed region has been yet found in humans (17–20). This miRNA is located at position 19q13.33 in the human genome.

3.1. MiR-150 in Lymphopoiesis and Lymphocyte Immune Functions

MiR-150 has a paramount role in B cell differentiation. It is expressed at high concentration in mature resting B cells, but not in their progenitors (26). Using techniques of homozygous deletion and ectopic expression of miR-150 in mice, Xiao et al. demonstrated that miR-150 deletion induces B1 cell expansion and an increase in the humoral response, while miR-150 ectopic expression in B cell progenitors induces a partial block of B cell development and a reduction in B1 numbers (27). c-Myb was identified as a target of miR-150, and the ectopic expression of miR-150 resulted in a phenotype very similar to that of c-Myb heterozygous deletion in B cell precursors. c-Myb is transcription factor that promotes survival of B cells by upregulating BCL2 protein levels (28, 29) and is also able to induce cell proliferation (30). Zhou et al. found that overexpression of miR-150 in hematopoietic stem cells impaired the transition from Pro-B to Pre-B cells (25), blocking the production of mature B cells.

The role of miR-150 in the immune response of mature B cells is yet unknown; expression of miR-150 is downregulated in germinal center B cells compared to postgerminal center memory B cells (7, 11). Expression of miR-150 can be induced by IgM stimulation (27), thus suggesting a role in B cell activation. Finally, miR-150 is highly expressed in CD8 positive T cells (12), probably having a role in their activation and/or function.

3.2. MiR-150 Involvement in Lymphoid Malignancies

Similar to miR-181a, miR-150 could be acting as a tumor suppressor in lymphoid malignancies, at least in part due to its ability to downregulate c-Myb. This transcription factor is involved in the pathogenesis of T cell acute leukemia, where it is involved in duplications and genomic rearrangements that cause its overexpression (31, 32). It is of note that miR-150 expression is generally decreased in lymphomas, i.e., diffuse large B-cell lymphoma (DLBCL) cell lines when compared to mature B cells (7), and even more in Hogdkin lymphoma compared to non-Hogdkin lymphoma (33). Consequently, c-Myb upregulation due to a decrease in miR-150 expression may contribute to the process of lymphomagenesis by inducing enhanced cell proliferation and decreasing apoptosis.

4. Cluster miR-17-92 and Paralog Clusters

This cluster of miRNAs is located at 13q31–q32, a region of the human genome that is frequently amplified in lymphomas (16). It is composed of 6 different miRNAs, some of which harbor related sequences (17–20). Furthermore, there are two paralog clusters to miR-17-92 in two different locations in the human genome: cluster miR-106b-25 located at 7q22.1 and cluster miR-106a-363 at Xq26.2. They share at least some functions with cluster miR-17-92, as was suggested by the more severe effects of the combined deletion of cluster miR-17-92 and cluster miR-106b-25 in mice (34). We have shown that the three clusters of this paralog group are upregulated in germinal center B cells (7) and follow a similar pattern of expression. This fact supports the hypothesis that these miRNA clusters are involved in related processes and suggests presence of coordinated miRNA regulation networks that may have important roles during lymphocyte differentiation.

4.1. Involvement in Lymphopoiesis

Cluster miR-17-92 is involved in B cell development. Targeted deletion of this cluster in mice induces an increase in expression of the proapoptotic protein BIM in B cells, leading to a decrease in cell survival and blocking the transition from pro-B to pre-B stage (34); these effects are similar to those observed following ectopic expression of miR-150 in B cell precursors.

Selective overexpression of cluster miR-17-92 in mouse lymphocytes induces increased proliferation and a decrease of activation-induced cell death, leading to lymphoproliferative disease and autoimmunity (35). These effects can be attributed to the ability of this miRNA cluster to target the antiproliferative factor PTEN and the proapoptotic factor BIM (35), though a regulatory loop between MYC, cluster miR-17-92, and E2F1 can also contribute to this phenotype, as will be explained in the following section.

4.2. Cluster miR-17-92 Involvement in Lymphoid Malignancies

Since cluster miR-17-92 targets tumor suppressors or proapoptotic proteins, it is not surprising that this cluster has an oncogenic role. In fact, it was described as the first "oncomiR" because it was found overexpressed in B cell lymphomas (16), particularly those with amplification of 13q31–q32, where this polycistron is located. This overexpression was associated with MYC overexpression in many cases, suggesting a possible cooperation between these genes in lymphomagenesis. In agreement with this notion, the development of lymphoid malignancies in Eμ-myc mice that overexpress MYC from B cell precursor stages was accelerated when cluster miR-17-92 was also overexpressed (16), exhibiting a synergistic effect and increasing the aggressiveness of tumors (36). It was demonstrated that MYC can induce E2F1 that contributes to its effects on the enhancement of transcription of cluster miR-17-92. It is well known that MYC can have either oncogenic or proapoptotic functions depending on the context; when MYC induces E2F1 function, the proapoptotic features of E2F1 can shift the balance to apoptosis, but if cluster miR-17-92 is also induced, proliferation is enhanced and apoptosis diminished (Fig. 2). Accordingly, NK-like homeodomain proteins that are overexpressed in T-ALL and are able to upregulate cluster miR-17-92 transcription, induce a decrease in apoptosis in etoposide-treated cells (37). Furthermore, miR-19a and miR-19b, that are part of miR-17-92 cluster, target SOCS1 inducing an increase in STAT3 signaling that promotes survival (38).

Cluster miR-17-92 is also overexpressed in several other types of cancer, including lung cancer (39), medulloblastoma (40) and anaplastic thyroid cancer (41) and its proliferative and antiapoptotic effects may contribute to their pathogenesis.

4.3. Redundant Functions of Paralog Clusters miR-17-92 and miR-106b-25

In agreement with the postulated cooperation between cluster miR-17-92 and its paralog clusters, cluster miR-106b-25 is also amplified in other cancers (esophageal neoplasias, gastric cancer (42, 43)) and exerts proliferative and antiapoptotic functions. Similar to cluster miR-17-92, the transcription of cluster miR-106b-25 is also

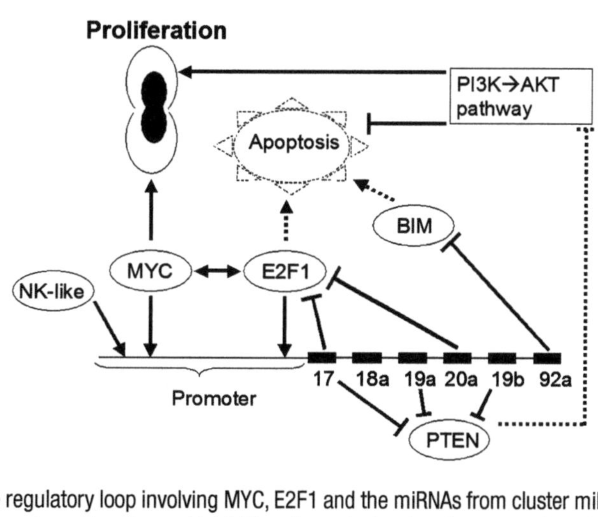

Fig. 2. The regulatory loop involving MYC, E2F1 and the miRNAs from cluster miR-17-92 is shifted towards proliferation and inhibition of apoptosis when the expression of this cluster is high. The *arrows* pointing out of the cluster correspond to regulation by individual miRNAs.

enhanced by E2F1 and MYC (43), and both clusters are able to target the same transcripts. MiR-106b and miR-93 of cluster miR-106b-25, as well as miR-17 and miR-20a of cluster miR-17-92, downregulate the expression of p21. Similarly, miR-25 from cluster miR-106b-25 targets BIM (42) and p57 (44), while miR-92a-1 from cluster miR-17-92 targets BIM. In the case of gastric cancer, these miRs may contribute to downregulation of these proteins, thus suppressing the function of the TGFβ antiproliferative signaling pathway and contributing to tumor progression (43).

In lymphoid malignancies, these two paralog clusters are overexpressed in multiple myeloma (38) and in B cell lymphomas (7). Taking into account the widespread involvement of MYC and the target genes of these miRNAs in lymphomas and leukemias, the role of these paralog clusters in the pathogenesis of many subtypes of these diseases is highly probable.

5. MiR-155

MiR-155 is located at chromosome 21q21.3 inside the BIC gene (45), which is a common site for insertion of proviral DNA in avian leukosis virus-induced lymphomas (46, 47). This miRNA is not included in any cluster and no other miRNA in the human genome has the same seed region (17–20). Nevertheless, Kaposi's Sarcoma-associated herpesvirus encodes an ortholog of miR-155 that is supposed to provide a survival advantage to the virus (48).

5.1. MiR-155 in Lymphopoiesis and Lymphocyte Immune Functions

Overexpression of miR-155 in murine Pro-B cells under the control of the immunoglobulin heavy chain Eμ enhancer induces increased proliferation of Pre-B cells, eventually leading to a leukemic malignancy (49).

Using strategies of loss of function and mature B cell restricted overexpression, Thai et al. demonstrated that miR-155 is a key factor in the regulation of germinal center sresponses (50). In miR-155 KO mice, the number of germinal centers in the spleen after chicken gamma globulin immunization was decreased compared to wild-type mice. Furthermore, the amount of B cells in the germinal centers was also reduced, as well as the titers of specific IgG_1 antibodies. Accordingly, in mice transgenic for miR-155 in B cells, all these indicators of germinal center response were increased. The reduction in specific IgG_1 production in miR-155-deficient mice can be explained, at least in part, by the ability of this miRNA to target SFPI1/PU.1 in B lymphocytes as overexpression of this transcription factor in B cells inhibits Ig class switching to IgG_1 (51). Another important target of miR-155 is AID, which is one of the key factors in Ig class switching (52) and the somatic hypermutation process that occurs in the germinal centers to induce mutations in the immunoglobulin genes (53, 54). These mutations allow the immunoglobulins to diversify and undergo antigen affinity maturation.

MiR-155 can also affect the germinal center reaction by regulating the production of cytokines by B and T cells. INPPD5 (SHIP) and NF-IL6 (CEBP/β) have been recently described as targets of miR-155, suggesting the role of this miRNA in IL-6 signaling during B cell maturation (55). Furthermore, in miR-155 KO mice the production of TNF-α and lymphotoxin-α by B cells was greatly reduced and T cell differentiation seemed to be biased towards a T_H2 phenotype, with increased IL-4, IL-5, and IL-10 secretion in detriment of IFNγ production in vitro (56). This cytokine profile would contribute to the impaired immune function observed in miR-155-deficient mice because IL-10 is known to dampen immune responses. In addition, FOXP3-driven expression of miR-155 contributes to the development of regulatory T cells (57), although it is not indispensable for their immune suppression function.

The multiple and pleotropic effects of miR-155 on the adaptive and innate (58) immune responses suggest that this miRNA is a key regulator of the immune system.

5.2. MiR-155 Involvement in Lymphoid Malignancies

Mir-155 has also an important role in lymphoid malignancies. Overexpression of miR-155 in murine B cell precursors leads to B cell leukemic malignancy (49), the first example of miRNA-induced cancer. MiR-155 is also overexpressed in Hogdkin lymphoma and some subsets of non-Hogdkin lymphomas (Primary Mediastinal B cell lymphoma and DLBCL) (59). In DLBCL, miR-155 is particularly overexpressed in the Activated B cell-like subtype, which is the most aggressive subtype of this disease (7, 60). High expression of miR-155 is also reported in CLL (61), in which a striking complementary pattern of expression between this miRNA and miR-150 is observed in the proliferation centers of leukemic cells in the lymph nodes. MiR-155 expression measured by in situ hybridization was associated with proliferation centers, from which miR-150 expression was practically excluded (62). The precise role of miR-155 in CLL and other malignancies is not well defined yet, but it could induce a decrease of caspase 3-dependent apoptosis as it does in prostate cancer cells by inhibiting TP53INP1 (63).

6. MiR-146

There are two microRNAs in the miR-146 family, miR-146a, and miR-146b; both share the same seed sequence (17–20) and are thought to participate in the regulation of the same proteins but are located in different sites in the human genome. MiR-146a is located at 5q33.3 and miR-146b at 10q24.32.

6.1. MiR-146 in Lymphopoiesis and Lymphocyte Immune Functions

MiR-146 is differentially expressed during several steps of B and T cell peripheral differentiation. Its expression is higher in postgerminal center B cells than in naïve B cells or centroblasts (7), and it is elevated in regulatory T cells (64) and in memory T cells (65). This is probably due to the induction of miR-146 expression by NFκB (66), a nuclear transcription factor important for the activation of lymphocytes and monocytes. Toll-Like Receptor (TLR) activation by LPS binding unleashes a signaling pathway that ends up in the activation of the transcription factor NFκB, which in turn induces the transcription of genes involved in the activation of B cells. It has been demonstrated that TLR stimulation amplifies the humoral response (67) though it is not indispensable for the germinal center reaction. Accordingly, mice deficient in NFκB show defective humoral responses and germinal center reactions (68).

What is the role of miR-146 in this context? It is involved in a regulatory negative feedback loop that attenuates NFκB induction after activation of TLRs. MiR-146 targets include IRAK1 and TRAF6, two proteins involved in the TLR signaling pathway downstream of the TLR (66, 69). The decrease in expression of these two proteins leads to the attenuation of this signaling pathway and results in the modulation of NFκB activation when it could become excessive. Although this regulation was initially described in monocytes, miR-146 is also expressed in B and T lymphocytes (70), probably exerting the same function.

6.2. MiR-146 Involvement in Lymphoid Malignancies

To date the data on miR-146 involvement in lymphoid malignancies is limited. MiR-146 is downregulated in Adult T cell Leukemia (ATL), consistent with an antioncogenic role. Nevertheless, this miRNA is overexpressed in the worst prognosis subtypes of CLL (71) and DLBCL (7, 60).

7. Conclusion

MiRNAs are molecules of paramount importance during lymphopoiesis and the immune response. The functions of miRNAs are explained by the inhibition of the expression of multiple targets that are commonly involved in the same or related signaling pathways. Although miRNAs usually fine-tune expression of their targets, the multiplicity of their effects on consequent members of the signaling cascades leads to marked regulation of multiple, frequently related intracellular processes, thus probably behaving as "hubs" in systems biology. Accordingly, they play a critical role in the regulation of the immune system and their deregulation is implicated in multiple neoplasms, including leukemias and lymphomas. The manipulation of miRNA expression in cancer cells is a promising new approach for cancer treatment that is predicted to be of particular interest in hematological malignancies.

References

1. Litman, G. W., Anderson, M. K., and Rast, J. P. (1999) *Annu Rev Immunol* **17**, 109–47.
2. Starr, T. K., Jameson, S. C., and Hogquist, K. A. (2003) *Annu Rev Immunol* **21**, 139–76.
3. Klein, U., and Dalla-Favera, R. (2008) *Nat Rev Immunol* **8**, 22–33.
4. Ambros, V. (2004) *Nature* **431**, 350–5.
5. Fazi, F., Rosa, A., Fatica, A., Gelmetti, V., De Marchis, M. L., Nervi, C., and Bozzoni, I. (2005) *Cell* **123**, 819–31.
6. Felli, N., Pedini, F., Romania, P., Biffoni, M., Morsilli, O., Castelli, G., Santoro, S., Chicarella, S., Sorrentino, A., Peschle, C., and Marziali, G. (2009) *Haematologica* **94**, 479–86.
7. Malumbres, R., Sarosiek, K. A., Cubedo, E., Ruiz, J. W., Jiang, X., Gascoyne, R. D., Tibshirani, R., and Lossos, I. S. (2009) *Blood* **113**, 3754–64.
8. Zhang, J., Jima, D. D., Jacobs, C., Fischer, R., Gottwein, E., Huang, G., Lugar, P. L., Lagoo, A. S., Rizzieri, D. A., Friedman, D. R., Weinberg, J. B., Lipsky, P. E., and Dave, S. S. (2009) *Blood* **113**, 4586–94.
9. Klein, U., Tu, Y., Stolovitzky, G. A., Keller, J. L., Haddad, J., Jr., Miljkovic, V., Cattoretti, G., Califano, A., and Dalla-Favera, R. (2003) *Proc Natl Acad Sci USA* **100**, 2639–44.
10. Basso, K., Sumazin, P., Morozov, P., Schneider, C., Maute, R. L., Kitagawa, Y., Mandelbaum, J., Haddad, J., Jr., Chen, C. Z., Califano, A., and Dalla-Favera, R. (2009) *Immunity* **30**, 744–52.
11. Tan, L. P., Wang, M., Robertus, J. L., Schakel, R. N., Gibcus, J. H., Diepstra, A., Harms, G., Peh, S. C., Reijmers, R. M., Pals, S. T., Kroesen, B. J., Kluin, P. M., Poppema, S., and van den Berg, A. (2009) *Lab Invest* **89**, 708–16.
12. Neilson, J. R., Zheng, G. X., Burge, C. B., and Sharp, P. A. (2007) *Genes Dev* **21**, 578–89.
13. Li, Q. J., Chau, J., Ebert, P. J., Sylvester, G., Min, H., Liu, G., Braich, R., Manoharan, M., Soutschek, J., Skare, P., Klein, L. O., Davis, M. M., and Chen, C. Z. (2007) *Cell* **129**, 147–61.
14. Calin, G. A., Dumitru, C. D., Shimizu, M., Bichi, R., Zupo, S., Noch, E., Aldler, H., Rattan, S., Keating, M., Rai, K., Rassenti, L., Kipps, T., Negrini, M., Bullrich, F., and Croce, C. M. (2002) *Proc Natl Acad Sci USA* **99**, 15524–9.
15. Cimmino, A., Calin, G. A., Fabbri, M., Iorio, M. V., Ferracin, M., Shimizu, M., Wojcik, S. E., Aqeilan, R. I., Zupo, S., Dono, M., Rassenti, L., Alder, H., Volinia, S., Liu, C. G., Kipps, T. J., Negrini, M., and Croce, C. M. (2005) *Proc Natl Acad Sci USA* **102**, 13944–9.
16. He, L., Thomson, J. M., Hemann, M. T., Hernando-Monge, E., Mu, D., Goodson, S., Powers, S., Cordon-Cardo, C., Lowe, S. W., Hannon, G. J., and Hammond, S. M. (2005) *Nature* **435**, 828–33.
17. Griffiths-Jones, S. (2004) *Nucleic Acids Res* **32**, D109–11.
18. Griffiths-Jones, S., Grocock, R. J., van Dongen, S., Bateman, A., and Enright, A. J. (2006) *Nucleic Acids Res* **34**, D140–4.
19. Griffiths-Jones, S., Saini, H. K., van Dongen, S., and Enright, A. J. (2008) *Nucleic Acids Res* **36**, D154–8.
20. Sanger-Institute, University of Manchester. (2009) miRBase, http://www.mirbase.org/
21. Chen, C. Z., Li, L., Lodish, H. F., and Bartel, D. P. (2004) *Science* **303**, 83–6.
22. Pekarsky, Y., Palamarchuk, A., Maximov, V., Efanov, A., Nazaryan, N., Santanam, U., Rassenti, L., Kipps, T., and Croce, C. M. (2008) *Proc Natl Acad Sci USA* **105**, 19643–8.
23. Pekarsky, Y., Santanam, U., Cimmino, A., Palamarchuk, A., Efanov, A., Maximov, V., Volinia, S., Alder, H., Liu, C. G., Rassenti, L., Calin, G. A., Hagan, J. P., Kipps, T., and Croce, C. M. (2006) *Cancer Res* **66**, 11590–3.
24. Shi, L., Cheng, Z., Zhang, J., Li, R., Zhao, P., Fu, Z., and You, Y. (2008) *Brain Res* **1236**, 185–93.
25. Zhou, B., Wang, S., Mayr, C., Bartel, D. P., and Lodish, H. F. (2007) *Proc Natl Acad Sci USA* **104**, 7080–5.
26. Monticelli, S., Ansel, K. M., Xiao, C., Socci, N. D., Krichevsky, A. M., Thai, T. H., Rajewsky, N., Marks, D. S., Sander, C., Rajewsky, K., Rao, A., and Kosik, K. S. (2005) *Genome Biol* **6**, R71.
27. Xiao, C., Calado, D. P., Galler, G., Thai, T. H., Patterson, H. C., Wang, J., Rajewsky, N., Bender, T. P., and Rajewsky, K. (2007) *Cell* **131**, 146–59.
28. Salomoni, P., Perrotti, D., Martinez, R., Franceschi, C., and Calabretta, B. (1997) *Proc Natl Acad Sci USA* **94**, 3296–301.
29. Taylor, D., Badiani, P., and Weston, K. (1996) *Genes Dev* **10**, 2732–44.
30. Nicolaides, N. C., Gualdi, R., Casadevall, C., Manzella, L., and Calabretta, B. (1991) *Mol Cell Biol* **11**, 6166–76.
31. Clappier, E., Cuccuini, W., Kalota, A., Crinquette, A., Cayuela, J. M., Dik, W. A., Langerak, A. W., Montpellier, B., Nadel, B., Walrafen, P., Delattre, O., Aurias, A., Leblanc, T., Dombret, H., Gewirtz, A. M.,

Baruchel, A., Sigaux, F., and Soulier, J. (2007) *Blood* **110**, 1251–61.

32. Lahortiga, I., De Keersmaecker, K., Van Vlierberghe, P., Graux, C., Cauwelier, B., Lambert, F., Mentens, N., Beverloo, H. B., Pieters, R., Speleman, F., Odero, M. D., Bauters, M., Froyen, G., Marynen, P., Vandenberghe, P., Wlodarska, I., Meijerink, J. P., and Cools, J. (2007) *Nat Genet* **39**, 593–5.
33. Gibcus, J. H., Tan, L. P., Harms, G., Schakel, R. N., de Jong, D., Blokzijl, T., Moller, P., Poppema, S., Kroesen, B. J., and van den Berg, A. (2009) *Neoplasia* **11**, 167–76.
34. Ventura, A., Young, A. G., Winslow, M. M., Lintault, L., Meissner, A., Erkeland, S. J., Newman, J., Bronson, R. T., Crowley, D., Stone, J. R., Jaenisch, R., Sharp, P. A., and Jacks, T. (2008) *Cell* **132**, 875–86.
35. Xiao, C., Srinivasan, L., Calado, D. P., Patterson, H. C., Zhang, B., Wang, J., Henderson, J. M., Kutok, J. L., and Rajewsky, K. (2008) *Nat Immunol* **9**, 405–14.
36. Tagawa, H., Karube, K., Tsuzuki, S., Ohshima, K., and Seto, M. (2007) *Cancer Sci* **98**, 1482–90.
37. Nagel, S., Venturini, L., Przybylski, G. K., Grabarczyk, P., Schmidt, C. A., Meyer, C., Drexler, H. G., Macleod, R. A., and Scherr, M. (2009) *Leuk Lymphoma* **50**, 101–8.
38. Pichiorri, F., Suh, S. S., Ladetto, M., Kuehl, M., Palumbo, T., Drandi, D., Taccioli, C., Zanesi, N., Alder, H., Hagan, J. P., Munker, R., Volinia, S., Boccadoro, M., Garzon, R., Palumbo, A., Aqeilan, R. I., and Croce, C. M. (2008) *Proc Natl Acad Sci USA* **105**, 12885–90.
39. Hayashita, Y., Osada, H., Tatematsu, Y., Yamada, H., Yanagisawa, K., Tomida, S., Yatabe, Y., Kawahara, K., Sekido, Y., and Takahashi, T. (2005) *Cancer Res* **65**, 9628–32.
40. Uziel, T., Karginov, F. V., Xie, S., Parker, J. S., Wang, Y. D., Gajjar, A., He, L., Ellison, D., Gilbertson, R. J., Hannon, G., and Roussel, M. F. (2009) *Proc Natl Acad Sci USA* **106**, 2812–7.
41. Takakura, S., Mitsutake, N., Nakashima, M., Namba, H., Saenko, V. A., Rogounovitch, T. I., Nakazawa, Y., Hayashi, T., Ohtsuru, A., and Yamashita, S. (2008) *Cancer Sci* **99**, 1147–54.
42. Kan, T., Sato, F., Ito, T., Matsumura, N., David, S., Cheng, Y., Agarwal, R., Paun, B. C., Jin, Z., Olaru, A. V., Selaru, F. M., Hamilton, J. P., Yang, J., Abraham, J. M., Mori, Y., and Meltzer, S. J. (2009) *Gastroenterology* **136**, 1689–700.
43. Petrocca, F., Vecchione, A., and Croce, C. M. (2008) *Cancer Res* **68**, 8191–4.
44. Kim, Y. K., Yu, J., Han, T. S., Park, S. Y., Namkoong, B., Kim, D. H., Hur, K., Yoo, M. W., Lee, H. J., Yang, H. K., and Kim, V. N. (2009) *Nucleic Acids Res* **37**, 1672–81.
45. Eis, P. S., Tam, W., Sun, L., Chadburn, A., Li, Z., Gomez, M. F., Lund, E., and Dahlberg, J. E. (2005) *Proc Natl Acad Sci USA* **102**, 3627–32.
46. Clurman, B. E., and Hayward, W. S. (1989) *Mol Cell Biol* **9**, 2657–64.
47. Tam, W., Ben-Yehuda, D., and Hayward, W. S. (1997) *Mol Cell Biol* **17**, 1490–502.
48. Skalsky, R. L., Samols, M. A., Plaisance, K. B., Boss, I. W., Riva, A., Lopez, M. C., Baker, H. V., and Renne, R. (2007) *J Virol* **81**, 12836–45.
49. Costinean, S., Zanesi, N., Pekarsky, Y., Tili, E., Volinia, S., Heerema, N., and Croce, C. M. (2006) *Proc Natl Acad Sci USA* **103**, 7024–9.
50. Thai, T. H., Calado, D. P., Casola, S., Ansel, K. M., Xiao, C., Xue, Y., Murphy, A., Frendewey, D., Valenzuela, D., Kutok, J. L., Schmidt-Supprian, M., Rajewsky, N., Yancopoulos, G., Rao, A., and Rajewsky, K. (2007) *Science* **316**, 604–8.
51. Vigorito, E., Perks, K. L., Abreu-Goodger, C., Bunting, S., Xiang, Z., Kohlhaas, S., Das, P. P., Miska, E. A., Rodriguez, A., Bradley, A., Smith, K. G., Rada, C., Enright, A. J., Toellner, K. M., Maclennan, I. C., and Turner, M. (2007) *Immunity* **27**, 847–59.
52. Muramatsu, M., Kinoshita, K., Fagarasan, S., Yamada, S., Shinkai, Y., and Honjo, T. (2000) *Cell* **102**, 553–63.
53. Dorsett, Y., McBride, K. M., Jankovic, M., Gazumyan, A., Thai, T. H., Robbiani, D. F., Di Virgilio, M., San-Martin, B. R., Heidkamp, G., Schwickert, T. A., Eisenreich, T., Rajewsky, K., and Nussenzweig, M. C. (2008) *Immunity* **28**, 630–8.
54. Teng, G., Hakimpour, P., Landgraf, P., Rice, A., Tuschl, T., Casellas, R., and Papavasiliou, F. N. (2008) *Immunity* **28**, 621–9.
55. Costinean, S., Sandhu, S. K., Pedersen, I. M., Tili, E., Trotta, R., Perrotti, D., Ciarlariello, D., Neviani, P., Harb, J., Kauffman, L. R., Shidham, A., and Croce, C. M. (2009) *Blood* **114**(7), 1374–82.
56. Rodriguez, A., Vigorito, E., Clare, S., Warren, M. V., Couttet, P., Soond, D. R., van Dongen, S., Grocock, R. J., Das, P. P., Miska, E. A., Vetrie, D., Okkenhaug, K., Enright, A. J., Dougan, G., Turner, M., and Bradley, A. (2007) *Science* **316**, 608–11.
57. Kohlhaas, S., Garden, O. A., Scudamore, C., Turner, M., Okkenhaug, K., and Vigorito, E. (2009) *J Immunol* **182**, 2578–82.

58. Dahlberg, J. E., and Lund, E. (2007) *Sci STKE* **2007**, pe25.

59. Kluiver, J., Poppema, S., de Jong, D., Blokzijl, T., Harms, G., Jacobs, S., Kroesen, B. J., and van den Berg, A. (2005) *J Pathol* **207**, 243–9.

60. Lawrie, C. H., Soneji, S., Marafioti, T., Cooper, C. D., Palazzo, S., Paterson, J. C., Cattan, H., Enver, T., Mager, R., Boultwood, J., Wainscoat, J. S., and Hatton, C. S. (2007) *Int J Cancer* **121**, 1156–61.

61. Fulci, V., Chiaretti, S., Goldoni, M., Azzalin, G., Carucci, N., Tavolaro, S., Castellano, L., Magrelli, A., Citarella, F., Messina, M., Maggio, R., Peragine, N., Santangelo, S., Mauro, F. R., Landgraf, P., Tuschl, T., Weir, D. B., Chien, M., Russo, J. J., Ju, J., Sheridan, R., Sander, C., Zavolan, M., Guarini, A., Foa, R., and Macino, G. (2007) *Blood* **109**, 4944–51.

62. Wang, M., Tan, L. P., Dijkstra, M. K., van Lom, K., Robertus, J. L., Harms, G., Blokzijl, T., Kooistra, K., van T'veer M. B., Rosati, S., Visser, L., Jongen-Lavrencic, M., Kluin, P. M., and van den Berg, A. (2008) *J Pathol* **215**, 13–20.

63. Gironella, M., Seux, M., Xie, M. J., Cano, C., Tomasini, R., Gommeaux, J., Garcia, S., Nowak, J., Yeung, M. L., Jeang, K. T., Chaix, A., Fazli, L., Motoo, Y., Wang, Q., Rocchi, P., Russo, A., Gleave, M., Dagorn, J. C., Iovanna, J. L., Carrier, A., Pebusque, M. J., and Dusetti, N. J. (2007) *Proc Natl Acad Sci USA* **104**, 16170–5.

64. Sonkoly, E., Wei, T., Janson, P. C., Saaf, A., Lundeberg, L., Tengvall-Linder, M., Norstedt, G., Alenius, H., Homey, B., Scheynius, A., Stahle, M., and Pivarcsi, A. (2007) *PLoS One* **2**, e610.

65. Wu, H., Neilson, J. R., Kumar, P., Manocha, M., Shankar, P., Sharp, P. A., and Manjunath, N. (2007) *PLoS One* **2**, e1020.

66. Taganov, K. D., Boldin, M. P., Chang, K. J., and Baltimore, D. (2006) *Proc Natl Acad Sci USA* **103**, 12481–6.

67. Meyer-Bahlburg, A., Khim, S., and Rawlings, D. J. (2007) *J Exp Med* **204**, 3095–101.

68. Franzoso, G., Carlson, L., Poljak, L., Shores, E. W., Epstein, S., Leonardi, A., Grinberg, A., Tran, T., Scharton-Kersten, T., Anver, M., Love, P., Brown, K., and Siebenlist, U. (1998) *J Exp Med* **187**, 147–59.

69. Kawai, T., and Akira, S. (2007) *Trends Mol Med* **13**, 460–9.

70. Nakasa, T., Miyaki, S., Okubo, A., Hashimoto, M., Nishida, K., Ochi, M., and Asahara, H. (2008) *Arthritis Rheum* **58**, 1284–92.

71. Bellon, M., Lepelletier, Y., Hermine, O., and Nicot, C. (2009) *Blood* **113**, 4914–7.

Chapter 10

Mouse Models for miRNA Expression: The *ROSA26* Locus

Stefano Casola

Abstract

In 1991, Soriano and coworkers isolated the ROSA26 locus in a gene-trap mutagenesis screening performed in mouse embryonic stem (ES) cells. The ubiquitous expression of ROSA26 in embryonic and adult tissues, together with the high frequency of gene-targeting events observed at this locus in murine ES cells has led to the establishment in the past 10 years of over 130 knock-in lines expressing successfully from the ROSA26 locus a variety of transgenes including reporters, site-specific recombinases and, recently, noncoding RNAs. Different strategies can be employed to drive transgene expression from the ROSA26 locus. This chapter provides an overview of the current methodologies used to generate ROSA26 knock-in lines and describes different approaches that exploit the ROSA26 gene to control expression of transgenes, including miRNAs, in a temporal, cell-type, and stage-specific fashion.

1. Introduction

1.1. The ROSA26 Gene

Located on mouse chromosome 6, the *Gt(ROSA)26Sor* (ROSA26) locus spans around 9 kb and consists of three exons. The ROSA26 gene generates three polyadenylated RNAs of which two, transcribed from the plus strand, lack an open reading frame. The third consists of an antisense transcript coding for a putative protein of 505 aminoacids (1) (see Fig. 1). The function of the ROSA26 gene remains to date unknown, as mutant mice are viable, age, and lack obvious signs of illness (Casola, unpublished results). Similarly to other housekeeping genes, *ROSA26* lacks a TATA box. The ROSA26 gene is moderately expressed with levels varying between different tissues in pre- and postnatal life.

1.2. Targeting the ROSA26 Locus in Mouse ES Cells

The first attempts to insert transgenes by homologous recombination into the ROSA26 locus of mouse ES cells revealed a high frequency of correctly targeted events and, most importantly stable

Silvia Monticelli (ed.), *MicroRNAs and the Immune System: Methods and Protocols*, Methods in Molecular Biology, vol. 667,
DOI 10.1007/978-1-60761-811-9_10, © Springer Science+Business Media, LLC 2010

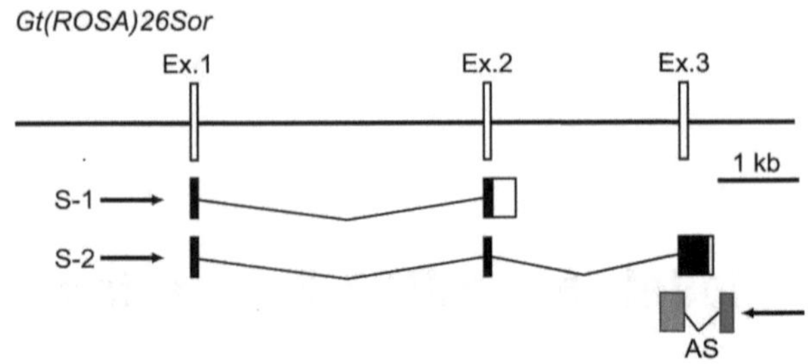

Fig. 1. Gt(ROSA)26Sor genomic locus drawn in scale. *Open rectangles* indicate ROSA26 exons. Sense (S) transcript-1 and transcript-2 (*black rectangles*) are transcribed from the ROSA26 promoter. Antisense (AS) transcript is composed of two exons (*gray*).

1.2.1. Basic Strategy

expression of the transgene in ES cells and in every tissue so far tested of the developing embryo and the adult mouse (1, 2). These results highlight the usefulness of the ROSA26 targeting approach to achieve stable expression of a single-copy transgene. The common strategy to introduce transgenes into the ROSA26 locus reproduces the gene-trap event that allowed the original identification of the locus (3). Specifically, in its simplest version, a splice acceptor sequence (such as that from the adenovirus major late transcript) followed by the coding sequence (cDNA) of the transgene of interest is inserted within the first intron of the ROSA26 gene in correspondence of an XbaI restriction site. The transgenic cDNA carries its own starting codon and is followed by a polyadenylation site (see Fig. 2). In this configuration, the transgene is placed under the transcriptional control of the ROSA26 promoter. The moderate strength of the ROSA26 promoter may in some instances result insufficient to achieve the desired levels of transgene expression. To overcome this limitation an exogenous promoter can be inserted into the ROSA26 intron 1, upstream of the transgene. The synthetic cytomegalovirus early enhancer/chicken β-actin (CAG) promoter represents a successful example of enhancer/promoter combination driving high transgene expression from the ROSA26 locus (4, 5) (see Fig. 2). When exogenous promoters are introduced into the ROSA26 locus a particular care should be given to the orientation of the transgenic transcriptional unit (6).

In order to achieve homologous recombination in ES cells, a copy of the transgenic cDNA is cloned into a targeting vector (TV) between two genomic fragments of the ROSA26 gene required to drive the recombination event. The pROSA26-G19 plasmid generated by the Soriano laboratory, represents a useful source of *ROSA26* genomic DNA (see Subheading 2.1). To enrich for ES clones undergoing homologous recombination events, a positive selection marker (e.g., neomycine resistance gene) flanked by loxP sites (to eliminate by Cre-mediated recombination the marker from the locus once correctly targeted clones have been identified) and a negative selection marker (e.g., minigene coding for Diphtheria toxin A-subunit) are commonly included into the ROSA26 TV.

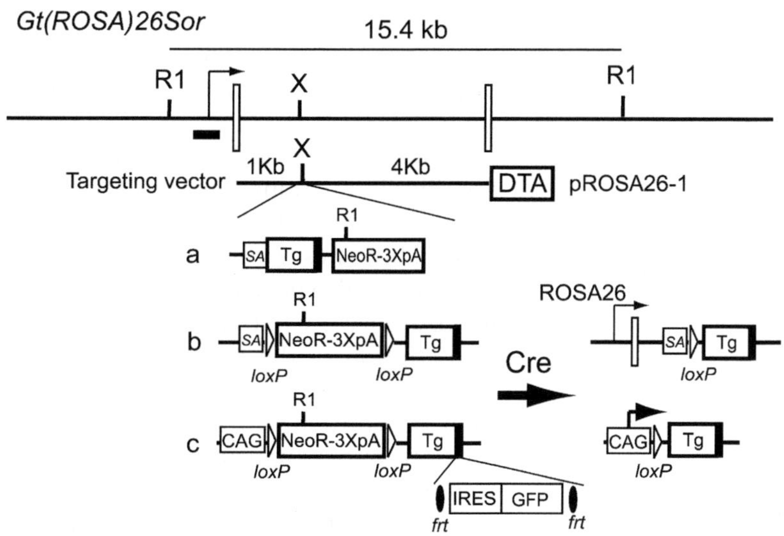

Fig. 2. Targeting strategy to insert single-copy transgenes (Tg) into the ROSA26 locus. Exons 1 and 2 of ROSA26 (*white rectangles*) are indicated. The pROSA26-1 is an example of targeting vector used to insert transgenes into intron 1 of the ROSA-26 gene. The basic vector contains 5 kb of ROSA26 genomic sequences to drive homologous recombination and the gene for the Diphtheria toxin A-subunit (DTA) as negative selection marker. The transgene in most cases preceded by a splice acceptor (SA) site is cloned into a unique Xba1 (X) site. Indicated are three different typologies of transgene: (**a**) expressed constitutively from the ROSA26 promoter, (**b**) conditional transgene expressed from the ROSA26 promoter upon Cre-mediated recombination, and (**c**) conditional transgene expressed from the CAG promoter upon Cre-mediated recombination. To monitor expression of the transgene in vivo an IRES-GFP cassette can be cloned downstream of the transgene of interest. Flanking the reporter cassette with frt sites allows if requested its future deletion in vivo crossing transgenic animals to the FLP deleter strain. The screening for homologous recombinant ES clones can be performed by Southern analysis using the indicated 5′ external probe (*black rectangle*) on genomic DNA digested with EcoR1 (R1). A neomycin resistance gene (NeoR) followed by three polyadenylation (pA) sites constitutes the STOP cassette (flanked by loxP sites) in ROSA26 conditional vectors. The same DNA cassette is used a positive selection marker in the generation of conventional ROSA26 transgenes.

The pROSA26-1 generated by the Soriano group represents an example of a ROSA26 TV, which allows in a single cloning step, the insertion of the transgene of interest (preceded by a splice acceptor site) at the XbaI site within intron 1 of the ROSA26 gene (*2*) (see Fig. 2). To optimize the efficiency of gene targeting, it is common practice to construct targeting vectors carrying ROSA26 homology sequences isogenic with the DNA of the ES cell line that is to be used for the targeting experiment. The frequency of homologous recombination events described for the ROSA26 locus in mouse ES cells can reach up to 20% of drug-resistant colonies.

1.2.2. Constitutive vs. Conditional ROSA26 Transgenes

The ubiquitous and constitutive expression of transgenes from the ROSA26 locus provides an advantage for lineage tracing experiments on animals both in pre- and postnatal life (*2*).

However, more often, temporal and cell-type specific control of transgene expression is required. Two main strategies have been successfully employed to generate conditional ROSA26 transgenes.

The first is based on the Cre/loxP recombination system. Specifically, the transgene is cloned into the ROSA26 locus downstream of a loxP-flanked stuffer DNA sequence (STOP cassette), which abrogates transgene expression (2) (see Fig. 2). Upon temporal and cell-type-specific induction of Cre (for a comprehensive list of available Cre transgenic lines see http://mshri.on.ca/cre), transcription of the transgene from the ROSA26 promoter (or from an exogenous one inserted into the ROSA26 locus) is induced as result of the deletion of the loxP-flanked STOP cassette. To trace expression of the transgene in vivo, it can be useful to introduce downstream of the transgene an Internal Ribosome Entry Site (IRES) followed by a reporter gene coding for a fluorescence protein or an enzyme (β-galactosidase) (2, 7). In this way, coexpression from a bicistronic mRNA of the transgene and the reporter gene is achieved upon induction of Cre-mediated recombination (see Fig. 2). A list of useful plasmids to construct in a single cloning step a conditional ROSA26 TV is provided in Subheading 2.1.

The Cre/loxP system can control transgene expression in a time- and cell-type specific fashion. However, once induced, the transgene cannot be silenced any longer. To overcome this limitation, the tetracycline (Tet)-controlled system can be applied to generate inducible ROSA26 transgenes. Specifically, the coding sequence for the Tet repressor in either its active or inactive form (before exposure to tetracycline/doxycycline) is inserted as a transgene into the ROSA26 locus under its transcriptional control (8). The latter animals are then crossed to mice carrying the transgene of interest under the control of a Tet-regulated promoter. Alternatively, the Tet-inducible transgene is cloned downstream of the Tet repressor on the same ROSA26 allele, minimizing the number of strains and crosses required to perform the desired experiments (9). A combination of the Tet and Cre/loxP systems has led to the successful generation of ROSA26 conditional alleles in which temporal modulation is associated with cell-type and stage-specific expression of the desired transgene (10).

1.2.3. Choosing the ES Line to Target the ROSA26 Locus

There are different sources of mouse ES cell lines that can be used to target the ROSA26 locus. Several ES cell lines derived from the 129/Ola strain have shown over the years a good rate of germ-line transmission (including the feederless HPRT-deficient E14Tg2a line) (11). They represent a good option especially when targeting vectors such as pROSA-1 (containing ROSA26 homology sequences derived from the 129 strain) are employed. Good rates of germ-line transmission are also obtained with hybrid ES cell lines (12). In many instances it is desirable to generate a ROSA26 knock-in line on a pure C57BL/6 genetic background, thereby avoiding subsequent time-consuming back-crossing. Several ES cells lines established from C57BL/6N mice have been recently described to support good germ-line transmission rates (13, 14). A recent improvement in the technology of ROSA26 gene targeting is based on the Recombination Mediated Cassette Exchange (RMCE) system. This method takes advantage of modified ES cells carrying a ROSA26 allele tagged by a single loxP (or frt) site. Introduction of the transgenic construct (carrying a single loxP or frt site) into the tagged ROSA26 locus is mediated by the appropriate site-specific recombinase, transiently expressed in the cells (8, 15). The significant increase in the frequency of recombination events permits the rapid and concomitant generation of several ES lines, each expressing a different transgene.

1.3. Control of miRNA Expression from the ROSA26 Locus

Successful transgenic miRNA expression has been recently achieved exploiting the ROSA26 system. In most cases, conditional targeting vectors have been employed to drive enforced expression of the desired miRNA in a cell-type and stage-specific manner (5, 16, 17). A DNA fragment harboring the miRNA core sequence flanked on average by 200 bp of 5′ and 3′ genomic sequence is amplified by PCR and cloned into the ROSA26 TV. In those instances where the miRNA is encompassed within an exon, the entire exon sequence, preceded by a splice acceptor site and followed by a polyadenylation site, are introduced into intron 1 of the ROSA26 gene (16). Given the moderate expression from the ROSA26 locus, promoters such as CAG are preferentially used to drive strong expression of the transgenic miRNA (5, 16, 17). The addition of an IRES-GFP cassette downstream of the miRNA sequence can be helpful to monitor in vivo sites of transgenic miRNA expression. The decision to use miRNA of the same rather than of a different species (e.g., human) will depend on the extent of conservation of the miRNA between species.

1.4. ROSA26 Regulatory Sequences Drive Gene Expression in Conventional or BAC Transgenic Lines

The utility of the ROSA26 system goes beyond its property to provide stable expression of a transgene upon its insertion into the endogenous locus. This is of particular relevance when technical limitations do not allow genetargeting experiments in ES cells. Two alternative strategies allow faithful expression of a transgene from the ROSA26 promoter. An 800-bp fragment of the ROSA26 promoter is sufficient to drive ubiquitous expression of a transgene once the DNA construct is injected into fertilized eggs to give rise to transgenic animals carrying multiple copies integrated randomly into the genome (18). An alternative is represented by bacterial artificial chromosome (BAC) transgenesis. In the latter case, a BAC carrying a 180–200-kb segment of mouse chromosome-6 encompassing the ROSA26 locus is modified in bacteria by homologous recombination to insert the transgene of interest into the first intron of the ROSA26 gene. Correctly targeted BACs are microinjected into fertilized eggs to generate transgenic founders. ROSA26 BAC transgenics have shown efficient ubiquitous expression of the transgene of interest (19). BAC transgenesis offers several advantages over conventional transgenesis. First, BAC transgenics minimize the risk of position-effect variegation commonly seen with conventional transgenics. Second, expression of transgenes from integrated BACs is more reproducible when different founders are compared to each other. This is dependent on the low number of integrations (usually between one and four) and the existence of the complete set of *cis* regulatory sequences (including putative enhancers) required to drive transgene expression. For a depository of murine BAC clones visit the CHORI website (http://bacpac.chori.org).

2. Materials

2.1. Plasmids

Except for pROSA26-DV1 and pROSA26-DV3 all plasmids can be obtained from Addgene.

1. pROSA26-G19: Plasmid containing a 12-kb genomic fragment encompassing most of the mouse ROSA26 gene.
2. pSAβGEO: Source for splice acceptor sequence.
3. pROSA26-1: Targeting vector to insert single-copy transgenes into the ROSA26 locus (2).
4. pROSA-5 : Plasmid from which it is possible to retrieve an external probe for Southern screening of homologous recombinants (2).
5. pSTOP-eGFP-ROSA26TV: ROSA26 conditional targeting vector. ROSA26 homology sequences flank a segment of DNA introduced into intron 1 of the ROSA26 gene consisting of: (1) a loxP-flanked neomycin resistance gene followed by three polyadenylation sites (STOP cassette), (2) a unique cloning site to introduce the transgene of interest, (3) an frt-flanked IRES-GFP cassette, and (4) a polyadenylation site. The vector carries also as a negative selection marker a minigene coding for the A-subunit of diphtheria toxin (7).
6. pCAG-STOP-eGFP-ROSA26TV: Similar to pSTOP-eGFP-ROSA26TV with the only difference that the CAG promoter is cloned into the first intron of the ROSA26 gene upstream of the loxP-flanked STOP cassette (5).

7. pROSA26-DV1 and pROSA26-DV3: Modified versions of conditional ROSA26 TVs allowing the cloning of the transgene of interest using the Gateway system. The two versions of the TV allow expression of the transgene, respectively, from the ROSA26 and CAG promoter (20).
8. pPGK-Cre-bpA: Expression vector for Cre recombinase.

2.2. Probe to Screen for ROSA26 Homologous Recombinants

Several probes have been used to identify events of homologous recombination at the ROSA26 locus by Southern blot analysis. In our experience, the best one consist of a genomic fragment lying upstream of the ROSA26 5′ homology arm which can be PCR-amplified from genomic DNA using the following primers: R26-5′Prb-fw: CAGCAATGTGGATATAAGCATTAAG; R26-5′Prb-rv: CATGTTACTTGTGTAACGTCTTCAC.

2.3. In Vitro Culture of Mouse Embryonic Fibroblasts

Mouse embryonic fibroblasts (MEFs) are isolated from day 14 DR-4 embryos expressing four drug-selectable marker genes (21). Drug-resistant MEFs can be isolated also from other transgenic sources.

1. MEFs are grown in EF medium lacking antibiotics: DMEM (high glucose without sodium pyruvate) plus 10% fetal calf serum, 1 mM sodium pyruvate, 2 mM l-glutamine. Store complete medium at 4°C.
2. Gelatin (cell-culture grade, from porcine, stock: 2%; Sigma). 0.1% working solution is prepared in PBS without Mg^{2+}/Ca^{2+} and stored at +4°C.
3. Phosphate-buffered saline without Mg^{2+}/Ca^{2+}. Store at room temperature.
4. Trypsin–EDTA (2.5% trypsin/10 mM EDTA, Invitrogen). Store stock solution at –20°C. Working solution (0.25% trypsin/1 mM EDTA) is diluted in PBS. Diluted trypsin–EDTA solution can be kept for up to 1 week at 4°C.
5. Mitomycin C (Sigma): Dissolve powder (2 mg/vial) in 2-ml PBS and consider it a 100-fold concentrated stock solution. Aliquot in freezing tubes and store at –70°C. MMC is light sensitive.
6. Tissue-culture dishes: 9-cm dishes, flat-bottomed 96-well plates and U-bottomed 96-well plates.
7. 50-ml and 15-ml conical tubes.
8. Cryogenic vials.
9. CO_2 incubator (37°C, 10% CO_2 and maximal humidity).
10. Freezing medium: 10% Dymethylsulfoxide in fetal calf serum.

2.4. In Vitro Culture and Targeting of ES Cells

1. ES cells are grown in antibiotic-free ES medium: DMEM (High glucose without sodium pyruvate) plus 15% fetal calf serum (ES-tested HyClone), 1 mM sodium pyruvate (store at 4°C), 2 mM l-glutamine (store at –20°C), 0.1 mM non-essential aminoacids (store at 4°C), 100 μM 2-β-mercapthoethanol (store at 4°C), 1,000 U/ml leukemia inhibitory factor (1:1,000 dilution of LIF present in 720 LIFD cell-conditioned media). CHO-transfected 720 LIFD cells are from Genetics Institute Cambridge, MA – store aliquots of LIF-containing supernatant at –70°C.
2. Trypsin–EDTA working solution (diluted in PBS) is completed with the addition of 1% chicken serum (Invitrogen) if working with C57BL/6 ES cells.
3. ES transfection is done using a Bio-Rad electroporator, at 230–240 V, 480 μF.
4. Electroporation cuvettes: 4-mm Gene pulser cuvettes (Bio-Rad).
5. ES transfection buffer: RPMI 1640 without phenol red (Invitrogen, 11835-030).
6. G418-Sulfate (neomycin or geneticin, Invitrogen). Resuspend in sterile water at a concentration of 100 mg/ml. Check specific activity when calculating the amount of G418 to give to ES cells. Store stock solution at –70°C. G418-containing ES medium is kept at 4°C.
7. Trypsinization, expansion and daily feeding of picked ES colonies in 96-well plates are performed using a 12-well multipipettor or 8-well multistepper pipette. Medium is aspirated from 96-well plates using a multiwell plate washer manifold (Sigma).
8. Freezing medium: 10% DMSO in ES-tested FCS.
9. ES cell lysis buffer: 10 mM NaCl, 10 mM Tris–HCl pH 7.5, 10 mM EDTA, 0.5% sarkosyl, and 1.0 mg/ml freshly added proteinase K (Roche, 1 g is resuspended in sterile water at a final concentration of 10 mg/ml. Stock solution is stored at -20°C).
10. Restriction enzyme mixture: 1 mM DTT, 1 mM spermidine (Sigma), 100 μg/ml BSA, 50 μg/ml Rnase A, and 20 U of restriction enzyme per sample.
11. 0.15 N HCl.
12. Transfer solution for Southern blotting: 0.4 N NaOH, 0.6 M NaCl.
13. Hybridization buffer: 1 M NaCl, 50 mM Tris–HCl, pH 7.5, 10% dextran-sulfate (Sigma), 1% SDS, and 250 μg/ml sonicated fish sperm (Roche, 10 mg/ml).

14. Sodium acetate: 2 M, pH 6.5.
15. Absolute and 70% ethanol.
16. CO_2 incubator (37°C, 10% CO_2 and maximal humidity).

3. Methods

3.1. Preparing MEF Cells for the Transfection of ES Cells

1. Day 0: Rapidly thaw two vials (3×10^6 cells/vial) of MEF at passage-0 and transfer cells into one 15-ml conical tubes containing 10 ml of EF medium.
2. Spin at 195 ×*g* for 10 min at 4°C.
3. Resuspend pellet in 6 ml of EF medium and distribute cells (1 ml of cells/dish) in six 9-cm gelatin-coated tissue-culture (TC) dishes containing 9 ml of EF medium (passage-1: MEF-1) (see Note 1). Incubate in a humidified incubator at 37°C. Feed cells daily with 10-ml EF medium.
4. Day 3: Four confluent MEF-1 plates are trypsinized; steps 5–14 (see Note 2).
5. Wash MEF-1 twice with 10 ml of PBS.
6. Add 3 ml of 1× trypsin–EDTA solution and incubate for 3–5 min at 37°C.
7. Pipet cells gently until single-cell suspension is obtained (do not incubate MEF in trypsin–EDTA solution for longer than 7–8 min).
8. Neutralize trypsin adding 5 ml of EF medium.
9. Count the number of viable cells by the trypan blue exclusion method and make aliquots of 3×10^6 cells/15-ml conical tube.
10. Spin cells at 195 ×*g* for 10 min at room temperature.
11. Resuspend pellet in 1 ml of freezing medium (kept at 4°C).
12. Rapidly transfer cells into labeled cryogenic vials.
13. Place freezing vials into appropriate Styropore boxes and transfer cells overnight to a –70°C freezer.
14. Next day allocate freezing vials into a liquid N_2 tank where they can be kept for indefinite time.
15. Day 3: One MEF-1 9-cm TC plate is treated with mitomycin C (MMC): steps 16–22 (see Note 3). These cells will represent the feeder layer for the ES cells that will be thawed for the transfection experiment.
16. Aspirate medium and wash cells twice with PBS.
17. Add to cells 4 ml of EF medium containing 40 μl of a 100× MMC solution.

18. Incubate cells with MMC for 3–6 h in the incubator at 37°C.
19. Wash cells three times with 10 ml of PBS.
20. Trypsinize the plate following the method in steps 4–14.
21. Resuspend the pellet in 10 ml of EF medium and plate on one 9-cm TC dish.
22. Day 3: one MEF-1 plate is trypsinized and the cells are expanded to three 9-cm TC dishes (MEF-2).

3.2. Preparing ES Cells for Transfection

1. Day 4: Thaw rapidly one vial of frozen ES cells ($2–3 \times 10^6$ cells) and dilute cells in 10 ml of ES cell medium, and spin cells at $195 \times g$ for 10 min at room temperature.
2. Resuspend the ES cell pellet in 10 ml of ES medium and plate the cells onto MMC-treated MEF-1 (as described in Subheading 3.1, steps 15–21).
3. Day 4: Thaw two vials of MEF-1 (as described in Subheading 3.1, steps 1–3) and plate the cells on seven gelatin-coated 9-cm TC dishes (MEF-2). Feed daily ES cells and MEFs with fresh medium.
4. Day 6: Treat three MEF-2 plates with MMC (see Subheading 3.1, step 22), trypsinize the cells and plate them in three 9-cm TC dishes.
5. Day 7: Trypsinize ES cells as described in Subheading 3.1, steps 4–14 (see Note 4), count viable cells (see Note 5) and plate 1×10^6 ES cells on each of three MMC-treated MEF-2 plates as described in step 4, this subheading (see Note 6).
6. Day 8: Treat four MEF-2 plates (described in step 4, this subheading) for 3 h with MMC, trypsinize and count the cells.
7. Plate 3×10^6 MEF-2 cells in each 9-cm gelatin-coated TC dishes (four plates). Six plates will contain MMC-treated MEF-2 that will be used to plate ES cells from two electroporation experiments. As control 3×10^6 MMC-treated MEFs cells plated on one 9-cm TC dish will receive 0.5×10^6 untransfected ES cells. This control plate will indicate the stringency of the G418 selection. Never start picking ES cells before this control plate is free of viable ES colonies.

3.3. Transfection of ES Cells

The following protocol is for one transfection experiment.

1. Day 8: Linearize targeting vector:
   (a) Digest in a microfuge tube 30 μg of high quality plasmid DNA for 3–5 h at the appropriate temperature (see Note 7).
   (b) Phenol (saturated in Tris–HCl, pH 8.0), chloroform (50% v/v) extraction of the linearized targeting vector.

(c) Precipitate the vector in one-tenth volume of sodium acetate (3 M, pH 5.2) and 2.5 volumes of absolute ethanol.

(d) Precipitate DNA at −20°C for at least 20 min.

(e) Spin at 15,700×*g* in a microcentrifuge for 20 min at 4°C.

(f) Discard the supernatant and wash the DNA pellet twice with cold (−20°C) 75% ethanol.

(g) Spin the microfuge tube at 15,700×*g* for 5 min at 4°C.

(h) After the second wash, discard the ethanol and fill up the tube once more with cold 75% ethanol/H_2O solution.

(i) Spin the microfuge tube at 15,700×*g* for 5 min at 4°C.

(j) Discard the supernatant carefully under a cell-culture hood.

(k) Air-dry the pellet for 30–40 min under sterile conditions

(l) Resuspend the pellet in 100 μl of transfection buffer.

2. Day 9: Feed the ES plates with fresh ES medium 2 h before transfection.
3. Day 9: Trypsinize ES cells (see Note 8):

(a) Count the cells and aliquot 1×10^7 ES cells in a 50-ml conical tube.

(b) Spin the ES cells at 195×*g*, room temperature for 10 min.

(c) Wash once the ES cell pellet in 45 ml of PBS.

(d) Spin the ES cells at 195×*g*, room temperature for 10 min.

4. Resuspend the ES cell pellet in 700 μl of transfection buffer.
5. Add the DNA solution (100 μl) to the ES cell suspension. Mix well avoiding bubbles.
6. Transfer the cells to an electroporation cuvette.
7. Electroporate the ES cells at a 230–240 V (depending on the ES cell line) (see Note 9).
8. Incubate the cells for 5–10 min at room temperature.
9. Transfer the electroporated ES cells to a 50-ml conical tube containing 30 ml of ES medium.
10. Plate 10 ml of the transfected ES cell suspension into each of three 9-cm TC dishes containing MMC-treated MEF-2 cells. Transfer the cells to a 37°C incubator.
11. Feed daily the ES cells throughout the entire transfection experiment with 10 ml of fresh ES medium.
12. Two days after transfection (day 11), start feeding transfected ES cells with G418-containing ES medium (see Note 10).

13. Six days after transfection (day 15) thaw one vial of MEF-2 and plate cells onto three gelatin-coated 9-cm tissue-culture dishes (MEF-3) (see Note 11).
14. Feed MEF-3 daily with EF medium.
15. By days 7–8 posttransfection (days 16–17) distinct G418, Diphtheria toxin double-resistant colonies should be visible selectively in those plates containing transfected ES cells.
16. The day before picking resistant ES colonies (day 17), treat MEF-3 (three plates described in step 13) with MMC, trypsinize, and count cells.
17. Transfer MMC-treated MEF-3 cells from three confluent 9-cm plates to four flat-bottomed 96-well plates (see Notes 12 and 13).

3.4. Picking ES Colonies

Start picking at day 9 posttransfection (day 18) and continue through day 10 (day 19).

The following protocol is for picking 96 colonies into one 96-well plate (see Note 14).

1. Feed-transfected ES plates 2 h before picking.
2. Prepare one 96-well plate (U-bottom) containing in each well 20 μl of a 2× trypsin–EDTA solution (containing 1% chicken serum in case C57BL/6 ES cells are employed).
3. Wash one 9-cm TC plate containing double-resistant ES colonies twice with 10 ml of PBS.
4. After the second wash aspirate PBS and add 10 ml of PBS to the plate.
5. Pick colonies under a tissue-culture hood, with the help of a stereomicroscope, using a 20-μl micropipettor setting the pipette to 20 μl and using sterile disposable tips.
6. Transfer each picked colony into one well of the U-bottomed 96-well plate containing 20 μl of 2× trypsin–EDTA solution.
7. Pick from one ES plate for 30–40 min. Check for the status of picked colonies under the microscope. If cells are not yet dissociated place the plate for 5 min in the incubator at 37°C.
8. Add 110 μl of ES medium to each well. Dissociate cells using a multichannel pipettor and sterile tips (change tips for each set of wells) pipetting vigorously.
9. With a multichannel pipettor, transfer cells (150 μl) of each well to the respective well of a 96-well plate (flat bottom) containing MMC-MEF-3 cells.

10. If additional colonies need to be picked from the same 9-cm tissue-culture plate, wash twice with PBS and feed plate with ES medium containing G418. Picking from the same plate can be done later in the day or the next day (see Note 15).
11. Feed picked colonies for the following 2–3 days using a multistepper pipettor, adding 150 μl of G418-containing ES medium to each well.
12. When cells reach confluence, wash 96-well plates twice with PBS and split 1:3:
    (a) Trypsinize colonies adding 50 μl of trypsin–EDTA working solution to each well.
    (b) Place 96-well plate in the incubator for 5 min at 37°C.
    (c) Dissociate cells by pipetting them vigorously.
    (d) Neutralize trypsin adding100 μl of complete ES medium to each well.
    (e) Divide the 150-μl cell suspension in three parts and transfer cells to the corresponding well (50 μl each) of three 96-well plates containing MEF-3 (each well having already 150 μl of G418-containing ES medium).
13. Feed 96-well plates daily with ES medium (containing G418).
14. Three to four days later freeze down one of the three 96-well replica plates (see Subheading 3.5, steps 1–6).
15. The second replica plate is frozen down the day after.
16. The third replica plate is trypsinized as described in step 13. Cells are plated to three 96-well plates coated with gelatin and fed daily with ES medium (containing G418). From these plates, as soon as ES clones are grown to confluence, genomic DNA is extracted and screened for the occurrence of homologous recombination.

3.5. Freezing ES Clones in 96-Well Plates

1. Grow ES cells to subconfluence.
2. Aspirate medium, wash each well twice with 100 μl of PBS using a multistepper pipette and trypsinize cells (described in Subheading 3.4, step 12).
3. Neutralize trypsin by adding 50 μl of 2× concentrated freezing medium in each well.
4. Dissociate the cells vigorously pipetting them several times with a multichannel pipettor.
5. Overlay each well with 100 μl of sterile mineral oil.
6. Seal the 96-well plates with Parafilm and store at –70° C until the screening is completed.

3.6. Rapid Screening of ES Clones by Southern Blot Analysis

The following is a modification of the protocol described in ref. *22*.

1. Grow ES colonies on gelatin-coated 96-well plates until they reach confluence.
2. Wash each well twice with 100 μl of PBS.
3. After the last wash, aspirate PBS and add to each well 50 μl of ES lysis buffer.
4. Wrap the 96-well plate with Parafilm, and lyse the cells at 56°C overnight (see Note 16).
5. Next day, cool the humidified box allowing it to stand for 1 h at room temperature.
6. Precipitate DNA adding to each well 100 μl of absolute ethanol and 1.5 μl of 5 M NaCl.
7. Incubate the plate on the bench for 2 h on a shaker.
8. Discard the supernatant inverting carefully the plate.
9. Wash the 96-well plate by adding to each well 100 μl of ice-cold 70% ethanol.
10. Repeat step 9 two more times, inverting the plates after each wash.
11. After the last ethanol wash, the plates are left on the bench for 20 min to air-dry (see Note 17).
12. Apply to each well 35 μl of the restriction digest mix.
13. Wrap the plate in saran wrap and incubate overnight at the appropriate restriction enzyme temperature.
14. Next day, block the enzymatic digestion by adding 9 μl of 5× loading buffer (see Note 18).
15. Digested DNA from each well is loaded with a multichannel pipettor onto a 0.8–1.1% agarose gel (1× TAE) prepared using gel chambers accommodating up to four sets of gel combs (with each gel comb set allowing the loading of 50 DNA samples). Gel is run overnight at a 40 V (see Note 19).
16. Denature DNA incubating the agarose gel for 20 min in 0.15 N HCl and subsequently for 1 h in transfer solution.
17. Transfer DNA onto positively charged nylon membranes (in transfer solution) following conventional upward alkaline capillary transfer protocols (completed in 16–24 h) or performing 1-h downward alkaline capillary transfer (23).
18. Crosslink DNA, baking membranes at 80°C for 1 h or by brief ultraviolet irradiation (254-nm wavelength).
19. Prehybridize the membrane (for 4 h to overnight) and hybridize overnight in hybridization buffer using a ROSA26 5′ external probe (see Note 20).

20. Wash the membrane (see Note 21) and finally expose overnight in an autoradiography cassette at −70°C.
21. Develop film.

3.7. Thawing ES Clones from 96-Well Plates

1. Prepare MMC-treated MEF-3 and plate onto 48-well plates.
2. Warm up some sterile distilled water to 37°C and pour it in a sterile Pyrex dish under the cell-culture hood.
3. Remove one frozen 96-well plate from the −70°C freezer and place it on the surface of the water until its content is thawed.
4. Transfer the correctly targeted ES clones into 15-ml conical tubes containing 5 ml of ES medium using a 1-ml disposable pipette (see Note 22).
5. Spin the ES cells 10 min at 195 × *g* at room temperature.
6. Aspirate supernatant and resuspend cell pellet in 0.5 ml of ES medium containing G418. Plate ES cells into one well of a 48-well plate.
7. Feed cells daily with fresh ES medium containing G418.
8. Passage ES cells when they reach subconfluence.

3.8. Testing for Rosa26 Transgene Expression in Targeted ES Cells

Taking advantage of the ubiquitous expression of the ROSA26 gene, it is possible to test whether the targeted locus expresses the transgene of interest in correctly targeted ES clones. In those cases where the ROSA26 transgene lacks time and/or cell-type inducibility, expression can be rapidly assessed in one or two correctly targeted ES clones by western blot and/or reverse transcription (RT)-PCR analyses. In the latter case, the forward primer is complementary to the first ROSA26 exon, whereas the reverse one anneals to the coding sequence of the transgene. If a conditional ROSA26 transgene is controlled by the Cre/loxP system, appropriate expression of the transgene can be tested upon Cre-mediated deletion of the loxP-flanked STOP sequence. For this purpose, transient expression of Cre is induced by transfection of targeted ES cells with a plasmid encoding for the recombinase (see Subheading 2.1).

1. Thaw a vial of targeted ES cells and expand cells as described in Subheading 3.2.
2. Feed cells daily with ES medium (+G418) until they reach a density of 1×10^7 cells.
3. The day before transfection, precipitate 30 μg of the Cre expression vector in a microfuge tube with one-tenth volume of Na acetate (3 M, pH 5.2) and 2.5 volumes of absolute ethanol, for at least 40 min at −20°C.
4. Spin the DNA in a microcentrifuge at 15,700 × *g* for 20 min at 4°C.

5. Wash the pellet twice with 75% ice-cold ethanol.
6. Remove the last wash, open the microfuge tube under the hood and air-dry the pellet for 20 min.
7. Resuspend the DNA using sterile disposable tips in 100 μl of transfection buffer.
8. On the day of transfection, trypsinize, count and aliquot 5×10^6 ES cells in a 50-ml conical tube.
9. Perform electroporation of ES cells as described in Subheading 3.3, steps 5–9.
10. Plate 5×10^6 transfected ES cells in one 9-cm tissue-culture plate containing MMC-treated MEF-2 or MEF-3. ES cells are fed with ES medium lacking G418 (in case the neomycin resistance gene is inserted within the loxP-flanked STOP cassette).
11. As soon as ES colonies are visible (usually 2 days after transfection), trypsinize ES cells and plate 1×10^3 cells each onto three 9-cm tissue-culture plates containing MMC-treated MEF-2 or MEF-3 cells.
12. Feed ES cells daily with fresh ES medium (without G418).
13. Three to four days after plating, ES colonies are picked following the same protocol described in Subheading 3.4, with one exception: after trypsinization each ES clone is directly divided into two flat-bottomed 96-well replica plates containing MMC-treated MEF-3 cells (see Note 23).
14. After 2 days, one 96-well plate is fed with ES medium containing G418, and the second plate is fed with only ES medium (see Note 24).
15. Feed daily the ES colonies present in the replica plates with the appropriate ES medium.
16. Expand the ES colonies from the 96-well plate fed with ES medium alone, choosing those clones that are clearly dying in the same well of the replica plate fed with the G418-containing medium.
17. Grow selected ES clones, extract DNA, and confirm the successful deletion of the selection marker by Southern blotting and, when possible, by flow cytometric analysis (see Notes 25 and 26).

4. Notes

1. Add enough 0.1% gelatin solution to cover the TC dish. Incubate at room temperature for 10–15 min. Aspirate gelatin and plate cells.
2. A plate of confluent EF cells can contain from 3 to 5×10^6 cells.

3. Handle with care. Mitomycin is a chemotherapeutic agent inhibiting DNA synthesis and crosslinking DNA.
4. Trypsinization of C57BL/6 ES cells requires the addition of chicken serum (1% final concentration) to the trypsin–EDTA working solution to protect cells during the trypsinization procedure (chicken serum lacks trypsin inhibitors).
5. To calculate the number of ES cells in a 9-cm tissue-culture plate subtract from the total number of counted cells, 3×10^6 that should correspond to the approximate number of feeder cells present in a confluent 9-cm tissue-culture dish.
6. Freeze down the rest of ES cells (2×10^6 ES cells per vial in 1-ml freezing medium).
7. For each transfection use 20–30 μg of linearized vector.
8. Follow the ES cells under the microscope while incubating in trypsin–EDTA working solution. Large cell clumps should be avoided since this will significantly reduce the transfection efficiency.
9. Good transfection efficiencies are associated with time constants of 6–9 ms.
10. The concentration of G418 to add to transfected ES cells should be first titrated on wild-type ES cells. In our experience, 180–220 μg/ml (100% activity) of G418 are sufficient by day 8 posttransfection to kill all nontransfected ES cells present in the control plate.
11. At confluence 3, 9-cm plates of MMC-treated MEF-3 are sufficient to prepare a feeder layer for picking and expanding 96 double-resistant ES colonies.
12. 2×10^6 MEF-3 cells are sufficient for one 96-well plate.
13. Of the four MEF-3 coated plates, the first will be used to accommodate the picked colonies, while the remaining three will be used for their expansion 3–4 days later. (see Subheading 3.3, step 14).
14. Given the high frequency of homologous recombination events, it is sufficient to pick 96 colonies. From these, one should expect between 5 and 10 homologous recombinants.
15. ES clones carrying properly targeted loci may sometime grow slower and thus, picking ES colonies on more than 1 day increases the chance to identify correctly targeted ones.
16. Place 96-well plates into sealed containers in which a humidified atmosphere is achieved by adding wet paper towels.
17. Do not allow plates to overdry, since this will affect the efficiency of DNA digestion.
18. At this point, samples can be either run on an agarose gel or frozen at – 20°C.

19. Depending on the size of the expected bands, gel can be also run over day at a maximum voltage of 70 V.
20. Several ROSA26 5′ external probes have been described in the literature to screen for homologous recombination. In our experience, the best probe consists of a genomic fragment of the ROSA26 locus amplified by the PCR with primers listed in Subheading 2.2.
21. Stringency of washing conditions varies from probe to probe. Usually start washing membranes in 2×SSC, 0.1% SDS at 65°C for 30–40 min.
22. Thaw also ES clones present in wells preceding and following the well containing the targeted clone. Sometimes screening by Southern of a large number of ES clones may accidentally lead to mistakes in loading samples onto the agarose gel.
23. When using the Cre/loxP system to delete the loxP-flanked STOP cassette, usually 50% of Cre-transfected ES cells become G418-sensitive. Thus, picking 70 ES colonies will be enough to obtain at least 3–4 G418-sensitive colonies (calculating a 10% efficiency of transfection).
24. In our experience increasing by 25% the amount of G418 given to the ES cells makes it easier to detect sensitive (dying) colonies.
25. Internal probes can also be used for this purpose. In this case choose for the Southern analysis a restriction enzyme that cuts once in the targeted region and once outside.
26. In case a GFP reporter gene is inserted into the ROSA26 locus together with the transgene of interest, it is possible to verify successful recombination of the STOP cassette mediated by Cre expression, by performing a flow cytometric analysis of on a fraction of ES cells obtained after trypsinization of few G418-sensitive clones

Acknowledgments

S. Casola is supported by the Giovanni Armenise/Harvard Career Development Award, the AIRC Foundation and by the European Research Council Starting Independent Researcher Grant, through the Italian Ministry of University and Research (progetto FIRB-IDEAS).

References

1. Zambrowicz BP, Imamoto A, Fiering S, Herzenberg LA, Kerr WG, Soriano P. (1997) Disruption of overlapping transcripts in the ROSA beta geo 26 gene trap strain leads to widespread expression of beta-galactosidase in mouse embryos and hematopoietic cells. *Proc Natl Acad Sci USA* **94**, 3789–3794.

2. Soriano P. (1999) Generalized lacZ expression with the ROSA26 Cre reporter strain. *Nat Genet* **21**, 70–71.
3. Friedrich G, Soriano P. (1991) Promoter traps in embryonic stem cells: a genetic screen to identify and mutate developmental genes in mice. *Genes Dev* **5,** 1513–1523.
4. Niwa H, Yamamura K, Miyazaki J. (1991) Efficient selection for high-expression transfectants with a novel eukaryotic vector. *Gene* **108**, 193–199.
5. Xiao C, Calado DP, Galler G, et al. (2007) MiR-150 controls B cell differentiation by targeting the transcription factor c-Myb. *Cell* **131**,146–159.
6. Strathdee D, Ibbotson H, Grant SG. (2006) Expression of transgenes targeted to the Gt(ROSA)26Sor locus is orientation dependent. *PLoS One* **1**, e4.
7. Sasaki Y, Derudder E, Hobeika E, et al. (2006) Canonical NF-kappaB activity, dispensable for B cell development, replaces BAFF-receptor signals and promotes B cell proliferation upon activation. *Immunity* **24**, 729–739.
8. Beard C, Hochedlinger K, Plath K, Wutz A, Jaenisch R. (2006) Efficient method to generate single-copy transgenic mice by site-specific integration in embryonic stem cells. *Genesis* **44**, 23–28.
9. Backman CM, Zhang Y, Malik N, et al. (2009) Generalized tetracycline induced Cre recombinase expression through the ROSA26 locus of recombinant mice. *J Neurosci Methods* **176**, 16–23.
10. Schonig K, Schwenk F, Rajewsky K, Bujard H. (2002) Stringent doxycycline dependent control of CRE recombinase in vivo. *Nucleic Acids Res* **30**, e134.
11. Hooper M, Hardy K, Handyside A, Hunter S, Monk M. (1987) HPRT-deficient (Lesch-Nyhan) mouse embryos derived from germline colonization by cultured cells. *Nature* **326**, 292–295.
12. Eggan K, Akutsu H, Loring J, et al. (2001) Hybrid vigor, fetal overgrowth, and viability of mice derived by nuclear cloning and tetraploid embryo complementation. *Proc Natl Acad Sci USA* **98**, 6209–6214.
13. Tanimoto Y, Iijima S, Hasegawa Y, et al. (2008) Embryonic stem cells derived from C57BL/6J and C57BL/6N mice. *Comp Med* **58**, 347–352.
14. Pettitt SJ, Liang Q, Rairdan XY, et al. (2009) Agouti C57BL/6N embryonic stem cells for mouse genetic resources. *Nat Methods* **6**, 493–495.
15. Seibler J, Kuter-Luks B, Kern H, et al. (2005) Single copy shRNA configuration for ubiquitous gene knockdown in mice. *Nucleic Acids Res* **33**, e67.
16. Thai TH, Calado DP, Casola S, et al. (2007) Regulation of the germinal center response by microRNA-155. *Science* **316**, 604–608.
17. Xiao C, Srinivasan L, Calado DP, et al. (2008) Lymphoproliferative disease and autoimmunity in mice with increased miR-17-92 expression in lymphocytes. *Nat Immunol* **9**, 405–414.
18. Kisseberth WC, Brettingen NT, Lohse JK, Sandgren EP. (1999) Ubiquitous expression of marker transgenes in mice and rats. *Dev Biol* **214**, 128–138.
19. Giel-Moloney M, Krause DS, Chen G, Van Etten RA, Leiter AB. (2007) Ubiquitous and uniform in vivo fluorescence in ROSA26-EGFP BAC transgenic mice. *Genesis* **45**, 83–89.
20. Nyabi O, Naessens M, Haigh K, et al. (2009) Efficient mouse transgenesis using Gateway-compatible ROSA26 locus targeting vectors and F1 hybrid ES cells. *Nucleic Acids Res* **37**, e55.
21. Tucker KL, Wang Y, Dausman J, Jaenisch R. (1997) A transgenic mouse strain expressing four drug-selectable marker genes. *Nucleic Acids Res* **25**, 3745–3746.
22. Ramirez-Solis R, Rivera-Perez J, Wallace JD, Wims M, Zheng H, Bradley A. (1992) Genomic DNA microextraction: a method to screen numerous samples. *Anal Biochem* **201**, 331–335.
23. Chomczynski P. (1992) One-hour downward alkaline capillary transfer for blotting of DNA and RNA. *Anal Biochem* **201**, 134–139.

Chapter 11

Regulation of Monocytopoiesis by MicroRNAs

Laura Fontana*, Antonio Sorrentino*, and Cesare Peschle

Abstract

MicroRNAs (miRNAs or miRs) are ~22 nt single-stranded noncoding RNAs that control gene expression in eukaryotes. miRNAs play an essential role in all basic cellular processes including cell development, proliferation, differentiation, and apoptosis. Importantly, miRNAs regulate hematopoietic progenitor cells differentiation toward the different hematopoietic lineages. This occurs through the regulation of key factors involved in hematopoiesis (e.g., transcription factors, growth factor receptors). We, hereby, describe how to investigate the role of miRNAs in monocytopoiesis.

1. Introduction

In adult humans, blood cells derive from differentiation of multipotential hematopoietic progenitor cells (HPCs) which, in turn, originate from hematopoietic stem cells (HSCs) in the bone marrow (1). In addition to the capability to differentiate into all blood cells, HSCs also have the ability to self-renew, thus allowing the maintenance of the HSC pool. This feature is almost completely lost in HPCs. Differentiation of HPCs occurs through their progressive restriction of lineage potential and their development into differentiated precursors up to mature cells. From HPCs derive a common myeloid progenitor (CMP), which in turn generates an erythromegakaryocytic progenitor (MEP), giving rise to erythrocytes and megakaryocytes and a granulomonocytic progenitor (GMP) that generates granulocytes and monocytes/macrophages (1). Bone marrow and circulating monocytes are recruited to peripheral sites in response to proinflammatory, metabolic, and immune stimuli. Once in the tissue, monocytes mature into macrophages which contribute to host defense and tissue homeostasis, showing a high degree of heterogeneity and specialized

Silvia Monticelli (ed.), *MicroRNAs and the Immune System: Methods and Protocols*, Methods in Molecular Biology, vol. 667,
DOI 10.1007/978-1-60761-811-9_11, © Springer Science+Business Media, LLC 2010

adaptive states reflecting their different anatomical locations (e.g., osteoclasts contribute to bone remodeling; alveolar macrophages are involved in clearing microorganisms, virus, and environmental particles in the lung; antigen-presenting cells expose foreign antigens on their cell surface) (2).

We have identified different miRNAs that regulate monocytic differentiation: this occurs through the modulation of two key transcription factors, acute myeloid leukemia 1 (AML1) and PU.1 (3, 4). In this chapter, we describe the experimental procedures as well as additional considerations regarding the study of miRNAs function in monocytopoiesis, including isolation of CD34+ HPCs for unilineage monocytic (Mo) culture, northern blotting analysis of miRNAs expression, and ectopic expression of miRNAs using oligonucleotide transfection or lentiviral transduction.

2. Materials

2.1. CD34+ HPCs Isolation

1. Heparin sodium (Sigma, St. Louis, MO) is dissolved in water at 50 mg/ml and stored at 2–8°C.
2. Penicillin–streptomycin solution (P/S) 1×10^4 U/ml–10 mg/ml (EuroClone, West York, UK).
3. MACS buffer: phosphate-buffered saline (PBS) solution without Ca^{++}/Mg^{++} pH 7.2 (Gibco BRL, Bethesda, MD), 0.5% (w/v) bovine serum albumin (BSA) (EuroClone), 2 mM EDTA (Gibco BRL).
4. Lympholyte (Cedarlane, Burlington, NC) for mononuclear cells (MNCs) isolation from cord blood (CB).
5. Ammonium chloride solution (StemCell Technologies, Vancouver, BC, Canada).
6. Iscove's modified Dulbecco's medium (IMDM) (Gibco BRL).
7. Vacuum filtration system Stericup-GP, 0.22 μm (Millipore, Billerica, MA).
8. MACS Columns and MACS Separator (Miltenyi Biotech, Bergisch Gladbach, Germany).
9. FcR blocking reagent (Miltenyi Biotech).
10. CD34 Microbeads (Miltenyi Biotech).
11. PE-conjugated CD34 antibody for FACS analysis (BD Biosciences, Franklin Lakes, NJ).

2.2. Unilineage Mo Culture Analysis

2.2.1. Unilineage Mo Culture

1. IMDM (Gibco BRL).
2. BSA (Sigma) is dissolved as a 10% (w/v) stock solution in IMDM and stored at –20°C.
3. Fe-saturated human apo-transferrin (Sigma) is dissolved in IMDM at 70 mg/ml and stored at –20°C.

4. Human low-density lipoprotein (Sigma) is dissolved at 5 mg/ml in IMDM, as a single use aliquot to be used immediately (see Note 1).
5. Insulin (Sigma) is dissolved in IMDM/1% (w/v) BSA at 1 mg/ml and stored at −20°C.
6. Sodium pyruvate (Sigma) is dissolved in IMDM at 10 mM and stored at −20°C.
7. L-glutamine (Sigma) is disolved in IMDM at 200 mM and stored at −20°C.
8. α-tiomonoglycerol is dissolved in IMDM at 10^{-2} M and stored at −20°C.
9. Inorganic elements: Na_2SiO_3, $MnSO_4$, $(NH_4)_6Mo_7O_{24}$, NH_4VO_3, $NiCl_2$, $SnCl_2$ (Merck, Whitehouse Station, NJ) supplemented with iron sulfate ($FeSO_4$) are prepared as a 4×10^{-6} M solution in IMDM and stored at −20°C.
10. Nucleosides (Sigma) are dissolved in IMDM at 1 mg each/ml.
11. Human recombinant growth factors (HGFs): Flt3 ligand, IL-6, are M-CSF (Peprotech, Rocky Hill, NJ) are prepared as 100 mg/ml, 1 mg/ml, and 1×10^5 U/ml stock solutions in PBS/0.1% (w/v) BSA, respectively, and stored at −20°C.
12. Serum-free medium for unilineage Mo culture is prepared as follows: freshly prepared IMDM is supplemented with BSA (10 mg/ml), Fe-saturated human apo-transferrin (700 μg/ml), human low-density lipoprotein (40 μg/ml), insulin (10 μg/ml), sodium pyruvate (10^{-4} M), L-glutamine (2×10^{-3} M), α-tiomonoglycerol (10^{-4} M), rare inorganic elements (Na_2SiO_3, $MnSO_4$, $(NH_4)_6Mo_7O_{24}$, NH_4VO_3, $NiCl_2$, $SnCl_2$) supplemented with iron sulfate (4×10^{-8} M), and nucleosides (10 μg/ml each). HGFs are freshly added at the following concentrations: Flt3 ligand 100 ng/ml, IL-6 1 ng/ml, and M-CSF 100 U/ml.
13. Trypan blue 0.4% solution (Sigma).

2.2.2. Phenotypic and Morphological Characterization of Unilineage Mo Culture

1. Superfrost glass slides (Thermo Fisher Scientific, Waltham, MA).
2. Wright-Giemsa stain, modified (Sigma).
3. Accustain-Giemsa stain, modified (Sigma).
4. FITC-conjugated or APC-conjugated anti-CD14 and PE-conjugated anti-CD34 antibodies, and conjugated isotype-matched Igs for FACS analysis (BD Biosciences).

2.3. miRNAs Analysis by Northern Blot

1. 2× RNA loading buffer: 89 mM Tris-HCl, 89 mM boric acid, 2 mM EDTA, pH 8, 12% (w/v) Ficoll, 0.01% (w/v) bromophenol blue, 0.02% (w/v) xylene cyanol, 7 mM urea.
2. 15% acrylamide urea-denaturing precast gel (Invitrogen, Carlsbad, CA).

3. 1× TBE running buffer.
4. Ethidium bromide (Et-Br).
5. 3 MM paper.
6. Trans-Blot Electrophoretic Transfer apparatus (Invitrogen).
7. Hybond-N+ membrane (Amersham Biosciences, Little-Chalfont, UK).
8. 20 bp Molecular ruler (BIO-RAD, Hercules, CA).
9. 20× SSC: 3 M NaCl, 0.3 M NaCitrate.
10. 20× SSPE: 3 M NaCl, 200 mM NaH2PO4, 20 mM EDTA.
11. Polynucleotide kinase (New England Biolabs, Ipswich, MA).
12. 32P-γATP.
13. G-25 MicroSpin Columns (Amersham Pharmacia, Piscataway, NJ).
14. Autoradiography film (Kodak, Rochester, NY).
15. Chemi Doc software (Minneapolis, MN, USA).

2.4. Transfection of Mo Culture with miRNAs

1. Lipofectamine 2000 (Invitrogen).
2. Optimem (Gibco BRL).
3. Stability enhanced miRNA (Dharmacon, Lafayette, CO). Dissolve miRNA at a concentration of 75 μM in the buffer provided by the manufacturer and store at –80°C (see Note 2).
4. 24-well plates (BD Falcon, Franklin Lakes, NJ).

2.5. Infection of Mo Culture with Lentivirus

1. Packaging vector: pCMVΔR8.74; Envelope plasmid: pMD.G; Transfer vector pRRL.cPPT-CMV-PGK-GFP-WPRE (Tween) (5).
2. 293T Packaging cell line [American Type Culture Collection (ATCC), Manassas, VA].
3. Dulbecco's modified Eagle medium (DMEM), fetal bovine serum (FBS), P/S, l-glutamine, PBS (Gibco BRL).
4. $CaCl_2$ solution: 2.5 M $CaCl_2$ in 100 ml of HPLC-purified H_2O. Filter through 0.22-μm filter. Aliquot in 10 ml tubes and freeze at –20°C. Keep one working tube at 4°C.
5. 2× HBS solution: 8.0 g NaCl, 0.37 g KCl, 0.19 g Na_2HPO_4 $7H_2O$, 1 g dextrose, and 5 g HEPES in 500 ml of HPLC-purified H_2O pH 7.1. Filter through 0.22-μm filter. Aliquot and freeze at –20°C.
6. Polybrene (hexadimethrine bromide, Sigma).
7. dNTPs (Invitrogen).
8. Vacuum filtration system Stericup-HV, 0.45 μm (Millipore).

3. Methods

3.1. CD34+ HPCs Isolation

1. CB is collected from healthy, full-term placentas according to institutional guidelines.
2. Dilute CB 1:4 in PBS + 1% penicillin–streptomycin. Lay 35 ml of diluted blood over 15 ml lympholyte in 50-ml Falcon tubes. Proceed to the density gradient centrifugation: centrifuge at 400 × *g* for 45 min with no brake and acceleration at 20°C.
3. Gently remove the low-density MNCs ring at the interphase of plasma (upper layer) and density medium (lower layer) and transfer it into a 250-ml disposable conical tube. Fill the tube with PBS. Centrifuge at 400 × *g* for 15 min at 20°C. If the pellet is well separated (the supernatant is not opaque), remove all but 5 ml of the supernatant. If the supernatant is opaque, replace one-third of supernatant with fresh PBS and repeat the wash.
4. If the cell pellet is white colored for overnight storage, remove all but 5 ml of supernatant, transfer into a 50-ml Falcon tube, add IMDM to a final volume of 50 ml, and keep at 2–8°C. For immediate CD34 staining and separation, add MACS buffer to the pellet to a final volume of 50 ml. If the cell pellet is red colored due to the presence of erythrocytes, resuspend in PBS up to 50 ml and proceed to the red cells lysis using ammonium chloride.
5. Ammonium chloride lysis: centrifuge at 400 × *g* for 10 min at 4°C, remove the supernatant, break up the pellet with ammonium chloride lysis solution 1:5, and incubate on ice or at 4°C for 10 min. Fill the tube with PBS and centrifuge. Remove the supernatant, which will be red in case of good lysis; if the supernatant is not red, repeat the lysis. Once the pellet is white colored, add MACS buffer to 50 ml and count the cells. Resuspend the cells in 300 μl for up to 10^8 cells and proceed with CD34+ magnetic separation.
6. For up to 10^8 cells (in 300 μl), add 100 μl of FcR blocking reagent and 10 μl of CD34 Microbeads, mix well, and refrigerate for 30 min at 2–8°C.
7. Wash cells by adding 5–10 ml of MACS buffer and centrifuge at 300 × *g* for 10 min. Remove supernatant, resuspend the cells in 500 μl of MACS buffer, and proceed with magnetic separation.
8. When using LS Columns, dilute up to 3 ml with MACS buffer. Apply cell suspension onto the column, collect the unlabelled fraction that pass through, and wash three times with 3 ml of MACS buffer (collect each of the unlabelled fractions).
9. Remove the column from the magnetic separator and change the collection tube. Add 5 ml to the column and firmly push

the plunger into the column to collect the labeled fraction. To increase the purity of the cells, proceed to a second round of isolation in a newly prepared column.

10. Keep the cells in ice for 30 min. To evaluate the purity of the isolated HPCs, stain with PE-conjugated CD34+ antibody and proceed to flow cytometry analysis (see Note 3).

3.2. Unilineage Mo Culture Analysis

3.2.1. Unilineage Mo Culture

1. CD34+ HPCs are cultured in a fully humidified 5% CO_2 5% O_2 atmosphere, in serum-free medium in the presence of various recombinant human cytokine combinations. Serum-free medium composition for unilineage Mo culture is described in the Subheading 2.
2. Cells are counted every 2–3 days and constantly kept at the optimal concentration of 2×10^5 cells/ml. Viable cells are counted using Trypan blue staining: briefly mix 0.2 ml of cells with 0.5 ml of Trypan blue 0.4% solution and 0.3 ml of PBS, wait for 5 min (no more than 15 min), and proceed to count. Under such selected conditions, highly purified HPCs proliferate significantly, reaching 100–400-fold cell expansion as shown in Fig. 1.

3.2.2. Phenotypic and Morphologic Characterization of Unilineage Mo Culture

1. Cell differentiation in unilineage Mo culture is monitored at each cell count: every 2–3 days proceed to single or double color staining for FACS analysis using CD34 and CD14 antibodies and the appropriate isotype-matched Igs. Pellet 5×10^4 cells, resuspend them in 90 μl of MACS buffer plus 10 μl of FcR blocking reagent, and incubate at 4°C for 30 min with 1–2 μg of antibody. Wash twice with PBS/0.1% BSA and analyze on a FACS instrument. Standard kinetics of CD34 and CD14 antigens' expression during unilineage Mo culture is displayed in Fig. 2a (see Note 4).

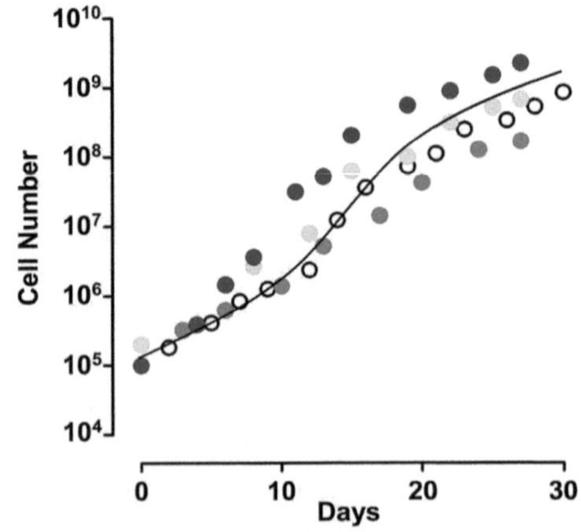

Fig. 1. Average cell proliferation in unilineage Mo culture of HPCs. Growth curve is represented as an absolute number of total viable cells (Trypan blue negative) at discrete days of culture.

2. To evaluate morphology and cell differentiation through the monocytic pathway, cells are harvested from day 2–3 to day 30. At each time point, collect 2×10^4 cells, wash in cold PBS/1% BSA, and resuspend in 200 μl of PBS/1% BSA. Pretreat glass slides and filters with PBS/1% BSA by centrifugation for 5 min at 400 rpm in a Shandon cytospin cytocentrifuge. Aliquot each sample into the corresponding well of the cytospin and centrifuge again for 5 min at 400 rpm in a Shandon cytospin cytocentrifuge. Dry the slides overnight under a laminar flow cabinet or in a desiccation chamber. The next day, proceed with staining: dip glass slides in diluted Giemsa stain (1:20, v/v) for 30 s. Wash with PBS and dip slides in undiluted Wright-Giemsa stain for 10 min, then, wash with H_2O, and let them air-dry in vertical position. Once the slides are dry, morphology is evaluated by conventional light field microscopy under magnification 400× (see Note 5). Count at least 500 cells per slide, and graph values as percentage of total cells (Fig. 2b).
3. The different stages of monocytic maturation from CD34+ HPCs are represented by the following cell types: blasts are immature, undifferentiated progenitor cells which gradually disappear in culture by day 10. Monoblasts are the first recognizable cells of the monocytic series: they measure from 13 to 20 μm in diameter and are characterized by a deep-blue cytoplasm and a large, eccentric, centrally indented nucleus with fine chromatin structure and one or two large nucleoli (Fig. 2c). Promonocytes emerge from day 6 to 8: they are larger cells with a lobated nucleus, slightly indented, and a clear blue cytoplasm containing few azurophilic granules (Fig. 2d). Monocytes represent approximately 50% of the cellular composition by day 15 and are recognizable by a reniform nucleus that occupies half of the cell volume and a finely granulated, gray-blue cytoplasm (Fig. 2e). The last step of maturation is represented by macrophages, which are large cells recognizable by an eccentric small nucleus and a highly vacuolated cytoplasm (Fig. 2f).

3.3. miRNAs Analysis by Northern Blot

1. Sample preparation: add 10–30 μg of RNA (diluted in H_2O up to 15–20 μl) to an equal volume of 2× RNA loading buffer. Denature at 70°C for 10 min.
2. Load the sample into the 15% polyacrylamide gel and run at 100–120 V for 80–90 min, until the xylene cyanol is 2–3 cm above the end of the gel.
3. Stain the gel with Et-Br (4 μg/ml) in 1× TBE for 10 min with shaking and take a picture with Chemi Doc software.
4. Blotting: equilibrate the gel and soak the membrane (Hybond-N+), filter paper, and fiber pads in transfer buffer (1× TBE) for 10 min. Assemble the gel sandwich as follows:

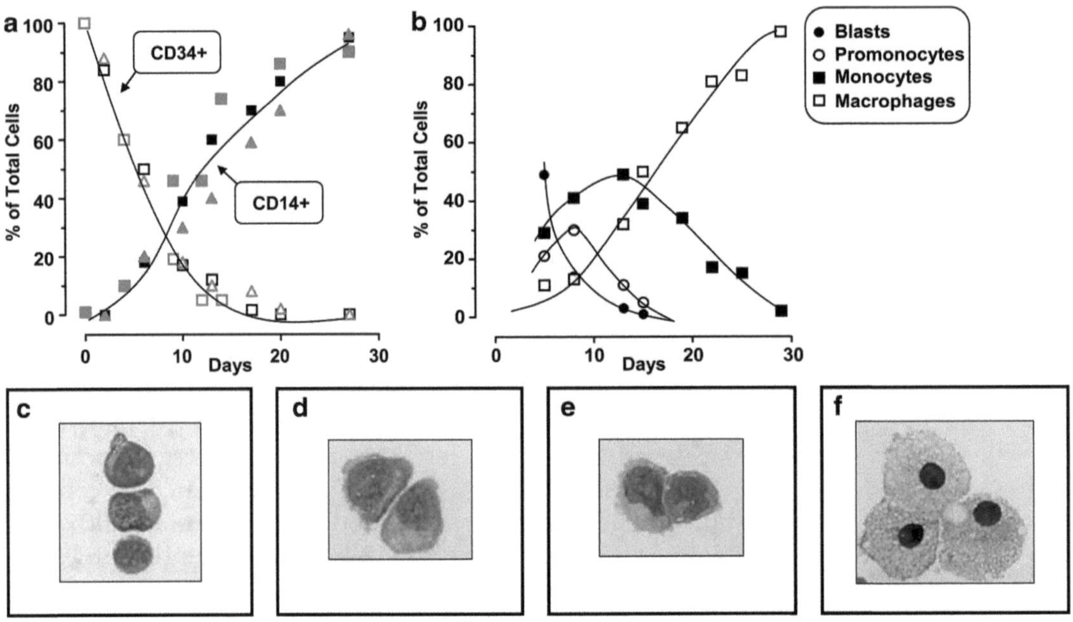

Fig. 2. Phenotypic and morphologic characterization of unilineage monocytic (Mo) culture. (**a**) Percentage of CD34 and CD14 positive cells at discrete sequential stages of unilineage Mo culture. The gradual decline in CD34+ positive cells correspond to the increase in CD14+ monocytic cells. (**b**) Schematic representation of Wright–Giemsa staining of unilineage Mo culture at various stages. Visibly, differentiation/maturation to the monocytic pathway proceed in sequential waves. Typical morphologic features of cells from unilineage Mo culture: (**c**) Monoblasts, (**d**) Promonocytes, (**e**) Monocytes, and (**f**) Macrophages (original magnification ×400).

- Cassette with negative side
- Prewetted fiber pad
- 3 MM filter paper (three sheets)
- Equilibrated gel
- Prewetted membrane
- 3 MM filter paper (three sheets)
- Prewetted fiber pad
- Cassette with positive side

Use a glass tube to gently roll air bubbles out. Run at 20 V overnight.

5. Cross-link the membrane at 80°C for 2 h.
6. Label the oligonucleotide by adding: 200 ng oligo, 6 μl ^{32}P-γATP, 4 μl 10× kinase buffer, 2 μl kinase enzyme, H_2O up to 20 μl (see Note 6). Incubate at 37°C for 1 h. Add 30 μl H_2O and purify the probe from unincorporated label with G-25 MicroSpin Columns (see Note 7).
7. Prehybridize the membrane in 6× SSC/0.1% SDS for at least 3 h at 37°C. Add the probe (40×10^6 cpm) to the prehybridization solution and incubate overnight at 37°C (see Note 8).

Wash the membrane at room temperature two times with 2× SSC/0.1% SDS and one time with 3× SSC (every wash lasts 15 min). Wet the membrane and expose with an autoradiographic film for at least an overnight (see Note 9).

8. The membrane can be hybridized with different probes (see Note 10). In this case, it has to be first dehybridized. Add in a beaker 500 ml of 0.1% SSPE/0.05% SDS and heat until the solution has reached 65°C. Add the membrane and leave until the solution arrives at room temperature. Wet the membrane and expose for an overnight. If you do not detect any signal you can proceed with the next hybridization (starting from the prehybridization step). Human tRNA for initiator methionine (tRNA-Met) is used as loading control. The sequence of the probe is: 5′-TGGTAGCAGAGGATGG TTTCGATCCATCGACCTCTG-3′.

3.4. Transfection of Mo Culture with miRNAs

1. CD34+ HPCs are transfected at day 5 of monocytic differentiation. Harvest cells needed for the experiment, centrifuge at 400 × *g* for 10 min, and resuspend in Mo medium w/o antibiotics at a density of 1.25×10^6 cells/ml. Add 500 ml of cell suspension into each well in a 24-well plate. Keep cells in the incubator.
2. Thaw the miRNA on ice. In a 1.5-ml Eppendorf tube, add 7.5 μl of 20 μM miRNA plus 50 μl of Optimem and mix well.
3. Prepare the Lipofectamine 2000 mix (if you have several samples prepare one mix for all the samples) by adding 1 μl of Lipofectamine 2000 plus 50 μl of Optimem. Mix well and incubate at room temperature for 5 min (the incubation should not be longer than 20 min).
4. Add 51 μl of the Lipofectamine 2000 mix to the miRNA previously diluted in Optimem and incubate at room temperature for 20 min.
5. Add the Lipofectamine 2000/miRNA mix to the cells and incubate at 37°C for 4 h.
6. Centrifuge cells at 400 × *g* for 10 min, remove the medium, and add complete Mo medium. Incubate cells at 37°C until further analysis.

3.5. Infection of Mo Culture with Lentivirus

1. Lentiviral production: lentiviral particles are generated by transient transfection in 293T cells using the three-plasmid system as described earlier (6). Plate 2.5×10^6 293T cells in a 150 × 25 mm Petri dish the day before transfection (see Note 11). On the day of transfection, replace with fresh medium at least 2 h before transfection. Thaw $CaCl_2$ and 2× HBS at room temperature. Mix in a 15-ml Falcon tube the DNA plasmids at the following concentrations in 900 μl of sterile H_2O:

Transfer vector	20 μg
Packaging vector	13 μg
Envelope vector	7 μg

2. Add 100 μl of $CaCl_2$ 2.5 M dropwise to the DNA solution. Mix by finger tapping. Add 1 ml of 2× HBS in dropwise fashion and mix by vigorously bubbling with an automatic pipettor for about 10–15 s. Add transfection mixture dropwise to the plate, gently swirl around, immediately put the plate back in the incubator at 37°C, and leave overnight (for about 16 h) (see Note 12).
3. Change medium after overnight incubation. Viral supernatant can be harvested 24 and 48 h post-transfection: filter supernatant using 0.45 μm membranes, snap-freeze aliquots, and store at −80°C. Viral supernatants concentration can be determined by infection of HeLa or 293T cells using serial dilutions of virus and analyzing cells at 48 h by FACS for the ratio of GFP+ cells. Average functional titers of viral vectors range from 8×10^7 to 7×10^8 particles/ml (see Note 13).
4. Lentiviral transduction: the day before transduction, isolate CD34+ HPCs and plate them in Mo medium at 2×10^5 cells/ml. Keep cells in the incubator overnight. The next day, centrifuge cells at $400 \times g$ for 10 min and place them in a six-well plate with the viral supernatant at 1×10^5 cells/ml and approximately 8×10^7 particles/ml (adjust volume with IMDM). Add polybrene at 4 μg/ml. Proceed with spin-inoculation (7): centrifuge cells at $1{,}000 \times g$ for 45 min at 32°C; place cells in incubator at 37°C for 1 h and 15 min. Following transduction, remove the medium containing viral particles, wash twice with warm PBS, and plate cells in Mo medium, supplemented with sterile dNTPs at a final concentration of 50 μM, in incubator at 37°C. 48 h post-transduction, sort GFP+ cells by flow cytometry. Average transduction efficiency measured as percentage of GFP+ cells range from 20 to 40% (see Note 14).

4. Notes

1. LDL is highly viscous. Do not freeze stock solution, always use freshly prepared.
2. From the 75 μM stock solution, prepare diluted aliquots at a concentration of 20 μM to be used for the experiments. Do not thaw the 20 μM aliquot more than three times.
3. Using freshly collected CB is mandatory for a suitable isolation of healthy CD34+. Collection of CB should be managed

in Falcon tubes containing PBS, 200 U/ml Heparin sodium, and 1% P/S solution in a total of 5 ml. When working with lympholyte (or Ficoll-Paque), keep in mind that Ficoll is light sensitive. While proceeding to the magnetic labeling, work fast and keep cells cold at each step to prevent nonspecific labeling; remove possible cell clumps that might form during this stage using a needle syringe, since it might clog the column. Everything must be sterile at any moment. It is critical for optimal unilineage culture to avoid initial contaminants: CD34+ cells must be >95% pure.

4. When analyzing GFP-transduced cells, make sure to use an APC-conjugated CD14 antibody due to saturation of the FITC channel by the GFP signal.
5. Cytocentrifugates for morphologic analysis can be prepared with fewer cells (down to 2×10^3 cells), but this will lead to a reduced statistical significance of the method.
6. When you label the oligonucleotide against the tRNA-Met, use 3 μl of enzyme.
7. The probe can be stored at −20°C for up to 1 week.
8. When using the probe against the tRNA-Met, add 5×10^6 cpm of labeled oligonucleotide.
9. If you do not see any signal after an overnight, expose for longer time (up to 1 week). When using the probe against the tRNA-Met expose the film for 1 h.
10. The membrane can be dehybridized for a maximum of three times. The probe against the tRNA-Met should be used as last probe.
11. 293T cells can be routinely used until the 15th passage (corresponding to roughly 1 month of continuous culture), as they dramatically lose the ability to produce virus with passaging. Never reach confluence when culturing.
12. Do not store 2× HBS in the fridge for more than 2 weeks; avoid thawing 2× HBS and $CaCl_2$ at 37°C. pH 7.1 for the 2× HBS is crucial for the reaction: following 2–3 h from the addition of the Calcium Phosphate–DNA complexes to the culture medium, when observing the cells under a microscope, one should observe evenly distributed small precipitates on the bottom of the flask. Too high pH will result in large precipitates, while too low pH will result in no precipitates. An imbalanced pH will result in cytotoxicity for 293T cells and will jeopardize the virus production.
13. In our experience with unilineage culture of HPCs, we advise against transduction using concentrated viral particles, as this generally leads to increase cytotoxicity. Cytokine prestimulation (8) greatly increases transduction efficiency but will alter

the course of the unilineage culture in terms of proliferation and differentiation timing: pretreatment with IL-3, SCF, Flt3 ligand, and TPO would accelerate Mo differentiation and increase the proportion of contaminants. When spin-inoculating, keep centrifuge at constant 32°C, as temperature is critical for the virus to enter the target cells. Adding dNTPs post-transduction increases the reverse transcriptase activity of the viral RNA.

14. GFP expression might gradually decrease during culture when using lentiviral vectors as transgene-delivery systems, as cells progressively condensate their chromatin during differentiation. Therefore, GFP expression should be monitored constantly when collecting and analyzing cells.

Acknowledgments

This work was supported by the Italy–USA Oncology Program and the Biotechnology Program, Istituto Superiore di Sanità, and Associazione Italiana per la Ricerca sul Cancro (AIRC) to C.P.

References

1. Orkin, S. H., and Zon, L. I. (2008) Hematopoiesis: an evolving paradigm for stem cell biology, *Cell 132*, 631–644.
2. Gordon, S., and Taylor, P. R. (2005) Monocyte and macrophage heterogeneity, *Nat Rev Immunol 5*, 953–964.
3. Fontana, L., Pelosi, E., Greco, P., Racanicchi, S., Testa, U., Liuzzi, F., Croce, C. M., Brunetti, E., Grignani, F., and Peschle, C. (2007) MicroRNAs 17-5p-20a-106a control monocytopoiesis through AML1 targeting and M-CSF receptor upregulation, *Nat Cell Biol 9*, 775–787.
4. Rosa, A., Ballarino, M., Sorrentino, A., Sthandier, O., De Angelis, F. G., Marchioni, M., Masella, B., Guarini, A., Fatica, A., Peschle, C., and Bozzoni, I. (2007) The interplay between the master transcription factor PU.1 and miR-424 regulates human monocyte/macrophage differentiation, *Proc Natl Acad Sci U S A 104*, 19849–19854.
5. Bonci, D., Cittadini, A., Latronico, M. V., Borello, U., Aycock, J. K., Drusco, A., Innocenzi, A., Follenzi, A., Lavitrano, M., Monti, M. G., Ross, J., Jr., Naldini, L., Peschle, C., Cossu, G., and Condorelli, G. (2003) "Advanced" generation lentiviruses as efficient vectors for cardiomyocyte gene transduction in vitro and in vivo, *Gene Ther 10*, 630–636.
6. Naldini, L., Blomer, U., Gallay, P., Ory, D., Mulligan, R., Gage, F. H., Verma, I. M., and Trono, D. (1996) In vivo gene delivery and stable transduction of nondividing cells by a lentiviral vector, *Science 272*, 263–267.
7. Bahnson, A. B., Dunigan, J. T., Baysal, B. E., Mohney, T., Atchison, R. W., Nimgaonkar, M. T., Ball, E. D., and Barranger, J. A. (1995) Centrifugal enhancement of retroviral mediated gene transfer, *J Virol Methods 54*, 131–143.
8. Geronimi, F., Richard, E., Redonnet-Vernhet, I., Lamrissi-Garcia, I., Lalanne, M., Ged, C., Moreau-Gaudry, F., and De Verneuil, H. (2003) Highly efficient lentiviral gene transfer in CD34+ and CD34+/38–/lin- cells from mobilized peripheral blood after cytokine prestimulation, *Stem Cells 21*, 472–480.

Chapter 12

MicroRNA Activity in B Lymphocytes

Virginia G. de Yébenes and Almudena R. Ramiro

Abstract

Gene expression regulation by miRNAs has been reported to control key aspects of B cell differentiation and function (Chen et al., Science 303:83–86, 2004; Xiao et al., Cell 131:146–159, 2007; O'Carroll et al., Genes Dev. 21:1999–2004, 2007; Koralov et al. Cell 132:860–874, 2008; Rodriguez et al., Science 316:608–611, 2007; Costinean et al., Proc Natl Acad Sci USA 103:7024–7029, 2006; Thai et al., Science 316:604–608, 2007; Vigorito et al., Immunity 27:847–859, 2007; Dorsett et al., Immunity 28:630–638, 2008; Teng et al., Immunity 28:621–629, 2008; de Yebenes et al., J Exp Med 205:2199–2206, 2008; He et al., Nature 435:828–833, 2005; Ventura et al. Cell 132:875–886, 2008; Xiao et al., Nat Immunol 9:405–414, 2008). In this chapter, we describe the methodology used to perform a functional screening of a miRNA library to identify miRNAs relevant for mature B cell function in primary mouse B cells. These procedures include the construction of a miRNA library and the expression of individual miRNA clones in spleen B cells, as well as the description of functional assays used to determine the impact of miRNA expression on several aspects of B cell function, such as proliferation, apoptosis, and class switch recombination.

1. Introduction

MicroRNAs (miRNAs) are ubiquitous small noncoding RNA molecules that regulate posttranscriptional gene expression by modifying the stability and/or the translation efficiency of their target mRNAs. The study of miRNA function in lymphocytes is of broad interest since miRNA-driven control has emerged as a key regulatory element in the development and function of T and B lymphocytes (reviewed in (1)). miRNA expression can be modified in B lymphocytes using different methodological strategies that involve the generation of animal models or in vitro assays to study miRNA function.

Animal models of genetic gain and loss of miRNA function are used to study the role of a particular miRNA in an in vivo context. Different animal models to study the function of miRNA

Silvia Monticelli (ed.), *MicroRNAs and the Immune System: Methods and Protocols*, Methods in Molecular Biology, vol. 667,
DOI 10.1007/978-1-60761-811-9_12, © Springer Science+Business Media, LLC 2010

in B lymphocytes have been reported: (1) miRNA transgenics that overexpress a miRNA in B cell precursors and/or mature B lymphocytes (2–4), (2) bone marrow (BM) chimera mouse models in which the mice are reconstituted with transduced BM precursors overexpressing a particular miRNA (5, 6), (3) miRNA knockouts in which the miRNA is depleted in B lymphocytes (3, 7–10), (4) global miRNA depletion in B cell precursors by specific deletion of dicer, the enzyme required for miRNA processing (11) or Ago2, a component of RNA-induced silencing complex (12), and (5) transgenics or knock-ins harboring a mutation in the binding site of a miRNA target allows to assess the effect of the loss of a specific mRNA–miRNA interaction (13, 14).

In spite of the usefulness of in vivo gain- and loss-of-function approaches, in vitro experiments can provide, in some cases, a more convenient and straightforward means to study miRNA function: (1) They allow the functional screening of a large number of miRNAs, such as miRNA collections cloned in expression libraries; this type of screening can, in turn, be used to identify candidate miRNAs for subsequent study through in vivo approaches. (2) They can be used to identify the specific mRNA sequence that is targeted by a miRNA. (3) They are considerably more time saving than the generation of mouse models. Gain of miRNA function in primary B cells and B cell precursors can be accomplished efficiently with retroviral transduction techniques (5, 15). Gain of function experiments in B cell lines can be done by retroviral and lentiviral transduction (16, 17) as well as by transfection with miRNA duplexes (18, 19). B cell lines have also been used for loss of miRNA function assays by transfection with anti-miRNA oligonucleotides (16, 18, 20).

In this chapter, we detail the methodology used to perform a functional screening of a miRNA library in primary B cells. When undertaking this kind of screening, the single most important factor to consider is the availability of in vitro assays that will allow testing of the functional aspects of interest in a simple, fast, and quantitative manner. Here, we describe the procedures to clone a miRNA library and express the individual miRNA clones in spleen B cells, as well as the readouts used to determine the impact of miRNA expression on several aspects of B cell function, including proliferation, apoptosis, and class switch recombination (CSR) (see an outline in Fig. 1).

2. Materials

2.1. miRNA Retroviral Constructs

1. Proteinase K buffer: 50 mM Tris-HCL pH 8, 200 mM NaCl, 10 mM EDTA, 1% SDS, 400 μg/ml proteinase K (Roche).
2. Phenol–chloroform–isoamyl alcohol 25:24:1 (Sigma).

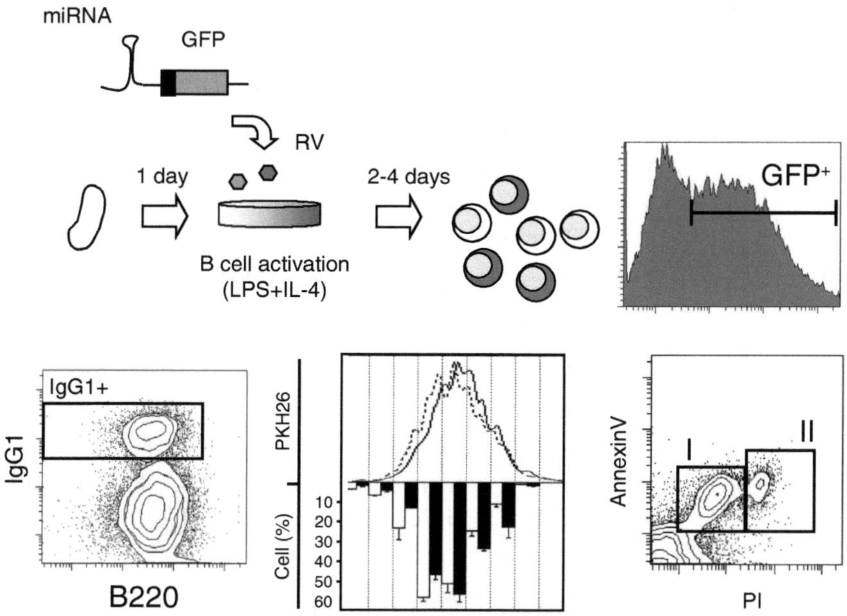

Fig. 1. Overview of procedures for the functional screening of a miRNA library in B cells. To asses miRNA function in primary B cells, retroviral supernatants from a miRNA library are used to transduce primary mouse spleen B cells. Transduced cells are identified by the expression of a reporter protein such as GFP. Several aspects of B cell function, such as CSR, proliferation, and apoptosis, can be used as readouts to determine the functional impact of miRNA expression. The figure shows a representative flow cytometry analysis of GFP expression (*top right histogram*), IgG1 CSR efficiency analysis (*bottom left contour plot*), PKH26 proliferation analysis (*bottom middle histogram and charts*), and apoptosis analysis (*bottom right contour plot*) in which early (AnnexinV$^+$ PI$^-$) and late (Annexin V$^+$PI$^+$) apoptosis cells subsets are identified (gates I and II, respectively).

3. Absolute ethanol.
4. Specific pre-miRNA primers.
5. PfuUltra high-fidelity polymerase (Roche).
6. DNTPs (Roche).
7. EcoR I (New England Biolabs).
8. Xho I (New England Biolabs).

2.2. Isolation and Culture of Primary Mouse B Lymphocytes

1. C57/BL/6J mice (Jackson Laboratory).
2. 70 μm nylon cell strainer (BD Falcon).
3. Phosphate-buffered saline (PBS).
4. Fetal calf serum (FCS).
5. AcK lysing buffer (BioWhittaker).
6. Mouse CD43 MicroBeads (Miltenyi Biotec).
7. MS Columns (Miltenyi Biotec).
8. MiniMACS separation unit (Miltenyi Biotec).
9. Antimouse B220-PE antibody (BD Pharmingen).

10. B cell medium: RPMI 1640 medium (Sigma) with 10% FCS, 50 μM β-mercaptoethanol, 10 mM HEPES, 10 ng/ml mouse IL-4 (Peprotech), and 25 μg/ml LPS (Sigma-Aldrich).
11. Flat-bottomed tissue culture multiwell plates.
12. PKH26GL labeling kit (Sigma-Aldrich).

2.3. Retroviral Transduction

1. 293T cells (ATCC).
2. Complete DMEM medium: DMEM with 10% FCS.
3. Complete RPMI medium: RPMI with 10% FCS.
4. Trypsin–EDTA.
5. Pre-miRNA and PCL-Eco (Imgenex) DNA preparations.
6. 2× HeBS: 280 mM NaCl, 10 mM KCl, 1.5 mM Na_2HPO_4, 12 mM (*d*)-glucose, 50 mM HEPES, pH 7.00 adjusted with 0.5 N NaOH in cell-culture grade H_2O.
7. 2.5 M $CaCl_2$.
8. Polybrene (Sigma-Aldrich).
9. 0.45 μm filters.

2.4. Quantification of Transduction and miRNA Processing Efficiency

1. Propidium iodide (PI).
2. Trizol (Invitrogen).
3. Chloroform.
4. Molecular biology-grade water.
5. SuperScript II reverse transcriptase (Invitrogen).
6. Random primers (Roche).
7. DNTPs (Roche).
8. RNaseOUT (Invitrogen).
9. Specific pre-miRNA primers.
10. Specific mouse GAPDH primers: forward-5′-TGAAGCAG-GCATCTGAGGG-3′ and reverse-5′-CGAAGGTGGAAGA-GTGGGAG-3′.
11. SYBR green PCR master mix (Applied Biosystems).
12. 96-well qPCR plates (Applied Biosystems).
13. Adhesive film for PCR plates (Applied Biosystems).
14. Real-time quantitative PCR system.
15. Specifc miRNA and small RNA endogenous control primers for reverse transcription and subsequent real time PCR (TaqMan MicroRNA Assays; Applied Biosystems).
16. TaqMan microRNA Reverse Transcription Kit (Applied Biosystems).
17. TaqMan 2× Universal PCR Master Mix, No AmpErase UNG (Applied Biosystems).

2.5. Effect of miRNA Overexpression in Mature B Cells

1. DAPI.
2. Annexin V-APC (BD Pharmingen).
3. Propidium iodide (PI).
4. Staining buffer: PBS 1×, 1% FCS, 1% BSA and 0.01% NaN_3.
5. Anti-mouse IgG1 biotin antibody (BD Pharmingen).
6. Anti-mouse B220-PE antibody (BD Pharmingen).
7. Streptavidin-APC (BD Pharmingen).
8. 7-AAD.
9. Flow cytometer with UV or violet, blue, and red laser lines.
10. ModFit flow cytometry analysis software (Verity Software House).

3. Methods

3.1. Design of Retroviral Constructs for miRNA Expression

To ectopically express miRNAs in primary mouse B cells, we have used a miRNA library comprising 150 individual microRNAs cloned in a retroviral vector that harbors GFP as a reporter protein. DNA fragments corresponding to 150 pre-miRNAs and their flanking 50-bp long genomic sequences were PCR-amplified and cloned in the pre-miRNA GFP plasmid (15). Using this experimental system, transduced B cells express constitutively the pre-miRNA precursor and GFP under the control of CMV and SV40 promoters, respectively.

When designing vectors for miRNA overexpression, several issues should be considered. An important aspect is choosing an appropriate reporter gene. GFP is currently the most frequently used reporter gene owing to its suitability for flow cytometry and fluorescent microscopy detection, although other fluorescent proteins such as YFP, Orange, and DsRed can be as well suited for these applications. The use of nonfluorescent reporters, such as truncated cell surface molecules, can be considered as an adequate alternative if the assays to be performed in the screening routinely involve isolation of transduced cells. The second factor that should be considered is the optimization of the pre-miRNA genomic context that is cloned in the vector. We and others (*5*) have observed that the position and size of genomic context can influence the expression and processing of the pre-miRNA precursor in a miRNA-specific fashion. Therefore, when possible it is advisable to design several constructs containing variations of the genomic context included in the retroviral vector and to check pre-miRNA expression in transduced cells (see Subheading 3.4) to identify the construct with the highest expression.

To generate miRNA pre-miRNA GFP retroviral constructs:

1. Design PCR primers to amplify the pre-miRNA of interest: obtain pre-miRNA sequences from Sanger miRNA Registry (http://microrna.sanger.ac.uk/sequences/), retrieve flanking genomic sequences (http://www.ncbi.nlm.nih.gov/Genomes/), and design primers with XhoI/EcoRI sites to amplify the appropriate fragments.
2. Prepare genomic DNA from mouse primary cells by standard procedures.
3. Amplify genomic DNA using XhoI/EcoRI primers and PCR with a high-fidelity polymerase.
4. Clone in pre-miRNA GFP XhoI/EcoRI sites. Verify cloning by sequencing.

3.2. Isolation and Culture of Primary Mouse B Lymphocytes

3.2.1. Isolation of Mouse Spleen B Lymphocytes by Magnetic Cell Sorting

This protocol describes the isolation of mouse spleen primary B cells using a magnetic depletion technique. Cell magnetic separation is based on the labeling of a cell surface antigen with a specific antibody that is coupled to magnetic beads. A mixture containing labeled and unlabeled cells is passed through a column placed within a strong magnetic field that will retain labeled cells. In the case of magnetic depletion, the cell surface antigen used for labeling is expressed in the cells that are to be removed. In the case of positive magnetic selection, the antigen used for magnetic labeling is exclusively expressed in the cell subset of interest. The former technique has the advantage that the cell subset of interest will not receive any unwanted signaling derived from the binding of an antibody to a cell surface molecule or receptor.

1. Prepare a single cell suspension of mouse splenocytes: isolate the spleen from a C57/Bl6 mouse (see Note 1). Place a 70 μm nylon cell strainer in a 60 × 15 mm petri dish with 3 ml of complete RPMI 1640. Place the spleen on the cell strainer and use the plunger of a 2-ml syringe to disgregate the spleen onto the medium. Transfer the cell solution to a 15-ml falcon tube.
2. *Removal of red blood cells from spleen suspension*: centrifuge for 10 min at 400 × *g*, remove supernatant, and resuspend in 1 ml of AcK lysis buffer for 4 min at room temperature. Stop the lysis reaction by adding 10 ml of complete RPMI 1640 medium, spin for 10 min at 400 × *g*, remove supernatant, and resuspend in 2 ml of complete RPMI 1640 medium. Count splenocytes using a hemocytometer (see Note 2).
3. *Labeling with CD43 magnetic beads*: resuspend splenocytes in 90 μl PBS-2% FCS per 10^7 total cells. Add 10 μl of CD43 MicroBeads per 10^7 total cells, mix well, and incubate for 15 min at 4°C with occasional shaking. Wash the cells by adding 10 ml of PBS-2% FCS and spin for 10 min at 400 × *g*. Remove supernatant and resuspend up to 10^8 cells in 500 μl of PBS-2% FCS (see Note 3).

4. Magnetic depletion of $CD43^+$ cells: place a MS column in the magnetic field of a miniMACS separator and start the flow of the column by adding 500 μl of PBS-2% FCS. Apply the CD43-labeled spleen cell suspension to the column, and collect the unlabeled $CD43^-$ cells that pass through. Wash the column adding 500 μl of PBS–2% FCS three times and collect the flow in the same tube. Remove the column from the separator and place it in a fresh 15-ml tube. Add 1 ml of PBS–2% FCS and apply the plunger provided with the column to collect $CD43^+$-labeled cells (see Note 4). Check the purity of the $CD43^-$ and $CD43^+$ purified fractions by flow cytometry after staining with an anti-mouse B220 labeled antibody. Typically, the $CD43^-$ fraction contains ≥95% $B220^+$ cells.
5. Culture primary spleen B cells: proceed to Subheading 3.2.2 to label the cells with a cell division tracking dye or culture at 1.3×10^6 cells/ml in B cell medium in flat-bottomed multiwell plates (see Notes 5 and 6).

3.2.2. Labeling B Lymphocytes with Cell Division Tracking Dyes

This protocol describes the usage of PKH26 labeling to monitor cell division. PKH26 labeling incorporates aliphatic reporter molecules into the cell membrane lipid bilayer so that subsequent cell division results in sequential halving of fluorescence. PKH26 is a red fluorochrome (maximum emission at 567 nm) that can be excited by a 488 nm laser line, enabling the simultaneous quantification of PKH26 labeling and GFP in conventional flow cytometers. When non-GFP reporter vectors are chosen for miRNA overexpression, labeling with 5-(and -6)-carboxyfluorescein diacetate succinimidyl ester (CFSE) is recommended, owing to the higher resolution of this dye in the quantitative analysis of cell division.

1. Wash cells in serum-free RPMI 1640 medium, spin for 10 min at $400 \times g$, and remove the supernatant.
2. Resuspend pellet in Diluent C (1 ml Diluent C per 2×10^7 cells). Add 2 μl of PKH26/ml of Diluent C.
3. Incubate for 4 min at room temperature.
4. Stop the labeling by adding an equal volume of serum and incubate 1 min at room temperature.
5. Dilute in an equal volume of complete RPMI 1640 medium. Spin for 10 min at $400 \times g$ and remove supernatant.
6. Resuspend in complete medium, transfer to a fresh 15-ml tube, and wash by adding 10 ml of complete RPMI 1640 medium, spinning for 10 min at $400 \times g$ and removing the supernatant. Repeat the wash three times.
7. Resuspend in complete RPMI 1640 medium and count cells using a hemocytometer.

8. Plate labeled cells at 1.3×10^6 cells/ml in B cell medium in flat-bottomed multiwell plates (see Notes 5 and 6).

3.3. Transduction with Retroviral Supernatants

This protocol describes the procedures for the transient production of retroviral supernatants in 293T cells. Cotransfection of the retroviral plasmid harboring the pre-miRNA together with PCL-Eco plasmid encoding the gag, env, and pol proteins required for assembling of retroviral particles enables the production of high-titer supernatants that allow efficient transduction of primary B lymphocytes. Independent transfections for each miRNA retroviral construct and for mock-retroviral construct should be carried out.

1. Plate 293T cells (day 1): plate 293T cells at 15–20% density in complete DMEM medium. Consider the volume of supernatant required for the assay to choose the adequate multiwell size for 293T plating (see Note 7). This protocol describes transfection in six-well plates; adjust quantities accordingly for other multiwell or plate sizes.
2. Transfect miRNA and pCL-Eco plasmids in 293T cells by calcium phosphate (day 2): Prepare an Eppendorf tube (A) with 2 μg of PCL-Eco plasmid, 2 μg of miRNA plasmid, and 10 μl of 2.5 M $CaCl_2$. Add Milli-Q deonized water to achieve a final volume of 100 μl. Prepare a second Eppendorf tube (B) with 100 μl of HeBS 2×. While generating bubbles with a pasteur pipette in Eppendorf B, add dropwise the solution from tube A. Incubate the mixture for 20 min at room temperature to allow for calcium phosphate precipitate formation. Add dropwise the 200 μl transfection mixture to the 293T plate while swirling the medium.
3. Remove transfection medium and plate primary B cells (day 3): 12–16 h after transfection, replace 293T calcium phosphate-containing medium with complete RPMI 1640.
4. Isolate and plate primary B cells in B cell medium as described in Subheading 3.2.
5. Transduce primary B cells (day 4): 24 h after plating primary B cells, collect the media from 293T transfected cells and pass it through a 0.45 μm filter. Add 50 μM β-mercaptoethanol, 10 mM HEPES, 10 ng/ml IL-4, 25 μg/ml LPS, and 8 μg/ml polybrene to the filtered retroviral supernatant media. Remove the maximum volume (approximately 80% of total volume) of media from the B cell cultures multiwell plates without disturbing the cells and replace it with the retroviral supernatant media. Save the LPS IL4-containing B cell culture media at 4°C. Centrifuge the B cell culture multiwell plates at $1,500 \times g$ at room temperature for 2.5 h. Culture the cells with the retroviral supernatant.

6. Remove retroviral supernatant medium (day 5): 16–20 h after transduction, remove the maximum volume (approximately 80% of total volume) of retroviral medium without disturbing the cells and replace it with 37°C preheated LPS- and IL4-containing B cell culture media that was saved on the previous day.

3.4. Quantification of Retroviral Transduction and miRNA Processing Efficiency

The usage of fluorescent proteins, such as GFP, as reporter proteins of retrovial transduction provides a fast and convenient way to identify transduced cells. However, miRNA processing is a complex multistep process that involves the sequential cleavage of a long primary transcript (pri-miRNA) into a stem–loop precursor of approximately 70 nucleotides (pre-miRNA), and finally into a 20–22 nucleotide long mature miRNA (reviewed in (21) and (22)). The efficiency of these processes can vary significantly among different pre-miRNAs and cellular contexts, and therefore, it is advisable to determine the pre-miRNA and mature miRNA processing efficiency in each specific assay condition. In the following procedures, we describe how to determine transduction efficiency by flow cytometry analysis and analyse the expression of pre-miRNA and mature miRNA in transduced cells by real-time PCR analysis.

3.4.1. Quantification of Transduction Efficiency by Gene Reporter Expression

Two days after transduction, remove a sample containing from 5×10^4 to 2×10^5 transduced B cells, spin for 10 min at $400\times g$, and resuspend in 500 µl of PBS with 2% FCS and 1 µg/ml propidium iodide. Incubate at room temperature for 5 min and determine the transduction efficiency by flow cytometry analysis of GFP expression in live (propidium iodide negative) cells (see Note 8). Typically, transduction efficiencies of primary mouse spleen B cells range from 20 to 40%.

3.4.2. Quantification of Pre-miRNA Processing Efficiency in Transduced B Cells

1. Design primers for pre-miRNA amplification. Use *Express Primer* software to design specific real-time PCR primers for pre-miRNA amplification. Complementary DNA (cDNA) normalization will be performed by using GAPDH, as an endogenous control (GAPDH primer sequences: forward-5′-TGAAGCAGGCATCTGAGGG-3′ and reverse-5′-CGAAGGTGGAAGAGTGGGAG-3′).
2. Sort transduced B cells: 48–72 h after retroviral transduction, collect 5×10^6 to 2×10^7 transduced B lymphocytes, spin 10 min at $400\times g$, and resuspend in PBS with 2% FCS at 1×10^7 cells/ml. Filter through a 70-µm filter and sort in a high-speed cell sorter with a 70-µM nozzle to isolate GFP^+ transduced B cells. Sort mock-GFP^+ transduced cells and miRNA-GFP^+ transduced samples.
3. Isolate RNA: Pellet 0.5×10^6 to 3×10^6 sorted GFP^+ B cells by centrifuging for 10 min at $400\times g$. Lyse cells in 1 ml of

TRIZol reagent by repetitive pipetting and incubate homogenized samples for 5 min at room temperature. Add 0.2 ml of chloroform. Cap sample tubes securely and shake vigorously for 15 s. Incubate at room temperature for 3 min and centrifuge at 12,000 × *g* for 15 min at 4°C. Transfer the upper aqueous phase to a fresh tube and precipitate the RNA by mixing with 0.5 ml of isopropyl alcohol. Incubate for at least 1 h at −20°C and centrifuge at 12,000 × *g* for 20 min at 4°C. Remove the supernatant and wash the RNA pellet once with 1 ml of cold 75% ethanol. Centrifuge at 7,500 × *g* for 10 min at 4°C, remove supernatant, and air-dry the RNA pellet for 5–10 min. Dissolve RNA in 10–30 μl of RNase-free molecular biology-grade water by passing the solution a few times through a pipette tip and incubating for 10 min at 55°C. Measure RNA concentration in spectrophotometer and check RNA integrity in a 0.8% agarose gel. RNAs should be stored at −80°C if not used immediately (see Note 9).

4. Retrotranscribe RNA into cDNA: add to a PCR tube 250 ng random primers, 0.5–5 μg of total RNA, 1 μl of dNTP mix (10 mM each), and ribonuclease-free water to a final volume of 12 μl. Incubate samples at 65°C for 5 min and then at 2°C for 1 min in a thermocycler. Transfer the tube to ice and add 4 μl of 5× First-Strand Buffer, 2 μl of 0.1 M DTT, and 1 μl (40 units/μl) RNAaseOUT. Mix the contents gently and incubate at 25°C for 2 min in a thermocycler. Then, add 1 μl (200 units) of SuperScript II Reverse Transcriptase and incubate at 25°C for 10 min, 42°C for 50 min, and 70°C for 15 min in a thermocycler. cDNAs should be stored at −20°C if not used immediately (see Note 10).
5. Analyze pre-miRNA expression by real-time RT-PCR: for each cDNA sample, prepare two different dilutions (typically 1/2 and 1/8 of original cDNA stock). Amplify each cDNA dilution with the specific pre-miRNA pair of primers and the endogenous control (GAPDH) pair of primers. Set all the reactions in duplicates. Prepare a mix for each amplification type containing 10 μl of SYBR green PCR master mix, 0.4 μM sense primer, 0.4 μM reverse primer, and molecular-grade water to reach a final reaction volume of 18 μl per reaction. Add 2 μl of the cDNA dilutions and 18 μl of the specific amplification mix per well in 96-well PCR plates. Cover the plate with an adherent film and centrifuge it for 15 min at 1,500 × *g* to eliminate any air bubbles. Run the reaction in a real-time quantitative PCR system using standard amplification conditions [50°C 2 min; 95°C 10 min; 40× (95°C 15 s; 60°C 1 min]. To analyze the data, first normalize the pre-miRNA amplifications by subtracting GAPDH Ct from premiRNA Ct (dCT = Ct-premiRNA–Ct-GAPDH).

Then, normalize amplifications of miRNA-transduced samples to mock-transduced samples (ddCT = dCT-miRNA RV sample–dCT-mock RV sample) and finally calculate fold expression levels in miRNA-transduced samples versus mock-transduced samples (=power(2, –ddCT)).

3.4.3. Quantification of Mature miRNA Processing Efficiency in Transduced B Cells

1. Sort transduced GFP^+ cells as described in Subheading 3.4.2 in step 2.
2. Prepare total RNA as described in Subheading 3.4.2 in step 3.
3. Retrotranscribe mature miRNA and an endogenous small RNA with specific primers. Use TaqMan microRNA assays from Applied Biosystems following the manufacturer's instructions.
4. Analyze by real-time RT-PCR mature miRNA expression in mock versus miRNA-transduced cells. Use TaqMan microRNA assays from Applied Biosystems following the manufacturer's instructions. Include the same PCR samples as in Subheading 3.4.2 in step 5.

3.5. Determination of the Functional Effect of miRNA Overexpression in Mature B Cells

Mature B cells are programmed to follow a complex maturation and differentiation program upon antigen recognition. This process involves cellular expansion and two molecular mechanisms named somatic hypermutation (SHM) and CSR, which serve to generate higher affinity antibodies with various functional specificities (reviewed in (23) and (24)). CSR can be induced in vitro in cultures of primary B lymphocytes by stimulation with different combinations of factors (see Note 6). We describe below the procedures to quantify the effect of miRNA overexpression in B cell proliferation, survival, or CSR in in vitro cultures of primary B cells. Analysis of other molecular process that occur upon B cell stimulation, such as Sμ and Sγ1 germline transcription, Sμ and Sγ1 mutation, and AID expression can be analyzed in sorted samples from mock and miRNA-transduced cells following previously reported experimental procedures (15, 25–27).

3.5.1. Determination of miRNA Impact on B Cell Proliferation

1. Remove cells for proliferation analysis at days 2, 3, and 4 after retroviral transduction of PKH26-labeled B cells. Include in the analysis mock-transduced cells and miRNA-transduced samples. Remove from the culture $\sim 1 \times 10^5$ cells, spin them for 10 min at $400 \times g$, and remove the supernatant.
2. Resuspend in 0.3 ml PBS with 2% FCS and 0.1 μg/ml DAPI to label dead cells. Incubate for 5 min at room temperature (see Note 8).
3. Analyze PKH26 florescence in transduced (GFP^+) live ($DAPI^-$) cells by flow cytometry. Laser line used for excitation/emission maxima: DAPI (UV or violet laser/blue emission

(max 461 nm)), GFP (blue 488 nm laser/green emission (max 509 nm)), and PKH26 (blue 488 nm laser/orange emission (max 567 nm)).

4. Include the following "single-color" control samples to set up flow cytometry compensation parameters: (1) nontransduced, DAPI-labeled cells; (2) transduced, nonPKH26 labeled samples; and (3) nontransduced, PKH26 labeled samples.
5. Analyze data with ModFit flow cytometry analysis software.

3.5.2. Determination of miRNA Impact on B Cell Apoptosis

1. Analyze cell death in in vitro cultures of spleen B cells at days 2, 3, and 4 after retroviral transduction. Include in the analysis mock-transduced and miRNA-transduced samples. Spin $\sim 1 \times 10^5$ cells for 10 min at $400 \times g$ and resuspend them in 1 ml of cold PBS. Repeat the washing step once more and then resuspend the cells in 100 μl of 1× AnnexinV binding buffer.
2. Transfer the solution to a 5-ml FACS tube and add 5 μl of AnnexinV-APC. Vortex gently and incubate for 15 min at room temperature in the dark.
3. Add 300 μl of 1× AnnexinV binding buffer and propidium iodide (PI) to 1 μg/ml final concentration. Incubate 15 min at room temperature in the dark.
4. Analyze by flow cytometry the percentage of early apoptotic (AnnexinV$^+$ PI$^-$) in transduced GFP$^+$ cells (see Note 11). Laser line used for excitation/emission maxima: GFP (blue 488 nm laser/green emission (max 509 nm)), PI (blue 488 nm laser/orange-red emission (max 617 nm)), and APC (red 633 nm laser line/red emission (max 660 nm)). Include single-stained samples to set up flow cytometry compensation controls.

3.5.3. Determination of miRNA Impact on CSR

1. Analyze IgG1 CSR efficiency in in vitro cultures of B cells at days 2, 3, and 4 after retroviral transduction. Include mock-transduced and miRNA-transduced samples in the analysis. Remove from the culture $\sim 1 \times 10^5$ cells, spin them for 10 min at $400 \times g$, and wash with cold PBS. Spin again for 10 min at $400 \times g$, remove the supernatant, and resuspend the cells in 100 μl of staining buffer with a 1/500 dilution of antimouse IgG1-biotinylated antibody. Incubate on ice for 20 min.
2. Wash by adding at least 100 μl of staining buffer, spinning for 10 min at $400 \times g$, and removing the supernatant. Resuspend the cells in 100 μl of staining buffer with 1/500 dilution of streptavidin-APC and 1/200 dilution of anti-B220-R-PE antibody. Incubate for 20 min on ice in the dark.
3. Wash by adding at least 100 μl of staining buffer, spinning for 10 min at $400 \times g$ and removing the supernatant. Resuspend the cells in 500 μl of staining buffer and transfer to a FACS tube.

4. Add 5 μl of 7-AAD and incubate for 20 min on ice to label dead cells.
5. Analyze by flow cytometry B220-R-PE versus IgG1-APC staining in GFP^+ transduced live (7-AAD^-) cells (see Note 8). Laser line used for excitation/emission maxima: GFP (blue 488 nm laser/green emission (max 509 nm)), R-PE (blue 488 nm laser/orange emission (max 578 nm)), 7-ADD (blue 488 nm laser/red emission (max 655 nm)), and APC (red 633 nm laser line/red emission (max 660 nm)). Include single-stained samples to set up flow cytometry compensation controls. The expected class-switch efficiencies to IgG1 in LPS+IL-4 cultures of primary transduced B cells range from 20 to 40% at day 4.

4. Notes

1. Spleen mouse isolation should be performed in clean semisterile conditions. Spray or submerge the sacrificed mouse in 70% ethanol and extract the spleen in a clean area, and whenever possible, under a laminar flow. After removing the spleen, all the procedures should be performed inside a tissue-culture laminar flow hood to preserve sterility.
2. The number of lymphocytes recovered from a spleen will typically range between 6 and 8×10^7 cells. Approximately 50% of splenocytes are B lymphocytes.
3. For magnetic selection procedures, keep cells on ice and use precooled solutions to prevent capping of antibodies on the cell surface and nonspecific cell labeling.
4. For selection of B lymphocytes from a single spleen (up to 8×10^7 total cells), use a MS column as indicated in the protocol. For selection of cells from more than one spleen, use one MS column per spleen or a single LS column (with up to 7×10^8 total cells), adapting the volumes as indicated in the manufacturer's instructions.
5. B cell viability is dependent on cell-to-cell interactions, and disturbance of these interactions after the initial setup of the cultures should be avoided. Plan in advance the different analysis time points of B cell cultures, and when possible, plate the cells in independent multiwells so that they will be used for individual analysis. Typically, we use a 96-well plate, plated with 2.5×10^5 B lymphocytes, for each analysis time point.
6. Different stimulation conditions can be used to promote CSR to other isotypes. Stimulation with LPS alone promotes class

switch to IgG3, stimulation with LPS, IL-4, and TGFβ promotes class switch to IgA, and stimulation with anti-CD40 antibodies and IL-4 can also be used to promote class switch to IgG1. When using alternative CSR stimuli, take into account that B cell proliferation, and therefore retroviral transduction, can vary across different stimulation conditions.

7. Consider the number of B cells to be transduced with each miRNA construct to plate the adequate number of multiwells with 293T cells. 6-, 12-, and 24-well plates will yield about 3 ml, 1.5 ml, and 0.8 ml of retroviral supernatant, respectively. For a screening assay in which a B cell function is assesed through a single end-point time flow cytometry analysis, a single 24-well plate of 293T cells transfected with each miRNA construct will yield enough retroviral supernatant.
8. Primary B cell cultures can be kept alive in culture for a maximum of 6–7 days. However, the percentage of dead cells in the cultures is significant from day 3 (≥50%) and will steadily increase at later time points. It is therefore important to include a cell-viability dye that enables live/dead discrimination by flow-cytometry analysis. Several dyes with different excitation/emission spectra (DAPI, propidium iodide, TO-PRO, or 7-AAD) can be used for this purpose.
9. When working with RNA, keep clean conditions to avoid degradation by ribonucleases. Clean working surfaces and pipettes with 70% ethanol and RNAse decontaminant (such as Ambion's RNaseZap), wear always clean gloves, use filter tips, and prepare ethanol dilutions with ribonuclease-free water. RNAs should be stored at −80°C and kept on ice during all working procedures. Repetitive RNA freezing and thawing cycles should be avoided.
10. Store cDNAs at −20°C. Thaw cDNAs on ice, and keep them on ice while working. Avoid repetitive freezing and thawing cycles.
11. GFP expression is partially lost as cells die due to cell membrane permeabilization. To accurately quantify the proportion of transduced cells in late apoptosis (AnnexinV$^+$ PI$^+$) either sort transduced GFP$^+$ cells prior to cell culture or use a modified GFP version, like farnesylated GFP, that is retained in the cell membrane as reporter gene of retroviral transduction.

Acknowledgments

We would like to thank Dr He for kindly sharing a miRNA library with us and for helpful discussion. This work was supported by grants from the Ministerio de Educación y Ciencia (SAF2007-63130), the Comunidad Autónoma de Madrid (DIFHEMAT-CM), and the European Research Council (BCLYM-207844). V. G. de Yebenes and A. R. Ramiro are supported by the Ramón y Cajal program from the Ministerio de Educación y Ciencia.

References

1. Xiao, C., and Rajewsky, K. (2009) MicroRNA control in the immune system: basic principles, *Cell* **136**, 26–36.
2. Costinean, S., Zanesi, N., Pekarsky, Y., Tili, E., Volinia, S., Heerema, N., and Croce, C. M. (2006) Pre-B cell proliferation and lymphoblastic leukemia/high-grade lymphoma in E(mu)-miR155 transgenic mice, *Proc. Natl. Acad. Sci. USA.* **103**, 7024–7029.
3. Thai, T. H., Calado, D. P., Casola, S., Ansel, K. M., Xiao, C., Xue, Y., Murphy, A., Frendewey, D., Valenzuela, D., Kutok, J. L., Schmidt-Supprian, M., Rajewsky, N., Yancopoulos, G., Rao, A., and Rajewsky, K. (2007) Regulation of the germinal center response by microRNA-155, *Science* **316**, 604–608.
4. Xiao, C., Srinivasan, L., Calado, D. P., Patterson, H. C., Zhang, B., Wang, J., Henderson, J. M., Kutok, J. L., and Rajewsky, K. (2008) Lymphoproliferative disease and autoimmunity in mice with increased miR-17-92 expression in lymphocytes, *Nat. Immunol.* **9**, 405–414.
5. Chen, C. Z., Li, L., Lodish, H. F., and Bartel, D. P. (2004) MicroRNAs modulate hematopoietic lineage differentiation, *Science* **303**, 83–86.
6. He, L., Thomson, J. M., Hemann, M. T., Hernando-Monge, E., Mu, D., Goodson, S., Powers, S., Cordon-Cardo, C., Lowe, S. W., Hannon, G. J., and Hammond, S. M. (2005) A microRNA polycistron as a potential human oncogene, *Nature* **435**, 828–833.
7. Xiao, C., Calado, D. P., Galler, G., Thai, T. H., Patterson, H. C., Wang, J., Rajewsky, N., Bender, T. P., and Rajewsky, K. (2007) MiR-150 controls B cell differentiation by targeting the transcription factor c-Myb, *Cell* **131**, 146–159.
8. Rodriguez, A., Vigorito, E., Clare, S., Warren, M. V., Couttet, P., Soond, D. R., van Dongen, S., Grocock, R. J., Das, P. P., Miska, E. A., Vetrie, D., Okkenhaug, K., Enright, A. J., Dougan, G., Turner, M., and Bradley, A. (2007) Requirement of bic/microRNA-155 for normal immune function, *Science* **316**, 608–611.
9. Ventura, A., Young, A. G., Winslow, M. M., Lintault, L., Meissner, A., Erkeland, S. J., Newman, J., Bronson, R. T., Crowley, D., Stone, J. R., Jaenisch, R., Sharp, P. A., and Jacks, T. (2008) Targeted deletion reveals essential and overlapping functions of the miR-17 through 92 family of miRNA clusters, *Cell* **132**, 875–886.
10. Vigorito, E., Perks, K. L., Abreu-Goodger, C., Bunting, S., Xiang, Z., Kohlhaas, S., Das, P. P., Miska, E. A., Rodriguez, A., Bradley, A., Smith, K. G., Rada, C., Enright, A. J., Toellner, K. M., Maclennan, I. C., and Turner, M. (2007) MicroRNA-155 regulates the generation of immunoglobulin class-switched plasma cells, *Immunity* **27**, 847–859.
11. Koralov, S. B., Muljo, S. A., Galler, G. R., Krek, A., Chakraborty, T., Kanellopoulou, C., Jensen, K., Cobb, B. S., Merkenschlager, M., Rajewsky, N., and Rajewsky, K. (2008) Dicer ablation affects antibody diversity and cell survival in the B lymphocyte lineage, *Cell* **132**, 860–874.
12. O'Carroll, D., Mecklenbrauker, I., Das, P. P., Santana, A., Koenig, U., Enright, A. J., Miska, E. A., and Tarakhovsky, A. (2007) A slicer-independent role for Argonaute 2 in hematopoiesis and the microRNA pathway, *Genes Dev.* **21**, 1999–2004.
13. Dorsett, Y., McBride, K. M., Jankovic, M., Gazumyan, A., Thai, T. H., Robbiani, D. F., Di Virgilio, M., San-Martin, B. R., Heidkamp, G., Schwickert, T. A., Eisenreich, T., Rajewsky, K., and Nussenzweig, M. C. (2008) MicroRNA-155 suppresses activation-induced cytidine deaminase-mediated Myc-Igh translocation, *Immunity* **28**, 630–638.
14. Teng, G., Hakimpour, P., Landgraf, P., Rice, A., Tuschl, T., Casellas, R., and Papavasiliou, F. N. (2008) MicroRNA-155 is a negative regulator of activation-induced cytidine deaminase, *Immunity* **28**, 621–629.
15. de Yebenes, V. G., Belver, L., Pisano, D. G., Gonzalez, S., Villasante, A., Croce, C., He, L., and Ramiro, A. R. (2008) miR-181b negatively regulates activation-induced cytidine deaminase in B cells, *J. Exp. Med.* **205**, 2199–2206.
16. Inomata, M., Tagawa, H., Guo, Y. M., Kameoka, Y., Takahashi, N., and Sawada, K. (2009) MicroRNA-17-92 down-regulates expression of distinct targets in different B-cell lymphoma subtypes, *Blood* **113**, 396–402.

17. Huppi, K., Volfovsky, N., Runfola, T., Jones, T. L., Mackiewicz, M., Martin, S. E., Mushinski, J. F., Stephens, R., and Caplen, N. J. (2008) The identification of microRNAs in a genomically unstable region of human chromosome 8q24, *Mol. Cancer Res.* **6**, 212–221.

18. Nie, K., Gomez, M., Landgraf, P., Garcia, J. F., Liu, Y., Tan, L. H., Chadburn, A., Tuschl, T., Knowles, D. M., and Tam, W. (2008) MicroRNA-mediated down-regulation of PRDM1/Blimp-1 in Hodgkin/Reed-Sternberg cells: a potential pathogenetic lesion in Hodgkin lymphomas, *Am. J. Pathol.* **173**, 242–252.

19. Kluiver, J., van den Berg, A., de Jong, D., Blokzijl, T., Harms, G., Bouwman, E., Jacobs, S., Poppema, S., and Kroesen, B. J. (2007) Regulation of pri-microRNA BIC transcription and processing in Burkitt lymphoma, *Oncogene* **26**, 3769–3776.

20. Sampath, D., Calin, G. A., Puduvalli, V. K., Gopisetty, G., Taccioli, C., Liu, C. G., Ewald, B., Liu, C., Keating, M. J., and Plunkett, W. (2009) Specific activation of microRNA106b enables the p73 apoptotic response in chronic lymphocytic leukemia by targeting the ubiquitin ligase itch for degradation, *Blood* **113**, 3744–3753.

21. He, L., and Hannon, G. J. (2004) MicroRNAs: small RNAs with a big role in gene regulation, *Nat. Rev. Genet.* **5**, 522–531.

22. Chang, K., Elledge, S. J., and Hannon, G. J. (2006) Lessons from Nature: microRNA-based shRNA libraries, *Nat. Methods* **3**, 707–714.

23. de Yebenes, V. G., and Ramiro, A. R. (2006) Activation-induced deaminase: light and dark sides, *Trends. Mol. Med.* **12**, 432–439.

24. Stavnezer, J., Guikema, J. E., and Schrader, C. E. (2008) Mechanism and regulation of class switch recombination, *Annu. Rev. Immunol.* **26**, 261–292.

25. Sernandez, I. V., de Yebenes, V. G., Dorsett, Y., and Ramiro, A. R. (2008) Haploinsufficiency of activation-induced deaminase for antibody diversification and chromosome translocations both in vitro and in vivo, *PLoS One* **3**, e3927.

26. Reina-San-Martin, B., Difilippantonio, S., Hanitsch, L., Masilamani, R. F., Nussenzweig, A., and Nussenzweig, M. C. (2003) H2AX is required for recombination between immunoglobulin switch regions but not for intra-switch region recombination or somatic hypermutation, *J. Exp. Med.* **197**, 1767–1778.

27. Nambu, Y., Sugai, M., Gonda, H., Lee, C. G., Katakai, T., Agata, Y., Yokota, Y., and Shimizu, A. (2003) Transcription-coupled events associating with immunoglobulin switch region chromatin, *Science* **302**, 2137–2140.

Chapter 13

Isolation and Characterization of MicroRNAs of Human Mature Erythrocytes

Carolyn Sangokoya, Gregory LaMonte, and Jen-Tsan Chi

Abstract

Human mature erythrocytes are terminally differentiated cells that have lost their nuclei and organelles during development. Even though mature erythrocytes lack ribosomal and other large-sized RNAs, they still retain small-sized RNAs. We have recently shown that there are abundant and diverse species of microRNAs in mature erythrocytes through the use of several different techniques, including northern blot, miRNA microarray, and real-time PCR. Furthermore, fractionation and genomic analysis has revealed that erythrocyte microRNA expression is different from that of reticulocytes or leukocytes and that mature erythrocytes contribute the majority of microRNA expression in whole blood. Therefore, global analysis of microRNA expression in circulating erythrocytes has the potential to provide mechanistic insights into erythrocyte biology and erythrocyte-related disorders. Here, we have provided the detailed methods for isolating and characterizing the microRNAs from human mature erythrocytes to enable such researches into human diseases involving erythrocytes.

1. Introduction

Human erythrocytes are end products of a highly regulated differentiation process that involves the gradual loss of cellular organelles, a decline in nucleic acid content, and a step-wise acquisition of erythrocyte characteristics (1). The nuclei are extruded as they become differentiated into reticulocytes. Cytoplasmic RNA and translation activities, while still detectable in reticulocytes, fall below detection limit as they become mature erythrocytes (2). The prevailing view that mature erythrocytes lack most RNAs primarily comes from their inability to stain with RNA-binding dyes (e.g., acridine orange, methylene blue), the basis of these dyes to distinguish reticulocytes from mature erythrocytes in clinical setting (3). Given the potential limitations and

Silvia Monticelli (ed.), *MicroRNAs and the Immune System: Methods and Protocols*, Methods in Molecular Biology, vol. 667, DOI 10.1007/978-1-60761-811-9_13,

biases of these methods, certain RNA species may not be detected. We have recently found that human mature erythrocytes, though largely lacking in ribosomal and large-sized RNA, possess diverse and abundant microRNAs (4). It is also important to note the recent discovery of microRNAs and proteins mediating microRNA function in platelets, another group of terminally differentiated anuclear blood cells (5). These erythrocyte microRNAs allow the application of DNA microarray technology to capture and extract the biological information to understand erythrocyte phenotypes during physiological and pathological adaptations in many human diseases affecting erythrocytes.

MicroRNAs are noncoding RNAs of 19–25 nt in size which mediate posttranscriptional regulation of target mRNAs through the formation of noncanonical base pairing with the 3′ UTR. MicroRNAs regulate a wide variety of biological processes (e.g., differentiation, apoptosis, and oncogenic transformation) (6). Many publications have highlighted the role of several microRNAs that have been implicated in the process of erythropoiesis, (7–16) as well as during in vitro erythroid differentiation (8, 17–19). Since erythroid cells lose their nuclei and active transcription during the reticulocyte stages of their development, posttranscriptional regulation of remaining mRNAs probably plays a very important role. Although microRNAs are likely to play a regulatory role in posttranscriptional regulation in erythroid cells, we have very limited information thus far. The genomic study of microRNAs in mature erythrocytes may provide a unique and accessible window to enhance our understanding of their regulatory roles in erythroid cells, both under normal circumstances and in pathological states, such as various anemic diseases (4) and polycythemia vera (14, 20). To facilitate the study of microRNAs in the human erythrocytes, we are providing the detailed methodology for the isolation and characterization of erythrocyte microRNAs.

2. Materials

1. Miltenyi MACS® Separators (autoMACS).
2. Miltenyi autoMACS® Columns, Miltenyi.
3. Miltenyi human CD71 microbeads, Miltenyi.
4. Blood samples (~20 mL) to be analyzed, collected from donors.
5. Human blood for the isolation of common reference RNAs used for microarrays.
6. Purecell Neo-leukoreduction filter (PALL Biomedical Products, East Hills, NY).

7. Phosphate-buffered saline (PBS), pH 7.4 (10× stock solution: 1.37 M NaCl, 27 mM KCl, 100 mM Na_2HPO_4, 18 mM KH_2PO_4).
8. Staining buffer: PBS with 2% of fetal bovine serum (FBS).
9. mirVana miRNA isolation kit (Ambion, Applied Biosystems, Foster City, CA).
10. Vac-Man® Laboratory Vacuum Manifold (Promega, WI).
11. miRCURY LNA™ microRNA Array (Exiqon, Denmark).
12. miRCURY LNA™ microRNA Hy3/Hy5 Power labeling kit (Exiqon, Denmark).
13. Qiagen RNeasy Mini Kit.
14. MAUI® SC mixer for microarray hybridization.
15. Wash Buffer A: For 1 L, 100 mL of 20× SSC, 20 mL 10% detergent, 880 mL water.
16. Wash Buffer B: For 1 L, 50 mL of 20× SSC, 950 mL water.
17. Wash Buffer C: For 1 L, 10 mL 20× SSC, 990 mL water.
18. 20× SSC:
    - (a) Dissolve 175.3 g of NaCl, 88.2 g of sodium citrate in 800 mL of distilled H_2O.
    - (b) Adjust the pH to 7.0 with a few drops of 1 M HCl.
    - (c) Adjust the volume to 1 L with additional distilled H_2O.
    - (d) Sterilize by autoclaving.
19. GenePix 4000B microarray scanner (Axon, Fremont, CA).

3. Methods

We have divided our discussion of the methods into four sections: (Subheading 3.1) the isolation of human mature erythrocytes using leukoreduction filters and autoMACS®, (Subheading 3.2) the purification all RNAs larger than 10 nt using the microRNA isolation kits, (Subheading 3.3) the labeling of erythrocyte microRNA, and (Subheading 3.4) the profiling of erythrocyte microRNA species using spotted Exiqon microRNA microarrays. The conventional wisdom that mature erythrocytes lack RNA may be due to a technical issue during traditional RNA isolation procedures (e.g., Trizol or Qiagen RNeasy or other column-based RNA isolation kit), during which the majority of small-sized RNAs are lost. Therefore, we modified an isolation protocol using Ambion's miRVana kit to capture all RNA larger than ten nucleotides (nt) for our analysis of erythrocytic microRNAs. To isolate the microRNA from mature erythrocytes, it is important to first remove other cell types in the human blood because the higher level of RNAs from contaminating cells has the potential to complicate the miRNA analysis. Finally, we label the erythrocyte microRNAs for interrogation by the microRNA microarrays. In the labeling procedures, we use a higher amount of ethanol in the Qiagen RNeasy kit to remove the unlabeled Cy-Dye while retaining the labeled microRNAs.

3.1. Purification of Mature Erythrocytes from Human Blood

1. Centrifuge whole blood sample and aspirate plasma and buffy coat layer for initial removal of plasma and leukocytes. Resuspend the cells in PBS (see Note 1).
2. Cut the outlet tubing of the Pall leukoreduction filter and insert into the filters with the pointed ends to allow the infusion of the whole blood from the top of the filter to allow filtration by simple gravity.
3. Pour the blood into the leukoreduction filter bag and then collect the filtrate which contains red blood cells. Use PBS to wash the filter, and collect filtrate into a 50-mL Falcon tube.
4. Wash the leukocyte-depleted blood with cold PBS and add 80 μL of CD71 (this protocol uses the presence/absence of CD71 to differentiate reticulocytes from erythrocytes) microbeads to each 20 mL of blood sample (see Note 2). We mix the sample gently by inverting the tubes and incubating for 20 min on ice to allow the binding of the beads to the CD71+ reticulocytes.
5. Wash the cells by adding staining buffer to the top once and centrifuge at $805 \times g$ in a table top centrifuge for 5 min without brake. Pipette off supernatant carefully and completely. The red cell pellet can be loose, therefore requiring extra caution.
6. Resuspend the cells in staining buffer again and bring the volume to less than 50% hematocrit in 25 or 50 mL of PBS. For each run on Miltenyi MACS® Separators, 25 mL is the highest capacity, so you may need two separate runs for some samples.
7. Apply the cell suspension onto the column, run negative selection (DEPLETES program) for mature RBC, collect both CD71+ and CD71− samples for the same patient samples. The cells in the CD71+ fraction will be in approximately 2 mL, while the CD71− fractions (the majority of the erythrocytes) will be in similar volume of starting sample volume.
8. After the completion of the separation, clean all the tubes and empty the waste, and then place new tubes and run sleep program of the autoMACS® Separator.
9. The purity of the resulting mature erythrocytes can be evaluated using flow cytometry (for the percentage of CD71+ cells, Fig. 1a), methylene blue stain (Fig. 1b), or RT-PCR for

a

Surface markers	Before Purification	After Purification
CD16	0.78%	0.00%
CD45	1.14%	0.12%
CD71	0.12%	0.00%
CD235a	93.0%	99.8%

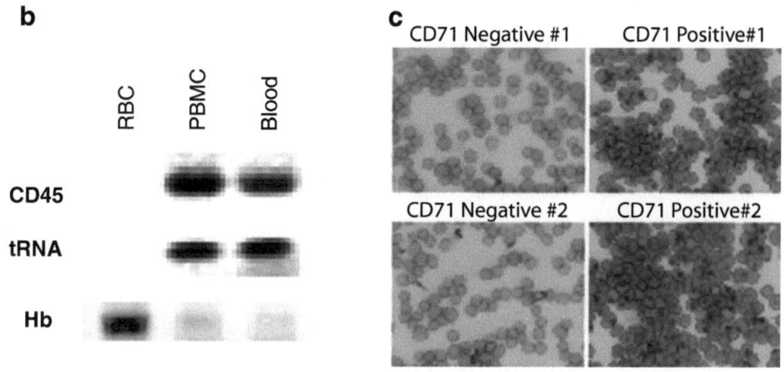

Fig. 1. (**a**) Assessment of the purified mature erythrocytes was performed by examining the surface expression of indicated lineage markers on whole blood (before purification) and purified erythrocytes (after purification) with flow cytometry to estimate the percentage of cells with surface expression of CD16 (leukocyte marker), CD45 (leukocyte marker), CD71 (reticulocyte marker), and CD235a (mature erythrocytes marker). (**b**) RT-PCR assay to evaluate the cell purity based on the abundance of indicated transcripts (CD45, tRNA and beta-hemoglobin) in the RNA from purified erythrocytes (RBC), peripheral blood mononuclear cells (PBMC) and whole blood. (**c**) New methylene blue stain of the CD71− erythrocytes (*left*) and CD71+ reticulocytes (*right*) from two independent isolations.

lineage-specific transcripts (Fig. 1c). Alternatively, the samples can be sent to a reticulocyte lab for similar determination using RNA-staining dye (e.g., acridine orange).

3.2. Isolation of MicroRNAs from the Purified Human Mature Erythrocytes

1. Pool all the CD71 cells together and fill the tube up to the top with cold PBS and centrifuge 805 × *g* without brake to pellet the red cells.
2. After centrifugation, remove the supernatant carefully due to the looseness of the red cell pellets.
3. The CD71+ population can be lysed using the recommended 500 μL of lysis buffer (in the Ambion miRVana RNA isolating kit). However, for the CD71− population (mature erythrocytes), you will need to lyse the cell pellet using 5 mL of lysis buffer in a 50-mL Falcon tube due to the large cell number and amount of protein in red cells (see Note 3). It is important to ensure complete lysis of the red cell pellet by repeated pipetting and thorough vortexing (at least 60 s). Since we mostly follow the recommended sample amount for

the CD71+ cells, we will emphasize the modifications we have made for CD71− population in the remaining protocol.

4. Add 50 μL (for the CD71+) and 500 μL (for the CD71−) homogenate additive in the Ambion miRVana RNA isolating kit to each sample, consistent with the one-tenth volume of the lysis buffer used in the previous step.
5. Leave the mixtures of lysed samples and homogenate additive on ice for 10 min.
6. Add acid phenol choloroform (5 mL) to the CD71− samples and vortex vigorously for 1–2 min to ensure thorough mixing and adequate protein extraction.
7. Separate the aqueous and organic phase by centrifuging the 50-mL Falcon tube for 5 min at 10,000 × *g* at room temperature with complete brake ON.
8. Collect the supernatant (aqueous) which contains RNA and transfer it to a fresh tube and repeat the phenol/chloroform extraction step until the supernatant becomes clear to indicate the completeness of the organic phase extraction.
9. Estimate the volume of the resulting supernatant and then add 1.25 volumes 100% ethanol and mix thoroughly by carefully inverting the tube several times.
10. The lysate/ethanol mixture from one sample will be passed through one or two RNA-binding filter cartridges provided by miRVana kits by vacuum manifold modified using the Promega Vacuum Manifold. The bottom of an Eppendorf tube is cut off and connected with the adaptor in the Vacuum Manifold through a 200 μL pipette tip sealed with parafilm to allow the vacuum. We pipette the sample continuously onto the membrane before the membrane becomes dry after the passing of the samples. (Note: It is important to ensure that the flow rate of the vacuum is not too high as this will decrease yields. Also, make sure to check the filters for small holes, which will also reduce yields.)
11. The RNA-binding filter cartridge with the erythrocyte RNAs will be removed from the vacuum manifold and placed in a fresh Eppendorf tube. The filter cartridge will be washed with 700 μL of the miRNA Wash Buffer A using a microcentrifuge as recommended in the kit.
12. Wash the filter cartridge with 500 μL Wash Buffer B/C twice.
13. Elute RNA with 100 μL DEPC-water at 95°C (in two washes of 50 μL each to increase RNA yield) and measure the concentration via Nanodrop. The size distribution of the isolated RNAs can be assessed by Agilent Bioanalyzer (Fig. 2a) or RNA gels (see Note 4).

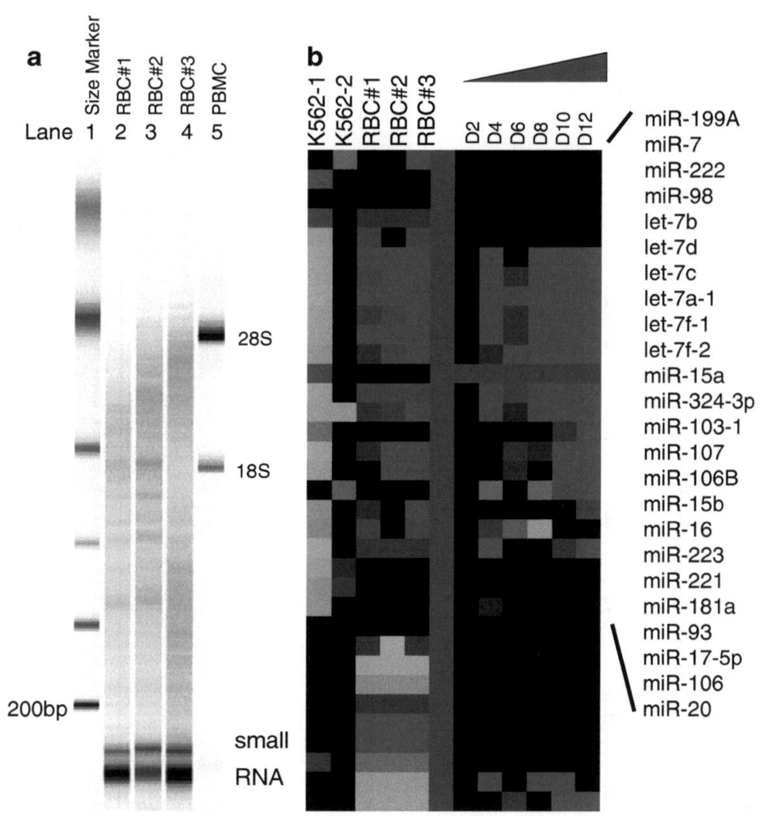

Fig. 2. (**a**) The size distribution of RNAs of three independent erythrocyte samples (*lanes 2–4* labeled RBC #1–3) and one PBMC sample (*lane 5* labeled as PBMC) were determined with Agilent Bioanalyzer with the indicated size markers (*lane 1* as indicated). (**b**) *Left*: the microRNA expression pattern obtained with microRNA microarrays of three mature erythrocyte samples was compared to that of two erythroleukemia K562 cell lines. *Right*: the expression of erythrocyte-specific microRNAs in the CD34+ erythroid progenitor cells at indicated stages of erythroid differentiation in a previously published study (14).

3.3. Profiling of Erythrocyte MicroRNAs Using MicroRNA Microarrays

1. Start with 5 μg of total RNA with the following sample sheet (Table 1).
2. Place all Exiqon labeling kit components on ice and thaw for 20 min. Add 29 μL of nuclease-free water to the supplied Cy-Dyes, mix by vortexing, and spin down. Keep the dyes covered since they are photosensitive.
3. Prepare the samples (table above) with total volume of RNA samples with water to 6 μL and prepare master mix for all samples and keep on ice until all the samples are ready.
4. Vortex and spin down, add 13 μL of premade master mix to each samples.
5. Use PCR machine to incubate all samples at 0°C for 1 h, followed by 15 min at 65°C, and then 4°C forever. But do not leave the completed samples on PCR machine for more than 30 min.

Table 1
Sample sheet for the assembly reagent for microRNA labeling for microarray experiments

	Amt Cy3	Amt Cy5	Cy3 Conc	Cy5 Conc	Cy3	LBI	H_2O	Cy5	Lbl	H_2O	Slides	Notes
1	5	5									miRNA-EX_01_	
2	5	5									miRNA-EX_01_	
3	5	5									miRNA-EX_01_	
4	5	5									miRNA-EX_01_	
5	5	5									miRNA-EX_01_	
6	5	5									miRNA-EX_01_	
7	5	5									miRNA-EX_01_	
8	5	5									miRNA-EX_01_	
9	5	5									miRNA-EX_01_	
10	5	5									miRNA-EX_01_	

Cy3 erythrocyte RNA samples from individual patients, *Cy5* common RNA reference isolated from one unit of blood, which will be used in all samples as normalization control (the dye choice for samples vs. reference is optional)

6. Place the labeling reaction in a Speedvac® and dry the sample to complete dryness or until the volume is less than 10 μL. It usually takes about 20 min.
7. Redissolve the dry sample in 5–10 μL nuclease-free water.
8. Add 350 μL buffer RLT (of the RNeasy Mini Kit from Qiagen) to the sample, and disrupt and homogenize immediately by vigorous vortexing.
9. Add 3.5 volumes of 100% ethanol (1,225 μL) and mix thoroughly by vortexing. Do not centrifuge. (Please note that here the large amount of ethanol is used to trap the small-sized RNAs.)
10. Pipette 700 μL of the sample, including any precipitate that may have formed, into an RNeasy Mini spin column placed in a 2-mL collection tube. Centrifuge for 15 s at ≥8,000 × *g* (≥10,000 rpm) and discard the flow through.
11. Repeat the loading of the samples onto the mini spin column until the whole sample has been pipetted into the spin column. Discard the flow-through each time.
12. Place the RNeasy Mini spin column into a new 2-mL collection tube. Pipette 500 μL buffer RPE into the spin column, and centrifuge for 15 s at ≥8,000 × *g* (≥10,000 rpm). Discard the flow-through.
13. Pipette another 500 μL buffer RPE (in the RNeasy kit) into the column and centrifuge for 15 s at ≥8,000 × *g* (≥10,000 rpm) again.
14. Centrifuge at full speed for 1 min finally.
15. Place the RNeasy Mini spin column into a 1.5-mL collection tube. Pipette 25 μL of RNase-free water directly onto the spin column membrane. Centrifuge for 1 min at ≥8,000 × *g* (≥10,000 rpm) to elute the labeled RNAs for the hybridization with microarrays.

3.4. Microarray Hybridization

1. Add 33 μL of 2× Exiqon hybridization buffer to make the total volume 66 μL.
2. Heat the sample tubes to 95° for 3 min and then spin briefly before adding them to the array.
3. Apply the samples to slides in MAUI® SC mixer – need 61–62 μL to load and hybridize at 60°C using nonevaporation trays covering slides. The hybridization depends on the melting temperature of the probes used on the microRNA microarrays.
4. Use glass stain dishes with metal slide holders for all washes.
5. Remove mixer with Wash Buffer A at 60°C.
6. Rinse the slides for 2 min wash at 60°C with Wash Buffer A.

7. Rinse the slides for 10 s at room temperature with Wash Buffer B.
8. Wash the slides for 2 min at room temperature with fresh Wash Buffer B.
9. Wash the slides for 2 min at room temperature with Wash Buffer C.
10. Spin dry the slides in the racks at 200–450 g at the table top centrifuge for 3 min.
11. Store the slides in a dark box until ready to scan using the Axon GenePix 4000B microarray scanner. It would be best to scan the arrays within a few hours before the signals decay. The obtained microRNA expression can be used to derive a biological conclusion (Fig. 2b).

4. Notes

1. For blood samples of each patient, collect 20 μL of whole blood for CBC analysis to determine the percentage of reticulocytes before and after purification procedures.
2. During the removal of CD71+ reticulocytes for the blood cells with high level of reticulocytes, the amount of CD71 beads may be limiting. Therefore, it is important to increase the amount of beads used to label the CD71+ cells to ensure efficient and successful immunodepletion.
3. Given the large amount of protein in the mature red cells relative to the RNAs, it is often important to increase the volume as well as the repetition of the phenol extraction to ensure the successful separation of the aqueous phase for RNA purification.
4. When the RNA gel or Bioanalyzer are used to analyze RNAs, the intactness and the 28S/18S rRNA ratio are usually used to indicate the integrity and quality of RNA. Given the fact that large-sized RNAs are often degraded in the mature erythrocytes, it is usual to observe only small-sized RNAs with significant degradation of the large-sized RNAs.

Acknowledgments

We thank the Duke microarray facility and members of the Chi lab for technical assistance and constructive feedback and the Telen lab for assistance with sample collection. This research was funded by NIH R21DK080994 and Roche Foundation for Anemia Research (RoFAR).

References

1. Hoffman R, Benz EJB, Shattil SJ, Furie B, Cohen HJ, et al. (2004) Hematology: Basic Principles and Practice: Churchill Livingstone, Edinburgh.
2. Goh SH, Lee YT, Bouffard GG, Miller JL (2004) Hembase: browser and genome portal for hematology and erythroid biology. *Nucleic Acids Res* **32**: D572–D574.
3. Linda G, Lee C-HCLAC (1986) Thiazole orange: a new dye for reticulocyte analysis. *Cytometry* 7: 508–517.
4. Chen SY, Wang Y, Telen MJ, Chi JT (2008) The genomic analysis of erythrocyte microRNA expression in sickle cell diseases. *PLoS One* **3**: e2360.
5. Landry P, Plante I, Ouellet DL, Perron MP, Rousseau G, et al. (2009) Existence of a microRNA pathway in anucleate platelets. *Nat Struct Mol Biol* **16**: 961–966.
6. Bartel DP (2004) MicroRNAs: genomics, biogenesis, mechanism, and function. *Cell* **116**: 281–297.
7. Felli N, Fontana L, Pelosi E, Botta R, Bonci D, et al. (2005) MicroRNAs 221 and 222 inhibit normal erythropoiesis and erythroleukemic cell growth via kit receptor down-modulation. *Proc Natl Acad Sci U S A* **102**: 18081–18086.
8. Wang Q, Huang Z, Xue H, Jin C, Ju XL, et al. (2007) MicroRNA miR-24 inhibits erythropoiesis by targeting activin type I receptor ALK4. *Blood* **111**: 588–595.
9. Yang GH, Wang F, Yu J, Wang XS, Yuan JY, et al. (2009) MicroRNAs are involved in erythroid differentiation control. *J Cell Biochem* **107**: 548–556.
10. Felli N, Pedini F, Romania P, Biffoni M, Morsilli O, et al. (2009) MicroRNA 223-dependent expression of LMO2 regulates normal erythropoiesis. *Haematologica* **94**: 479–486.
11. Fu YF, Du TT, Dong M, Zhu KY, Jing CB, et al. (2009) Mir-144 selectively regulates embryonic alpha-hemoglobin synthesis during primitive erythropoiesis. *Blood* **113**: 1340–1349.
12. Pase L, Layton JE, Kloosterman WP, Carradice D, Waterhouse PM, et al. (2009) miR-451 regulates zebrafish erythroid maturation in vivo via its target gata2. *Blood* **113**: 1794–1804.
13. Dore LC, Amigo JD, Dos Santos CO, Zhang Z, Gai X, et al. (2008) A GATA-1-regulated microRNA locus essential for erythropoiesis. *Proc Natl Acad Sci U S A* **105**: 3333–3338.
14. Bruchova H, Yoon D, Agarwal AM, Mendell J, Prchal JT (2007) Regulated expression of microRNAs in normal and polycythemia vera erythropoiesis. *Exp Hematol* **35**: 1657–1667.
15. Masaki S, Ohtsuka R, Abe Y, Muta K, Umemura T (2007) Expression patterns of microRNAs 155 and 451 during normal human erythropoiesis. *Biochem Biophys Res Commun* **364**: 509–514.
16. Wang Q, Huang Z, Xue H, Jin C, Ju XL, et al. (2008) MicroRNA miR-24 inhibits erythropoiesis by targeting activin type I receptor ALK4. *Blood* **111**: 588–595.
17. Georgantas RW, 3rd, Hildreth R, Morisot S, Alder J, Liu CG, et al. (2007) CD34+ hematopoietic stem-progenitor cell microRNA expression and function: a circuit diagram of differentiation control. *Proc Natl Acad Sci U S A* **104**: 2750–2755.
18. Zhan M, Miller CP, Papayannopoulou T, Stamatoyannopoulos G, Song CZ (2007) MicroRNA expression dynamics during murine and human erythroid differentiation. *Exp Hematol* **35**: 1015–1025.
19. Choong ML, Yang HH, McNiece I (2007) MicroRNA expression profiling during human cord blood-derived CD34 cell erythropoiesis. *Exp Hematol* **35**: 551–564.
20. Bruchova H, Yoon D, Agarwal AM, Swierczek S, Prchal JT (2009) Erythropoiesis in polycythemia vera is hyper-proliferative and has accelerated maturation. *Blood Cells Mol Dis* **43**: 81–87.

Chapter 14

Stable Overexpression of miRNAs in Bone Marrow-Derived Murine Mast Cells Using Lentiviral Expression Vectors

Ramon J. Mayoral and Silvia Monticelli

Abstract

MicroRNAs (miRNAs) constitute a class of molecules regulating gene expression in many different cell types, including cells of the mammalian immune system. Indeed, changes in miRNA expression patterns have been implicated in various physiological and pathological processes. Mast cells (MCs) are hematopoietic cells that originate in the bone marrow and migrate into the tissues, where they mature and reside. They have an important immunoregulatory and effector role in IgE-associated allergic disorders, as well as in certain innate and adaptive immune responses. An effective way to explore the functions of miRNAs in murine MCs includes the modification of miRNA expression in primary bone marrow-derived mast cells (BMMCs), followed by the analysis of the phenotypic consequences of such perturbation. In this chapter, we describe how to differentiate BMMCs and transduce them with lentiviruses. As an example, we expressed miR-221 and miR-222, which showed stable expression in BMMCs and acted as post-transcriptional regulators of c-Kit expression.

1. Introduction

Mast cells (MCs) are long-lived cells that originate as progenitors in the bone marrow, but terminate their maturation only in the vascularized tissues, where they will ultimately reside. MCs are mostly found near sites of contact with the external environment such as skin and the vascular and mucosal barriers (1), which are a prime location for the initiation and modulation of innate immune responses. Differentiated MCs normally express on the surface as major receptors the high-affinity IgE receptor (FcεRI) and c-Kit, which have important roles in the differentiation, survival, proliferation, and function of MCs. Even though MCs are best known as main effector cells in IgE-mediated allergic responses (2, 3), recent studies also indicate that these cells can contribute to diseases such as multiple sclerosis, rheumatoid

Silvia Monticelli (ed.), *MicroRNAs and the Immune System: Methods and Protocols*, Methods in Molecular Biology, vol. 667,
DOI 10.1007/978-1-60761-811-9_14,

arthritis, atherosclerosis, aortic aneurysm, cancer, obesity, and diabetes (4–9). In fact, MCs can also enhance the adaptive immune response by releasing cytokines and other mediators that recruit neutrophils, eosinophils, and T lymphocytes on a site of infection (10, 11). Dysregulation of their proliferation and functions can also lead to diseases like mastocytosis (12).

MicroRNAs (miRNAs) constitute a family of small noncoding RNAs that have emerged as key posttranscriptional regulators in a wide variety of organisms (13–15). Their mode of action consists in binding, through partial complementarity, to sites in the 3′ UTR of target mRNAs. The importance of miRNAs in fine-tuning gene expression is highlighted by the finding that changes in the abundance of a single miRNA can affect the levels of expression of hundreds of proteins (16, 17). It is, therefore, not surprising that a single dysregulated miRNA can have profound effects on the state of the cell. Indeed, we have recently shown that a family of miRNAs expressed in murine MCs has an important role in regulating their proliferation and cell cycle (18, 19).

Here, we describe how to differentiate murine MCs in vitro starting from precursors from the bone marrow. Since IL-3 is an essential cytokine for BMMC proliferation and survival, we also explain a relatively fast and inexpensive way to produce it. Finally, we describe how to stably express any miRNA gene of interest using self-inactivating lentiviruses (20–22). Lentiviral particles are less prone to transcriptional silencing compared to oncoretroviral vectors; therefore, they are better suited for long-term cultures like the ones needed when working with BMMCs. Lentiviral vectors stably integrate into the target cell genome; therefore, the miRNA gene of interest is transmitted to the progeny of a transduced cell in an expanding BMMC population (23, 24).

As an example, we validated this method by expressing miR-221 and miR-222, two miRNAs expressed in BMMCs at basal levels, but upregulated upon activation (19). We demonstrated that the effect of these miRNAs in BMMCs is specific and dependent on the complementarity of the miRNA with the target mRNAs.

2. Materials

2.1. Plasmids

1. Plasmids TWEEN and pAPM (*25, 26*): these are the transfer vectors containing the miRNA sequence. These vectors have deleted parts of the HIV-1 genome and *cis*-acting elements necessary for transgene encapsidation, reverse transcription, and integration. They are self-inactivating (SIN), therefore,

they lose transcriptional capacity of the viral long terminal repeat (LTR) once they are transferred into the target cells, minimizing the risk of emergence of replication and avoiding problems linked to promoter interference. Their CMV, hPGK, and SFFV promoters are functional in a broad spectrum of cells and provide various levels of expression in BMMCs. A schematic representation of both lentiviral vectors is shown in Fig. 1a.

2. Plasmid psPAX2 (Addgene plasmid 12260): this is the packaging vector containing the CAG promoter (a combination of chicken β-actin promoter and CMV enhancer) driving the expression of packaging proteins.
3. Plasmid pMD2.G (Addgene plasmid 12259): this vector expresses the envelope protein-G of vesicular stomatitis virus (VSV-G), which has a high stability and confers broad tropism to the virus.

2.2. Growth and Maintenance of Cell Cultures

1. Fetal bovine serum (FBS).
2. Solution of 0.25% trypsin and 1 mM EDTA.
3. IMDM complete medium: Iscove's modified Dulbecco's medium (IMDM) supplemented with 10% (v/v) heat-inactivated fetal bovine serum, 2 mM L-glutamine, 100 U/mL penicillin, 100 μg/mL streptomycin, 0.1 mM nonessential amino acids, and 50 μM β-mercaptoethanol.
4. DMEM complete medium: Dulbecco's modified Eagle's medium (DMEM) with 4.5 g/L glucose and no pyruvate, supplemented with 10% (v/v) heat-inactivated fetal bovine serum, 2 mM L-glutamine, 100 U/mL penicillin, 100 μg/mL streptomycin, 0.1 mM nonessential amino acids, and 50 μM β-mercaptoethanol.
5. WEHI-3 myelomonocytic leukemia mouse cells (ATCC code: TIB 68); maintained in IMDM complete medium at 37°C in a 5% CO_2 incubator.
6. BMMC medium: a 1:1 solution of WEHI3 conditioned supernatant (containing IL-3) and IMDM complete medium.
7. Human embryonic kidney cells 293 T; maintained in DMEM complete medium at 37°C in a 5% CO_2 incubator.

2.3. Transfection of HEK 293 T Cells to Produce Lentiviral Particles and Transduction of BMMCs

1. Modified Eagle's minimum essential medium (Opti-MEM)
2. Polyethylenimine (Polysciences, Inc): polyethylenimine (PEI) powder is dissolved to a concentration of 1 mg/mL in nuclease-free water pre-warmed to 80°C. After allowing the solution to cool down to room temperature, the pH is adjusted to 7.2 with HCl 5 M. The solution is filter sterilized, aliquoted, and stored at −80°C.

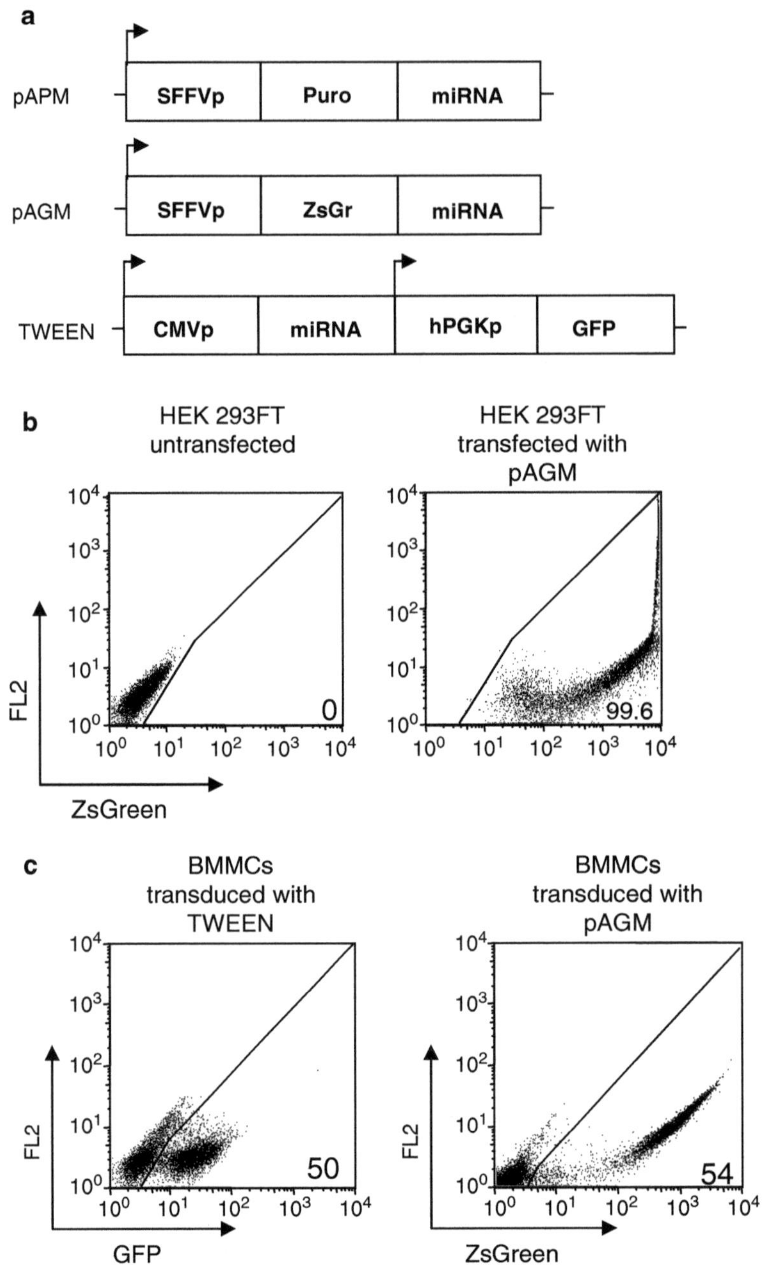

Fig. 1. Lentiviral vectors can be used to effectively transduce primary murine BMMCs. Schematic diagram of the lentiviral vectors used. The pAPM vector contains the spleen focus-forming virus promoter (SFFVp) driving expression of the selective agent, a Pac gene encoding puromycin N-acetyl-transferase, followed by a miRNA gene. To easily check the yield of transfection of HEK 293 T cells and transduction of BMMCs we use in parallel a variant of this vector containing a ZsGreen fluorescent protein reporter gene instead of the selective agent. The TWEEN vector contains two independent promoters: the cytomegalovirus promoter (CMVp), driving the expression of the miRNA gene of interest, and the human phosphoglycerate kinase promoter (hPGKp), driving the expression of the green fluorescent protein (GFP) reporter gene (**a**). Expression levels of reporter ZsGreen after transfection of HEK 293 T cells with the pAGM lentiviral vector. Using the transfection method described in this chapter, we routinely achieve an efficiency of transfection close to 100% (*right panel*) as compared to untransfected cells (*left panel*) (**b**). Efficiency of transduction of BMMCs. Using the transduction conditions described in this chapter, we routinely achieve ~50% efficiency of transduction, as assessed by GFP (*left panel*) or ZsGreen (*right panel*) expression. FACS analysis for reporter gene expression was performed 5 days after BMMC transduction. The efficiency of transduction is comparable for both the TWEEN (*left panel*) or pAGM (*right panel*) vectors (**c**).

3. TNES solution: 10 mM Tris-HCl, pH 7.5, 100 mM NaCl, 1 mM EDTA, 25% sucrose. Sterilize by filtering.
4. Polybrene (Sigma)
5. Transfection medium: DMEM complete medium with no antibiotics.

3. Methods

3.1. Production of IL-3 Conditioned Medium Using WEHI-3 Cells

1. Set up T-175-cm^2 flasks with 100 mL IMDM complete medium and WEHI-3 cells at a concentration of 10^5 cells/mL (see Note 1).
2. Incubate them without feeding until the concentration reaches at least 1×10^6 cells/mL (usually 6–7 days).
3. Spin down the cell culture at $300 \times g$ for 7 min and transfer the supernatant to a new tube.
4. Clear the supernatant of the remaining cell debris by filtering it through a 0.45 μm low-binding protein filter into a sterile bottle and store at −20°C or lower for later use (see Note 2).

3.2. Differentiation of Murine Bone Marrow-Derived Mast Cells

1. Flush the marrow from femurs and tibias of donor mice (4–12 weeks old) using IMDM complete medium and a small syringe.
2. Spin down the cells at $300 \times g$ for 7 min and wash them once with IMDM complete medium. Plate them in BMMC medium at a concentration of 5×10^5 cells/mL.
3. The next day, discard the adherent cells by changing the flask. Repeat the same procedure every 2 days until there are no more adherent cells in culture. This allows the elimination of irrelevant adherent cells, as MCs grow in suspension. Feed the cells by adding fresh medium 2–3 times a week (see Note 3).
4. Three weeks after differentiation, the population should be homogeneous, with ~95% of the cells in culture being c-Kit$^+$ and FcεRI$^+$ at surface staining and testing positive for toluidine blue staining (see Note 4).

3.3. Transient Transfection of HEK 293 T Cells and Production of Lentiviral Particles

1. A transient co-transfection of three plasmids is used to generate recombinant viral particles. The first plasmid, TWEEN or pAPM, provides the sequence of the miRNA of interest; the second plasmid, pMD2.G, the envelope protein VSV-G; the third plasmid, pSPAX2, the packaging proteins.
2. Day 1. Seed 4×10^6 HEK 293 T cells in a T-75-cm^2 flask using DMEM complete medium; the cells should be at least 80% confluent at the day of transfection. Never let the cells

grow to 100% confluence, as it can lead to reduced efficiency of transfection and reduced virus production.

3. Day 2. Rinse the cultures of HEK 293 T cells with PBS and add 16 mL of DMEM complete medium without antibiotics. Prepare the DNA cocktail using the following ratio and volume: 5 μg of pMD2.G, 15 μg of psPAX2, and 20 μg of lentiviral vector in 2 mL of Opti-MEM. After incubating the cocktail for 5 min at RT, add 90 μL of PEI solution pipetting up and down and mixing rapidly. Incubate the mixture at least 10 min at RT before adding it dropwise to the cell culture (see Notes 5 and 6). Figure 1b shows a typical result of HEK 293 T cells transfected using this method.
4. Day 3. Change the transfection medium by gently rinsing the cells with PBS and adding DMEM complete medium (with antibiotics if desired).
5. Day 4. Collect the lentivirus-containing supernatant of the transfected HEK 293 T and remove the remaining cells by centrifuging at 300 × *g* for 7 min; filter it through a 0.45 μm low-binding protein filter to eliminate cell debris. Viral particles are concentrated using a Beckman Coulter Optima LE-80 K ultracentrifuge and a SW-32-Ti swinging bucket rotor, compatible with large 129.1 and small 139.5 buckets. Centrifugation is carried out at 6°C for 2 h at maximum accel/decel. When using the 139.5 buckets, add 13 mL of supernatant to the tube and underlay it with 2 mL of TNES buffer, adding the remaining supernatant on top; spin at 25,000 rpm (~77000 × *g*). If large buckets are used, add 30 mL of virus and underlay with 6.5 mL of TNES buffer; spin at 24,300 rpm (~73000 × *g*). After centrifugation, remove the supernatant and aspirate as much sucrose as possible before resuspending the pellet of viral particles in fresh BMMC medium. Starting from a T-75-cm^2 flask and finally resuspending the pellet in 250 μL usually yields a concentration of viral particles of about 3×10^5 TransductionUnits/μL (see Note 7).
6. Day 5. Perform a second harvest of the retroviral supernatant following exactly the same procedure as described in point 5. Eliminate the transfected cells.

3.4. Transduction of BMMCs with Lentiviral Particles

1. Using 12-well plates, plate $0.5–1 \times 10^6$ BMMCs differentiated for 3–10 weeks in 750 μL of BMMC medium and add 250 μL of the concentrated virus from **step 5** of the Subheading 3.3. Adding polybrene at a concentration of 1 μg/mL can increase the efficiency of transduction. When plating 0.9×10^6 BMMCs and using the concentrated viral supernatant produced from one T-75-cm^2 flask, the multiplicity of infection (TransductionUnits/cell) is about 100.

Transduction efficiency of BMMCs under these conditions should normally be around 50% as shown in Fig. 1c.

2. Twenty-four hours later, transfer the transduced cells to a six-well plate and add the second harvest of lentiviral particles (from **step 6** of the Subheading 3.3) together with 750 μL of fresh BMMC medium, so that the total final volume is 2 mL.
3. Keep expanding the cells and transfer them to a T-25-cm^2 flask after 1–2 days, and either sort or select them depending on the selective agent of the lentiviral construct used (see Note 8).

4. Notes

1. For routine maintenance of WEHI-3 cells, spin down the cells at $300 \times g$ and resuspend them in IMDM complete medium at a concentration of 10^5 cells/mL. Check the cell counts and feed them at least twice a week.
2. Each batch of WEHI-3 conditioned medium can be tested by evaluating cell survival of BMMCs or any other IL-3 dependent mast cell type like the MC/9 cell line (ATCC code: CRL 8306). This is based on the fact that upon IL-3 withdrawal, murine MCs undergo apoptosis (27). Therefore, an assay can be easily set up by adding different volumes of WEHI-3 supernatant into complete IMDM medium and analyzing cell viability by trypan blue exclusion. When cultured in optimal conditions, more than 95% BMMCs should be alive.
3. Always maintain BMMCs at a concentration between 10^5 and 10^6 cells/mL. When feeding cells, spin down 1/3 or 1/2 of the culture and resuspend the cells in fresh medium. We find that cells are healthier and grow faster if not more than half of the medium is replaced, or if the cells are not diluted to more than 1:2.
4. Mature BMMCs are metachromatic because of the high content of acidic radicals in the heparin glycosaminoglycans found in cytoplasmatic granules. Toluidine blue is a basic aniline dye that changes color turning purple upon encountering these acidic radicals. This dye can be therefore used to identify mature BMMCs, whose cytoplasm will turn dark purple as opposed to the pale blue of the nuclei and other cell types. A toluidine blue stock solution is prepared by dissolving 0.5 g of powder in 70% (v/v) ethanol. The working solution is prepared fresh by mixing the stock solution with 1% NaCl,

pH 2.3, using a ratio of 1:9. Cells are washed once with PBS and cytospun on a glass slide. They are then stained for 2–3 min with the working solution of toluidine blue. After rinsing the slide with PBS, the stained cells are covered with Clarion mounting medium (Sigma) and a cover slide, prior to observation under the microscope.

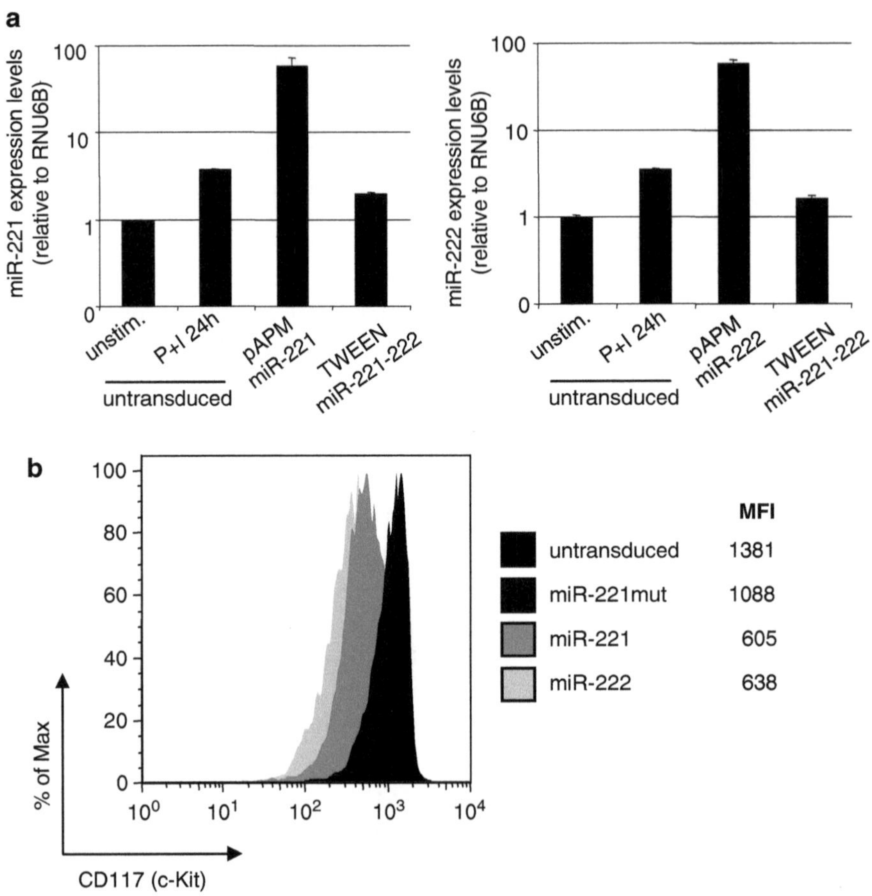

Fig. 2. MiR-221 and miR-222 are overexpressed in transduced BMMCs and they are functional on endogenous targets. Real-time RT-PCR showing the levels of miR-221 (*left panel*) and miR-222 (*right panel*) expression in BMMCs 10 days after transduction. Cells were either left untransduced or transduced with a TWEEN vector expressing both miR-221 and miR-222 or with a pAPM vector expressing either miR-221 (*left panel*) or miR-222 (*right panel*). As a control, the untransduced cells were left resting or stimulated with 20 nM PMA and 1 μM Ionomycin for 24 h, as this treatment increases the endogenous levels of expression of both miR-221 and miR-222 (19). RNU6B was used as endogenous control for PCR normalization (**a**), Immunostaining of CD117 (c-Kit), a validated target for miR-221 and miR-222 in BMMCs. BMMCs differentiated in vitro for 4 weeks were either left untreated or transduced with pAPM vectors expressing miR-221, miR-222, or a mutant version of the miR-221 expressing vector (miR-221mut) that contains a four-nucleotide substitution in the seed region of miR-221, which should therefore abrogate target specificity of this miRNA. As shown also by the mean fluorescence intensity (MFI) numbers on the right, levels of c-Kit expression on the cell surface are significantly reduced in BMMCs expressing either miR-221 or miR-222, but not in cells expressing the miR-221mut version, demonstrating that the miRNAs expressed from these vectors are functional and specific for their targets (**b**).

5. Polyethylenimine (PEI) is a stable cationic polymer with ethylenimine motifs responsible for the positively charged backbone. PEI ensnares the negatively charged DNA, and the whole complex binds to the cell surface (28). Uptake of the DNA occurs via endosomal vesicles, which release the plasmid to the cytoplasm after osmotic swelling (29).
6. For scaling up or down this transfection, the ratio of DNA:PEI should be kept constant. For example, if transfecting HEK 293 T cells in a 10-cm round plate, a total DNA amount of 8 μg should be used, with 4 μg of transfer vector carrying the transgene, 3 μg of packaging vector (psPAX2), and 1 μg of VSVg Envelope (pMD2.G).
7. Concentrated virus can be frozen in aliquots at −80°C for later use. Multiple freeze—thaw cycles can cause a two to fourfold drop in viral titers per cycle, and should therefore be avoided.
8. Levels of miR-221 and miR-222 expression and functional analysis of one of their validated targets are shown in Fig. 2.

Acknowledgements

We would like to thank Dr. Thomas Pertel and Dr. Desiree Bonci for the pAPM and TWEEN lentiviral vectors, respectively. RJM is the recipient of a pre-doctoral fellowship from the San Raffaele University, Milan, Italy. This work is supported in part by a Ceresio Foundation fellowship and a Swiss National Science Foundation grant to SM.

References

1. Vliagoftis H, Befus AD. Mast cells at mucosal frontiers. Curr Mol Med 2005;5:573–89.
2. Bingham CO, Austen KF. Mast-cell responses in the development of asthma. J Allergy Clin Immunol 2000;105:S527–34.
3. Robbie-Ryan M, Brown M. The role of mast cells in allergy and autoimmunity. Curr Opin Immunol 2002;14:728–33.
4. Secor VH, Secor WE, Gutekunst CA, Brown MA. Mast cells are essential for early onset and severe disease in a murine model of multiple sclerosis. J Exp Med 2000;191:813–22.
5. Lee DM, Friend DS, Gurish MF, Benoist C, Mathis D, Brenner MB. Mast cells: a cellular link between autoantibodies and inflammatory arthritis. Science 2002;297:1689–92.
6. Sun J, Sukhova GK, Wolters PJ, et al. Mast cells promote atherosclerosis by releasing proinflammatory cytokines. Nat Med 2007; 13:719–24.
7. Sun J, Sukhova GK, Yang M, et al. Mast cells modulate the pathogenesis of elastase-induced abdominal aortic aneurysms in mice. J Clin Invest 2007;117:3359–68.
8. Coussens LM, Raymond WW, Bergers G, et al. Inflammatory mast cells up-regulate angiogenesis during squamous epithelial carcinogenesis. Genes Dev 1999;13: 1382–97.
9. Liu J, Divoux A, Sun J, et al. Genetic deficiency and pharmacological stabilization of mast cells reduce diet-induced obesity and diabetes in mice. Nat Med 2009; 15(8):940–45.
10. Marshall JS. Mast-cell responses to pathogens. Nat Rev Immunol 2004;4:787–99.

11. Malaviya R, Georges A. Regulation of mast cell-mediated innate immunity during early response to bacterial infection. Clin Rev Allergy Immunol 2002;22:189–204.
12. Akin C, Metcalfe DD. Systemic mastocytosis. Annu Rev Med 2004;55:419–32.
13. Ambros V. The functions of animal microRNAs. Nature 2004;431:343–9.
14. Baulcombe D. RNA silencing in plants. Nature 2004;431:356–63
15. He L, Hannon GJ. MicroRNAs: small RNAs with a big role in gene regulation. Nat Rev Genet 2004;5(7):522–31.
16. Selbach M, Schwanhäusser B, Thierfelder N, Fang Z, Khanin R, Rajewsky N. Widespread changes in protein synthesis induced by microRNAs. Nature 2008;455:58–63.
17. Baek D, Villén J, Shin C, Camargo FD, Gygi SP, Bartel DP. The impact of microRNAs on protein output. Nature 2008;455:64–71.
18. Monticelli S, Ansel KM, Xiao C, et al. MicroRNA profiling of the murine hematopoietic system. Genome Biol 2005;6(8);R71.
19. Mayoral RJ, Pipkin ME, Pachkov M, van Nimwegen E, Rao A, Monticelli S. MicroRNA-221-222 regulate the cell cycle in mast cells. J Immunol 2009;182(1):433–45.
20. Follenzi A, Ailles LE, Bakovic S, Geuna M, Naldini L. Gene transfer by lentiviral vectors is limited by nuclear translocation and rescued by HIV-1 pol sequences. Nat Genet 2000;25(2):217–22.
21. Van den Driessche T, Thorrez L, Naldini L, et al. Lentiviral vectors containing the human immunodeficiency virus type-1 central polypurine tract can efficiently transduce nondividing hepatocytes and antigen-presenting cells in vivo. Blood 2002;100(3):813–22.
22. Zufferey R, Dull T, Mandel RJ, et al.Self-inactivating lentivirus vector for safe and efficient in vivo gene delivery. J Virol 1998; 72(12):9873–80.
23. Miyoshi H, Smith KA, Mosier DE, Verma IM, Torbett BE. Transduction of human CD34+ cells that mediate long-term engraftment of NOD/SCID mice by HIV vectors. Science 1999;283:682–6.
24. Pfeifer A, Ikawa M, Dayn Y, Verma IM. Transgenesis by lentiviral vectors: lack of gene silencing in mammalian embryonic stem cells and preimplantation embryos. Proc Natl Acad Sci USA 2002;99(4):2140–5.
25. Ricci-Vitiani L, Pedini F, Mollinari C, et al. Absence of caspase 8 and high expression of PED protect primitive neural cells from cell death. J Exp Med 2004;200:1257–66.
26. Bernasconi R, Pertel T, Luban J, Molinari M. A dual task for the Xbp1-responsive OS-9 variants in the mammalian endoplasmic reticulum: inhibiting secretion of misfolded protein conformers and enhancing their disposal. J Biol Chem 2008;283(24):16446–54.
27. Mekori YA, Oh CK, Metcalfe DD. IL-3-dependent murine mast cells undergo apoptosis on removal of IL-3. Prevention of apoptosis by c-kit ligand. J Immunol 1993;151(7):3775–84.
28. Boussif O, Lezoualc'h F, Zanta MA, et al. A versatile vector for gene and oligonucleotide transfer into cells in culture and in vivo: polyethylenimine. Proc Natl Acad Sci USA 1995;92:7297–301.
29. Sonawane ND, Szoka FC, Verkman AS. Chloride accumulation and swelling in endosomes enhances DNA transfer by polyamine-DNA polyplexes. J Biol Chem 2003; 278: 44826–31.

Chapter 15

Monitoring MicroRNA Activity and Validating MicroRNA Targets by Reporter-Based Approaches

Alessia Baccarini and Brian D. Brown

Abstract

An essential requirement for discovering microRNAs that may be relevant to an immune cell's function is to identify the microRNAs that are active in the cell and the genes they target. As several chapters in this volume describe, there are a number of technologies available for profiling microRNA expression, including oligonucleotide array-based approaches, real-time PCR, and, now, deep-sequencing. A complementary approach to expression profiling is the use of a microRNA reporter vector for assaying microRNA activity. In their simplest form, these vectors are comprised of a reporter gene tethered to tandem repeats of a sequence that is complementary to a specific microRNA. This technology enables the activity of a microRNA to be detected, and at single-cell resolution, and provides a means to help identify microRNAs that may have a role in cell function. This is particularly relevant for studying microRNAs in the highly heterogeneous cellular network of the immune system. Reporter vectors have also proved useful for validating microRNA target sites and 3′ untranslated regions (UTR) that are under microRNA control. This chapter describes how to construct, produce, and use a reporter vector for assaying microRNA activity, and for validating a microRNA target.

1. Introduction

MicroRNA regulation plays an important role in the function of the immune system (1, 2). This is evident from studies showing that disruption of the microRNA pathway in certain cells of the immune system can lead to immune pathology (3, 4). Intense investigation is underway to identify the specific microRNAs, and the role they play, in regulating immune cell development and function, and already a number of relevant microRNAs have been identified. For example, miR-155 has been shown to control the homeostasis of regulatory T cells (5), and miR-150 is involved in B cell differentiation (6).

Small RNA cloning and other techniques have provided a powerful method for detecting the presence of hundreds of

Silvia Monticelli (ed.), *MicroRNAs and the Immune System: Methods and Protocols*, Methods in Molecular Biology, vol. 667,
DOI 10.1007/978-1-60761-811-9_15, © Springer Science+Business Media, LLC 2010

different microRNAs in various cells of the immune system (3, 7–9). However, there are limitations with these approaches. Of particular relevance, detection of a microRNA does not provide meaningful information about its activity in a particular cell. For example, a microRNA may be detected, but its expression may be too low to mediate significant target regulation (10, 11). Moreover, because expression profiling is performed on bulk populations, which are often heterogeneous, the expression of the microRNA may be predominately occurring in a subset of the profiled population. To address some of these issues, microRNA reporter or "sensor" vectors can be used (12–16). These are gene transfer vectors that express a reporter gene that contains binding sites for a specific microRNA. The inclusion of these binding sites means that if the cognate microRNA is active in a cell, the expression of the reporter gene will be suppressed, whereas in cells where the microRNA is not active, the reporter gene will be expressed at normal levels. This provides an invaluable means for monitoring the activity of a microRNA in a cell.

A similar technology can also be used to determine that a particular sequence or 3′UTR is regulated by a specific microRNA (12, 17–20). The putative microRNA target site or the 3′UTR is placed downstream of the reporter gene in a viral or nonviral gene transfer vector, and the vector is introduced into cells where the microRNA is overexpressed. A suppression of reporter gene expression compared to a control sample provides an indication that the target site or 3′UTR is subject to regulation by the particular microRNA. This approach has been used to validate targets predicted by algorithm, or found to be differentially expressed in transcriptome or proteome analysis (21, 22), and has the benefit of distinguishing a direct target of a microRNA from an indirect target (gene that is regulated by a microRNA).

Here, we describe how to construct, produce, and utilize one type of microRNA reporter, based on a dual florescence bidirectional lentiviral vector system, and a reporter assay for validating a microRNA target site.

2. Materials

2.1. Plasmid Construction

1. The following plasmids, or equivalents of, encoding the lentiviral vector genome: pCCL.sin.cPPT.pA.PL13.eGFP.minCMV.hPGK.mCherry.Wpre, pCCL.sin.cPPT.hPGK.mCherry.Wpre, pCCL.sin.cPPT.hPGK.eGFP.Wpre.
2. The following plasmids, or equivalents of, encoding the lentiviral vector packaging genes: pVSV-G, pMFLg/pRRE, pREV.
3. Annealing buffer (10×): 100 mM Tris–HCl (pH 7.5), 1 M NaCl, 10 mM EDTA in ddH_2O.

4. AgeI (5,000 U/ml) and NheI (10,000 U/ml).
5. QIAquick Gel Extraction Kit (Qiagen, Chatsworth, CA).
6. T4 Polynucleotide Kinase and T4 DNA Ligase reaction buffer.
7. Shrimp Alkaline Phosphatase (SAP).
8. Quick Ligation Kit: Quick T4 DNA Ligase, 2× Quick Ligation Reaction Buffer.
9. One Shot Top10 Chemically Competent *Escherichia coli* (Invitrogen, Carlsbad, CA).
10. SeaKem GTG Agarose for the recovery of nucleic acids (Cambrex Bio Science, Rockland, ME).
11. SeaKem LE Agarose for gel electrophoresis (Cambrex).
12. Agar plates with ampicillin.
13. Luria Broth Media.
14. Ampicillin and carbenicillin stock solutions are made by dissolving 5 g of the powder with endotoxin-free grade water, 0.22 μM filtered and stored in aliquots at −20°C.
15. Qiagen Endotoxin-free Plasmid Maxi Kit.
16. GFPsense primer: 5′-ATGGTCCTGCTGGAGTTCGTGA-3′ (desalt purification).

2.2. Vector Production

1. Human Embryonic Kidney 293T cells.
2. Iscove's Modified Dulbecco's Medium (IMDM) supplemented with 10% (heat inactivated) fetal bovine serum (FBS; Gibco), 5% of 10,000 μg of streptomycin (base)/ml and 10,000 U of penicillin (Gibco, Invitrogen).
3. Phosphate buffered saline (PBS; Gibco).
4. Trypsin–EDTA solution 0.25%, stored in aliquots at −20°C.
5. 2× HBS pH 7.05–7.09 solution is made by mixing 281 mM NaCl, 100 mM Hepes, 1.5 mM Na_2HPO_4, and dH_2O endotoxin-free (Sigma, St. Louis, MO), 0.22 μM filtered and stored in aliquots at −20 or −80°C.
6. 0.1× TE buffer: 10 mM Tris-HCl (pH 8.0), 1 mM EDTA (pH 8.0) diluted 1:10 with dH_2O, 0.22 μM filtered and stored at 4 C°. Before use, the 0.1× TE buffer is diluted 2:1 with dH_2O (two parts of 0.1× TE:one part of dH_2O).
7. 2.5 M calcium chloride is made by dissolving calcium chloride powder in Sigma tissue culture grade water, 0.22 μM filtered and stored in aliquots at −20°C.
8. Stericup PVDF (polyvinylidene fluoride) filter units (0.22 μM; 500, 250, and 150 ml size).
9. Polyallomer centrifuge tubes for ultracentrifugation (25 mm × 89 mm; Beckman Coulter, Brea, CA).

10. L-70 Ultracentrifuge (Beckman Coulter).
11. SW28 swinging bucket rotor (Beckman Coulter).

2.3. Cell Culture

1. Complete RPMI-1640 (1×): RPMI-1640 Medium containing 25 mM HEPES buffer, 1% l-glutamine, 10% FBS (Gibco), 5% of 10,000 μg of streptomycin (base)/ml and 10,000 U of penicillin (Gibco, Invitrogen), 20 μg/ml of granulocyte macrophage colony stimulating factor (GM-CSF; PeproTech), sodium pyruvate, 1 mM Hepes solution, and 50 μM β-mercaptoethanol.
2. Enrichment of Murine Hematopoietic Progenitors Kit (StemCell Technologies, Vancouver, BC).
3. StemSpan SFEM expansion medium (StemCell Technologies): 50 ng/ml SCF, 10 ng/ml IL-3, 10 ng/ml Flt3l, and 20 ng/ml IL-6 (PeproTech).
4. Interleukin-4 (IL-4) (PeproTech).
5. Lipopolysaccharide (LPS, 1 μg/ml).
6. BD Falcon 100 μm cell strainer.
7. Dual-Luciferase® Reporter Assay System (Promega).

2.4. Flow Cytometry

1. 5 ml BD Falcon polystyrene round-bottom fluorescence-activated cell sorter (FACS) tube.
2. FACS washing buffer: 500 ml of PBS (pH 7.2), 0.5% of BSA, 2 mM EDTA, stored at 4°C.
3. Trypsin solution 0.25%.
4. Antibodies: Anti-mouse CD11c– PE-Cy7 conjugated (0.2 mg/ml; BD Biosciences), anti-mouse MHC class II APC conjugated diluted 1:10 (0.2 mg/ml; BD Biosciences), anti-mouse CD86 PE conjugated (0.2 mg/ml; BD Biosciences), and anti-mouse CD16/32 (blocks Fc binding, 1 mg/ml; eBiosciences).
5. 4′,6-Diamidino-2-phenylindole, dihydrochloride (DAPI) stock solutions made by dissolving DAPI at 100 μM in deionized water and stored at 4°C protected from light.
6. 1% paraformaldehyde: Made from diluting 16% paraformaldehyde stock solution in PBS.
7. LSR II FACS (BD Biosciences).

3. Methods

Assaying the activity of a microRNA or validating a target site using a reporter vector requires: (1) construction of a vector encoding sequences with the microRNA target site downstream of a reporter transgene such as GFP or luciferase, (2) production of the vector, (3) introduction of the vector into the cell types of interest, and (4) an assay to measure changes in reporter expression. The microRNA reporter vector is delivered into cells or tissues by viral or nonviral means, and the expression of the reporter is assayed and normalized to an internal reporter, to control for transfection/transduction efficiency, and the results are compared to those obtained with a control vector that does not contain the microRNA target sites. A reduction in the level of microRNA reporter expression compared to the control indicates microRNA-mediated regulation of the target.

There are several aspects of the reporter vector, and the protocol for its use, that are critical for ensuring that the assay is sensitive enough to detect the activity of an endogenous microRNA. One critical variable is the possibility of saturating the microRNA by overexpression of the target bearing transcript (23–25). For this reason, we highly recommend designing the target sequences to be perfectly complementary to the microRNA, to use a weak or moderately expressed promoter to drive transgene expression, and to introduce a low vector copy into cells (26). Additionally, if target validation is the goal, and not to monitor endogenous microRNA activity, overexpression of the microRNA can be used to increase the level of target regulation and improve detection (21, 27).

Plasmid-based reporters can and have been used to effectively monitor microRNA activity. However, because it can be difficult to control the level of reporter expression that occurs by plasmid transfection, and plasmid transfection can be inefficient in many primary cell types, we utilize a lentiviral vector-based system as a microRNA reporter for studying microRNA activity in the hematopoietic system.

3.1. Construction of MicroRNA Reporter/Sensor Vectors

3.1.1. Generating MicroRNA Target Sites

1. For validating that the 3′UTR of a gene is regulated by a microRNA, the 3′UTR is amplified by PCR using primers that span the 3′UTR or a region of the 3′UTR that is predicated to contain the target site. Restriction sites for NheI or XbaI are added to the forward primer, whereas restriction sites for AgeI or XmaI/SmaI are added to the reverse primer. An additional six to eight nucleotides of random sequence are added to the 5′ end of each primer to improve restriction digestion. PCR can be performed on either genomic DNA or cDNA. The PCR product is purified by gel extraction or PCR purification kit. The concentration of the purified product is measured by spectrophotometer, and at least 1 μg of PCR product is digested with the appropriate restriction enzymes and purified by PCR purification kit to remove the digested ends. The product containing the 3′UTR of a gene and sticky ends can now be ligated into the reporter vector backbone.

2. For monitoring microRNA activity, the microRNA target sites are generated by synthesizing oligonucleotides that can be ligated together to create tandem repeats of a sequence that is perfectly complementary to the mature microRNA (for monitoring microRNA activity) or recapitulates a putative target site from a natural 3′UTR (for validating a target site) (see Note 1). For improved sensitivity, four to six target sites are recommended. The oligonucleotides are designed to anneal together and form sticky ends that can be annealed and ligated to restriction sites in the reporter vector. For example, the following oligonucleotides can be ordered to create target sites for hsa-miR-142-3p (5′ UGUAGUGUUUCCUACUUUAUGGA):

Sense1 5′-CTAGCATCCATAAAGTAGGAAACACTACAA GATTCCATAAAGTAGGAAACACTACA

Sense2 5′-ACGCGTTCCATAAAGTAGGAAACACTACAA CACTCCATAAAGTAGGAAACACTACAA

Antisense1 5′-ACGCGTTGTAGTGTTTCCTACTTTATG GAATCTTGTAGTGTTTCCTACTTTATGGATG

Antisense2 5′-CCGGTTGTAGTGTTTCCTACTTTATGG AGTGTTGTAGTGTTTCCTACTTTATGGA

3. The oligonucleotides are annealed by mixing (see Note 2):

2 μl	10× anneal buffer
1 μl	100 μM senseX oligonucelotide
1 μl	100 μM antisenseX oligonucleotide
16 μl	Water

Heat to 95°C for 5 min and cool to room temperature. This generates the duplex shown in Fig. 1, which can be stored at −20°C (Fig. 1).

4. The annealed oligonucleotides are phosphorylated by:

3 μl	10× T4 DNA Ligation reaction buffer (contains ATP)
1 μl	T4 polynucleotide kinase (10 U/μl)
20 μl	Annealed S/AS oligonucleotides
6 μl	Water

Incubate at 37°C for 30 min followed by 65°C for 20 min. Store at −20°C.

3.1.2. Vector Construction

1. These instructions assume the use of a reporter vector based on a third-generation self-inactivating bidirectional lentiviral vector system (pCCL.sin.cPPT.pA.PL13.eGFP.minCMV.

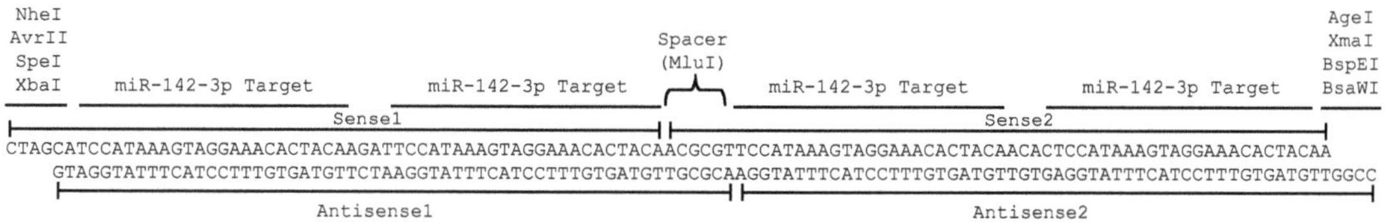

Fig. 1. Duplex structure of the annealed oligonucleotides containing the synthetic microRNA target sites for miR-142-3p.

hPGK.mCherry.Wpre, available upon request) (28). This vector encodes two florescent reporter transgenes, eGFP and monomeric cherry florescent protein (mCherry), that are expressed as separate transcripts from a single promoter, the human phosphoglycerate kinase (hPGK) promoter (Fig. 2, see Note 3). Alternatively, for studies aimed at validating a microRNA target site or 3′UTR, a luciferase reporter can be used, encoding firefly luciferase and mCherry or renilla luciferase (pCCL.sin.cPPT.pA.PL13.Firefly.minCMV.hPGK.mCherry.Wpre or pCCL.sin.cPPT.pA.PL13.Firefly.minCMV.hPGK.Renilla.Wpre available upon request). MicroRNA target sites can be incorporated into one of the two transgenes, and the other transgene can serve as an internal control for transfection/transduction. We clone microRNA target sites or 3′UTR between NheI and AgeI sites in the 3′UTR of the eGFP or firefly transgene.

2. The vector is digested with NheI and AgeI restriction enzymes, and the 9,001-bp backbone is gel purified from 1% low-melt agarose using gel extraction columns. 0.1–1 μg of gel-purified backbone is dephosphorylated using Shrimp Alkaline Phosphatase to prevent religation of any single-cut backbone.
3. Dilute the annealed and phosphorylated oligonucleotides (S1/AS1 and S2/AS2), which have sticky ends compatible with NheI and AgeI, 1/100 in water. Ligate 1 μl of 1/100 diluted S1/AS1 and 1 μl of 1/100 S2/AS2 into 50 ng of the digested vector backbone using Quick Ligase. Ligation mixture (1–3 μl) is transformed into competent bacteria.
4. The following day, colonies are selected, grown, and screened for the insert. This can be done by a restriction digest with NheI and AgeI, which cuts the insert. Plasmids with the insert will have bands at 9,001 and 128 bp, whereas plasmids with no insert will have bands at 9,001 and 16 bp.
5. Sequence plasmids using a GFPsense or Fireflysense primer to confirm that the sequence of the target sites are correct.
6. Prepare a maxi preparation of the plasmid using Endotoxin-free Maxi Prep Kit (see Note 4). The plasmid's concentration must be at least 1 μg/ml. In addition to using a spectrophotometer to measure the plasmid's concentration, the quality

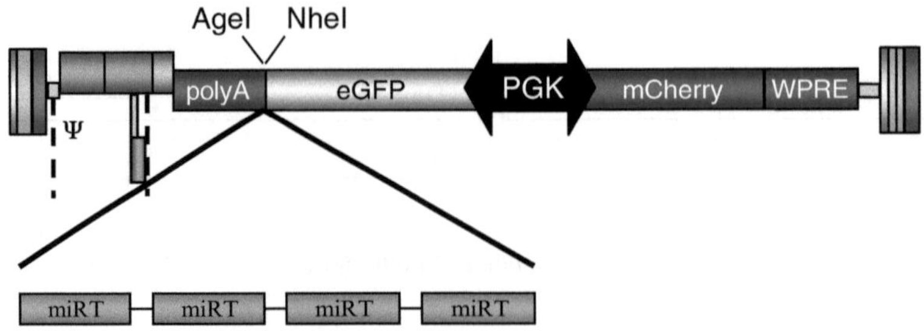

Fig. 2. Schematic of a microRNA sensor/reporter vector. Scheme of the dual florescence lentiviral vector-based microRNA reporter (based on pCCL.sin.cPPT.pA.PL13.eGFP.minCMV.hPGK.mCherry.Wpre). A modified version of the moderately expressed PGK promoter is used to coordinately drive transcription of two transgenes as distinct transcripts. microRNA target (miRT) sites, comprised of sequences with perfect complementarity to the sequence of a mature miRNA, are placed in the 3′UTR of the eGFP transgene. Because the mCherry gene does not contain the miRT, its transcript is unaffected by microRNA regulation. PolyA is from the Simian Virus 40, and the WPRE is from the woodchuck hepatitis virus.

of the plasmid should be checked by running 1–2 μg on a 1% agarose gel. The supercoiled form should be the predominant form and there should be no RNA or genomic DNA.

3.2. Lentiviral Vector Production by Transient Transfection

1. Day 0: Seed 9×10^6 293T cells in 20 ml complete IMDM in a 15-cm cell culture plate approximately 24 h before transfection and incubate at 37°C, 5% CO_2. Use low-passage cells that have never been grown to confluence. For transducing primary cells it is recommended to concentrate the lentiviral vector, and thus at least two 15-cm plates per vector are needed.
2. Day 1:
   (a) Change the cell medium 2 h before transfection with 18 ml of complete IMDM. The medium should be prewarmed to 37°C before adding to the cells. The cell density at the time of transfection is critical. The cells should be 60–70% confluent throughout the entire plate, with minimal cell-to-cell contact and no dense clusters of cells. If the cells are too confluent on the day of the transfection or appear to be loosely adherent, abort production. Repeat the cell seeding for the next day using less cells or with a new stock of 293T cells.
   (b) Prepare the mixture of plasmids and $CaCl_2$ for transfection in a 15-ml conical tube. The following volumes are for transfection in a 15-cm dish, using the third-generation lentiviral vector packaging system, and a transfer genome based on the bidirectional lentiviral vector platform.

7.00 μg	pVSV-G
12.50 μg	pMFLg/pRRE
6.25 μg	pREV
32.00 μg	Transfer plasmid (see Note 5)

The plasmid solution is made up to a final volume of 1,125 μl with 0.1× TE/dH_2O (2:1).

(c) Add 125 μl of 2.5 M $CaCl_2$ to the plasmid mixture, vortex, and leave at room temperature for 5 min.

(d) Place the 15-ml conical tube containing the 1,250-μl plasmid/$CaCl_2$ mixture plasmid on a vortex at high speed, and in a slow and dropwise manner add 1,250 μl of 2× HBS solution. The complete mixture should be added to the 293T cells immediately following the addition of the 2× HBS. Add the mixture to the side of the plate to prevent the cells from detaching. Incubate the cells at 37°C, 5% CO_2 overnight.

3. Day 2: 12–14 h after transfection, replace the medium with 16–18 ml of fresh, complete IMDM (prewarmed to 37°C). If the vector contains a transgene encoding a fluorescent reporter, such as GFP or mCherry, it is possible to assess the transfection efficiency of the cells under a fluorescent microscope. If <90% of the cells are transfected, this indicates that the transfection procedure was not optimal and will likely result in poor vector titer.
4. Day 3: Collect the cell supernatant 30 h after changing the medium and filter through a 0.22-μm PVDF disk filter to remove cell debris and other potential contaminants. There should be approximately 16 ml of supernatant per 15-cm plate. To concentrate the vector, add 35–38 ml of the filtered supernatant (from two 15-cm plates) to an ultracentrifuge tube. Ultracentrifuge at 50,000 × *g* for 2 h 20 min at room temperature in a swinging bucket rotor. Gently pour off the supernatant and resuspend in PBS. Approximately 80–100 μl of PBS per tube is recommended to concentrate the vector ~300–400-fold. Leave to resuspend for 30 min at room temperature. Make aliquots and freeze at −80°C.

3.3. Vector Titering (see Note 6)

1. One day prior, seed 5×10^4 293T cells per well in a 6-well plate.
2. The following day, prepare serial tenfold dilutions of the concentrated vector. In a 24-well plate, add 1 ml of IMDM to one well of a row and 900 μl of IMDM to the remaining wells. Add 2 μl of concentrated vector to the first well (containing 1 ml of medium) to create a 1/500 dilution of the vector (2×10^{-3} dilution). Mix by pipetting up and down. Transfer 100 μl of the 2×10^{-3} dilution to the next well containing 900 μl of medium to dilute the vector 2×10^{-4}-fold. Repeat this two more times so that there is a 2×10^{-3}, 2×10^{-4}, 2×10^{-5}, 2×10^{-6} dilution of the concentrated vector. If you are titering unconcentrated vector stock, you should add 800 ml of IMDM in the first well of the 24-well dilution plate

and 200 μl of the unconcentrated vector preparation and continue with the serial tenfold dilutions as described above (to get 2×10^{-1}, 2×10^{-2}, 2×10^{-3}, 2×10^{-4}).

3. Aspirate the medium from each well of the 6-well plate where 5×10^4 293T cells were seeded the previous day and add 0.5-ml fresh IMDM. Because 293T cells double approximately every 24 h, there should be $\sim 1 \times 10^5$ 293T cells per well.
4. Add 0.5 ml of one of the serial dilutions to each well. Because this is a further ½ dilution (0.5-ml medium + 0.5-ml vector/medium), the final vector dilutions are: 1×10^{-3}, 1×10^{-4}, 1×10^{-5}, 1×10^{-6}.
5. After 24 h, aspirate the medium and wash the wells with 2 ml of PBS. Replace with 2 ml of fresh IMDM.
6. Passage the cells for a minimum of 5–7 days after transduction to ensure that nonintegrated vector and pseudotransduction are minimized.
7. After >5 days, prepare the cells for FACS analysis. Aspirate the medium, wash the cells with PBS, and trypsinize. Stop the trypsinization with 2 ml PBS/10% FBS. Mechanically break up the cells by pipetting up and down and transfer 500 μl of cells to an FACS tube.
8. Centrifuge at $300 \times g$ for 5 min at room temperature. Aspirate the supernatant and add 1 ml of PBS/2% FBS/1% paraformaldehyde to the cell pellet.
9. Analyze mCherry and GFP expression in the cells by FACS. The vector titer is calculated at dilutions in which 0.5–20% of cells are positive for the florescent marker. The following formula is used to calculate titer:

$$\text{Transducing units/ml} = \#\text{Cells transduced} \times \frac{\%\,\text{mCherry} + (\text{or GFP} +)\,\text{cells}}{100} \times \text{Dilution factor}$$

Thus, if 2% of the cells are mCherry positive at the 10^{-6} dilution, then:

$$\begin{aligned}\text{Transducing units/ml} &= 10^5\,\textit{cells} \times \frac{2.0\%}{100} \times 10^6 \\ &= 2.0 \times 10^9\ \text{TU/ml}\end{aligned}$$

3.4. Monitoring Endogenous MicroRNA Activity by Reporter Vector In Vitro

1. These instructions assume the use of a reporter vector based on a third-generation self-inactivating bidirectional lentiviral vector system (pCCL.sin.cPPT.pA.PL13.eGFP.minCMV.hPGK.mCherry.Wpre) as described above.

2. Lentiviral vectors can efficiently transduce and stably integrate into most mouse and human hematopoietic cell lines and primary hematopoietic cells including hematopoietic progenitors cells, T cells, B cells, and monocytes. As an example of how the microRNA reporter vector can be used in primary cell culture to assay the activity of a microRNA, we describe a protocol for engineering mouse dendritic cells with the vector.
3. One day prior to transduction, mouse hematopoietic progenitor cells are collected from the bone marrow of adult mice by flushing the femurs with cold PBS. The cells are passed through a 0.45-μm nylon strainer, centrifuged at $300 \times g$ for 8 min, resuspended in Complete RPMI supplemented with GM-CSF, and placed in a 10-cm nonadherent cell culture dish.
4. The following day, cells are collected, counted, and 1.5×10^5 cells are seeded in a 24-well plate in 350-μl complete RPMI/GM-CSF or 7×10^4 cells are seeded in a 48-well plate in 150-μl complete RPMI/GM-CSF.
5. The vector is diluted to 2×10^7 TU/ml in complete RPMI/GM-CSF (see Note 7).
6. The cells are maintained in culture for at least 8 days to allow them to differentiate into dendritic cells (CD11c + MHCII+). The cells can be challenged with an appropriate stimulus, such as LPS, to induce dendritic cell maturation.
7. Expression of the fluorescent markers can be detected using an inverted, fluorescent microscope. All transduced cells will express mCherry, whereas the presence and level of GFP will depend on the expression of microRNA in the cells. This allows microRNA activity to be indirectly monitored as the cells differentiate.
8. After 8 days or a desired time point, the cells are collected into a 15-ml conical tube on ice, or a small volume of cells is placed into a well of a V-bottom 96-well plate. To remove adherent cells, the wells can be washed, trypsinized for 5 min at 37°C, 5% CO_2, and transferred to the tubes containing the nonadherent cells in complete medium.
9. The tubes or 96-well plate containing the cells are centrifuged at $300 \times g$ for 8 min at 4°C. The supernatant is removed, and the cells are resuspended in blocking solution (PBS pH 7.2, 0.5% BSA, 2% FBS, 2 mM EDTA, 0.5 mg/ml anti-mouse CD16/32 antibody).
10. After blocking on ice for 10 min, the cells are stained with fluorescently conjugated antibodies for the dendritic cells markers CD11c and MHCII, as well as for any other desired

markers. Importantly, fluorescent molecules that have spectral overlap with GFP and mCherry are not used.

11. To indirectly assess the activity of the microRNA in the cells, the expression of GFP tethered to the microRNA target sites can be compared to the expression of GFP in the control vector (Fig. 3). mCherry expression is used as a way to normalize values between different vectors because mCherry does not contain microRNA target sites. For each vector, the ratio of GFP mean florescence (MFI) to mCherry MFI (GFP MFI/mCherry MFI) is determined. The percentage of normal expression is determined by comparing the ratio between the microRNA target bearing vector and the control vector.

3.5. Monitoring Endogenous MicroRNA Activity by Reporter Vector In Vivo

1. The use of a lentiviral vector system permits the analysis of microRNA activity to be performed in vivo using genetically modified hematopoietic stem cell transplantation. This allows microRNA activity to be detected at single-cell resolution in the entire hematopoietic system.
2. Cells are collected from the bone marrow of adult CD45.1 C57BL/6 mice by flushing the femurs with PBS using a syringe and a 26-gauge needle. The cells are passed through a 0.45-μm nylon strainer, and the lineage negative cells, which are enriched for hematopoietic stem and progenitor cells, are

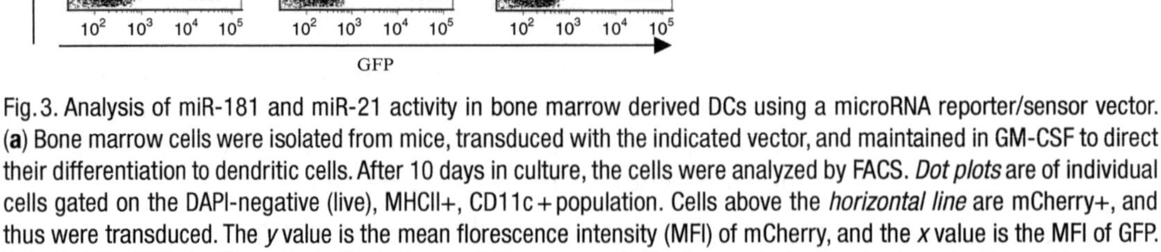

Fig. 3. Analysis of miR-181 and miR-21 activity in bone marrow derived DCs using a microRNA reporter/sensor vector. (**a**) Bone marrow cells were isolated from mice, transduced with the indicated vector, and maintained in GM-CSF to direct their differentiation to dendritic cells. After 10 days in culture, the cells were analyzed by FACS. *Dot plots* are of individual cells gated on the DAPI-negative (live), MHCII+, CD11c+population. Cells above the *horizontal line* are mCherry+, and thus were transduced. The *y* value is the mean florescence intensity (MFI) of mCherry, and the *x* value is the MFI of GFP. Note that the MFI of mCherry is similar between all three groups indicating equivalent vector transduction and transcriptional activity, whereas the MFI of GFP is drastically different between the three vectors, providing an indication of the activity of the cognate microRNA in BM-DCs. (**b**) The level of reporter regulation mediated by the cognate microRNA can be calculated using this type of formula. For example, the miR-181 reporter is expressed at 35% of the control, which indicates a 2.8-fold suppression, whereas the miR-21 reporter is expressed at <2% of the control. Thus, both miR-181 and miR-21 are active in BM-DCs, with miR-21 having significantly higher activity. In addition to the overall level of suppression, this analysis indicates that the microRNA is working in the whole population. It is worth noting that GFP was expressed in a small percentage of BM-DCs transduced with the miR-21 sensor, suggesting that miR-21 may not be as highly expressed in a small subset of the population.

purified by lineage negative selection using the Enrichment of Murine Hematopoietic Progenitors Kit.

3. Purified lineage negative cells are counted and brought to a concentration of 1×10^6 cells/ml in StemSpan SFEM expansion medium with this murine cytokine cocktail: 50 ng/ml SCF, 10 ng/ml IL-3, 10 ng/ml Flt3l, and 20 ng/ml IL-6.
4. 1 ml of cells (10^6 cells/ml) are added to one well of a 6-well plate, and the cells are transduced with 10^7–10^8 TU/ml of lentiviral vector. In addition to the microRNA sensor vector, a transplant should also be performed with a control vector that contains a scrambled microRNA target site or a target site for a microRNA that is not expressed in hematopoietic cells such as miR-122.
5. 18–24 h later, the cells are washed, and 5×10^5–1×10^6 cells are injected with a 28-gauge needle intravenously via tail vein or retro-orbitally into 6–8-week-old lethally irradiated CD45.2 C57BL/6 mice.
6. After a minimum of 6–8 weeks, when the hematopoietic compartment has been largely reconstituted with donor cells, the mice are euthanized. Blood, bone marrow, and lymphoid organs are collected and processed into single-cell suspensions and stained with appropriate markers for cell types of interest.
7. The cells are analyzed by FACS for GFP and mCherry expression, along with cell-type specific markers (see above for staining protocol).
8. There are several parameters that can be analyzed using this methodology. To determine if a microRNA is active in a specific cell population, a change in the GFP expression in cells engineered with the microRNA-target bearing vector can be compared with the GFP expression in cells engineered with the control vector (*see* Subheading 3.4). The mCherry expression in both vector groups serves as a way to normalize the data between the two groups.

3.6. Validating a MicroRNA Target by Reporter Vector

1. To validate that a particular sequence element or 3′UTR is regulated by a specific microRNA, the sequence of interest is cloned into a vector downstream of a reporter transgene, as described in Subheading 3.1. A plasmid or lentiviral vector-based reporter can be used for these studies (see Note 8). These instructions assume the use of a plasmid-based reporter.
2. Unlike the experimental design for assaying microRNA activity in a cell, validating that a natural sequence is a microRNA target site generally involves codelivering an oligonucleotide mimic of the microRNA or a vector capable of expressing the pre-microRNA (see Note 9). There are several commercially

available sources for microRNA mimics (synthetic oligonucleotides that mimic the structure of a pre-microRNA) or microRNA expression vectors (vectors that express a pre-microRNA). Alternatively, the microRNA gene can be cloned into an expression vector under the control of a strong promoter, such as the U6 or H1 promoters, or the CMV promoter. The appropriate microRNA mimic or microRNA expression vector, along with a control oligonucleotide or vector that encodes an unrelated microRNA, or a mutant version of the microRNA, must be acquired prior to the experiment (see Note 10). These instructions assume the use of a plasmid-based vector system for microRNA overexpression.

3. Day 0: Seed 1×10^5 293T cells (see Note 11) in 500 μl of complete IMDM in a 24-well plate, 24 h prior to transfection. Incubate at 37°C, 5% CO_2. Each condition is performed in triplicate and therefore the necessary number of wells must be seeded.
4. Day 1:
   (a) Replace the medium in each well with 500 μl of pre-warmed complete IMDM, 1–2 h prior to transfection.
   (b) In a 1.5-ml tube, prepare the DNA mixture with:
      - 10 ng of microRNA reporter plasmid (encoding the microRNA target site or 3′UTR and firefly luciferase).
      - 10 ng of transfection control plasmid (encoding renilla luciferase).
      - 300 ng of the microRNA expression plasmid (encoding a pre-microRNA) or 300 ng of a control expression plasmid (encoding an unrelated pre-microRNA or a mutant pre-microRNA).
      - Bring the amount of DNA to 1,000 ng with an empty plasmid (preferably promoterless) such as pBluescript.
      - Bring the total volume up to 17.5 μl with 0.1× TE/dH_2O (2:1).
   (c) Add 2.5 μl of 2.5 M $CaCl_2$ to the DNA mixture. Vortex for 5–10 s to ensure a good mixture and leave for 10 min at room temperature.
   (d) Pla dd 20 μl of 2× HBS solution. The complete mixture should be added to the 293T cells immediately following the addition of the 2× HBS and mixed gently in the well.
   (e) Incubate the cells at 37°C, 5% CO_2 overnight.
5. Day 2: Replace the medium in each well with 500 μl of pre-warmed complete IMDM.

6. Day 3: 48 h after transfection, harvest the cells and measure firefly and renilla luciferase activity using a dual luciferase reporter assay.
7. To determine whether the target site was suppressed by the microRNA, we calculate the mean (±standard deviation) of firefly and renilla luciferase expression from the three biological replicates, and use the following formula (see Note 12):

$$\frac{\text{Firefly microRNA reporter}}{\text{Renilla microRNA reporter}} \div \frac{\text{firefly control reporter} \times 100}{\text{renilla control reporter}} = \%\text{ of normal expression}$$

4. Notes

1. Four separate oligonucleotides (two sense and two antisense) are used instead of one long sense and one long antisense oligonucleotide because smaller oligonucleotides can be made with few errors and at smaller scale. However, modification in the design of the oligonucleotides can be made so that a single set of oligonucleotides (sense and antisense) with two tandem repeats of the target sequence can be concatemerized. This reduces cost but extends the cloning time.
2. The Sense1 and Antisense1 oligonucleotides are annealed together in one reaction, and the Sense2 and Antisense2 oligonucleotides are annealed together in a separate reaction.
3. A dual luciferase lentiviral vector is also available that expresses firefly and renilla luciferase as separate transcripts. This system may be preferable for detecting changes in gene expression in a narrow range, such as for validating a target site; however, the luciferase system cannot be used for single-cell analysis by FACS.
4. For good transfection efficiency of vector production, it is important to use an endotoxin-free kit for preparing the plasmid.
5. The transfer plasmid refers to the plasmid that encodes the genome to be packaged, and in this case refers to pCCL.sin.cPPT.pA.PL13.eGFP.minCMV.hPGK.mCherry.wpre containing the microRNA target sites. Control vectors that encode only one of the fluorescent transgenes should also be produced as they will be necessary for subsequent studies. The pCCL.sin.cPPT.hPGK.eGFP.wpre and pCCL.sin.cPPT.hPGK.mCherry.wpre can be used and are also available upon request.
6. The following protocol describes how to determine the number of vector particles that are capable of transducing (i.e.,

entering, stably integrating, and expressing) a model cell line. An additional parameter to measure is the concentration of p24 antigen, a component of the vector, in the preparation. This provides an estimate of the total number of physical vector particles, which includes particles capable of transduction and particles that are not capable of transduction for one reason or another. A high TU/ml:p24 ratio means a better quality preparation (more infective:noninfective particles) and a vector that will better infect cells.

7. Every primary cell type will have a slightly different protocol for transduction. For BM-derived dendritic cells and FLT3 Ligand-derived dendritic cells, we can transduce >50% of cells with a vector concentration $\geq 10^7$ TU/ml and a multiplicity of infection (MOI, transduction units: number of cells) >1. For higher transduction efficiency, we transduce the cells with a vector concentration between 10^7 and 10^8 TU/ml, and an MOI >10.
8. The use of a viral vector is not necessary for these studies if the assay is done in cell lines, such as 293T or HeLa cells, which are easy to transfect with a plasmid. Virtually, any expression plasmid can be used as a reporter, provided there are cloning sites available downstream of the reporter transgene and upstream of the polyA signal. There are several commercially available plasmid-based reporters that can be used for target validation, including pMIR-REPORT™ system or the pmirGLO Dual-Luciferase miRNA Target Expression Vector. For validating a target in primary cell types, or when overexpression of the microRNA is not being used, the use of a lentiviral vector-based reporter is recommended because of the ability to titrate the levels of target expression to physiological levels.
9. Overexpression of the microRNA, either by introduction of an oligonucleotide mimic or by expression from a vector, allows the assay to be better controlled, and because the level of regulation mediated by an endogenous microRNA on a natural target site is often modest (<50% change), introducing a high concentration of the microRNA into the cells can prevent the microRNA from being saturated by the reporter transcript. Overexpression of the microRNA will also increase the extent of target regulation and improve the sensitivity of the assay. The drawback of this approach is that at supraphysiological concentrations of the microRNA, interactions that are not favored at physiological concentrations may occur between the microRNA and a sequence element, and this can introduce a false positive in the assay.
10. Fluorescently tagged mimics or vectors encoding a reporter are useful to determine and optimize the transfection efficiency. However, it is important to note that a high transfection

efficiency does not ensure that the mimic or vector-derived microRNA is adequately processed into a mature microRNA. Thus, in addition to assessing transfection efficiency, it is recommended to directly determine the concentration of the mature microRNA in the cell by a quantitative reverse transcriptase PCR approach, such as real-time PCR or by northern blot.

11. Alternatively, the 293T cells transduced with the lentiviral vector-based microRNA reporter (generated during vector titering, Subheading 3.3) can be used for these experiments. In this case, the 293T cells that stably express GFP or firefly luciferase tethered to a 3′UTR or putative microRNA target site are transfected with the microRNA mimic/microRNA-encoding vector or control mimic/vector. A decrease in GFP or firefly expression indicates that the target site or 3′UTR is a direct target of the microRNA. This approach tends to provide more consistent results because transfection efficiency is minimized as a variable and more sensitive because single reporter gene copy/cell can be used.
12. The level of microRNA reporter suppression generally ranges between 30 and 60% of the control reporter and varies depending on a number of factors, such as the concentration of the overexpressed microRNA or the number of microRNA target sites in the 3′UTR.

Acknowledgments

Many of the protocols described here were developed in the Naldini laboratory (San Raffaele Scientific Institute, Milan, Italy) (29, 30), and we would like to thank members of the lab for their contributions. BDB is supported by the National Institutes for Health (NIH) Diabetes Pathfinder Award (DP2DK083052-01).

References

1. Xiao, C. and Rajewsky, K. (2009) MicroRNA control in the immune system: basic principles. *Cell* **136,** 26–36.
2. Li, Q. J., Chau, J., Ebert, P. J., Sylvester, G., Min, H., Liu, G., Braich, R., Manoharan, M., Soutschek, J., Skare, P., Klein, L. O., Davis, M. M., and Chen, C. Z. (2007) miR-181a is an intrinsic modulator of T cell sensitivity and selection. *Cell* **129,** 147–61.
3. Cobb, B. S., Hertweck, A., Smith, J., O'Connor, E., Graf, D., Cook, T., Smale, S. T., Sakaguchi, S., Livesey, F. J., Fisher, A. G., and Merkenschlager, M. (2006) A role for Dicer in immune regulation. *J Exp Med* **203,** 2519–27.
4. Cobb, B. S., Nesterova, T. B., Thompson, E., Hertweck, A., O'Connor, E., Godwin, J., Wilson, C. B., Brockdorff, N., Fisher, A. G., Smale, S. T., and Merkenschlager, M. (2005) T cell lineage choice and differentiation in the absence of the RNase III enzyme Dicer. *J Exp Med* **201,** 1367–73.
5. Lu, L. F., Thai, T. H., Calado, D. P., Chaudhry, A., Kubo, M., Tanaka, K., Loeb, G. B., Lee,

H., Yoshimura, A., Rajewsky, K., and Rudensky, A. Y. (2009) Foxp3-dependent microRNA155 confers competitive fitness to regulatory T cells by targeting SOCS1 protein. *Immunity* **30,** 80–91.

6. Xiao, C., Calado, D. P., Galler, G., Thai, T. H., Patterson, H. C., Wang, J., Rajewsky, N., Bender, T. P., and Rajewsky, K. (2007) MiR-150 controls B cell differentiation by targeting the transcription factor c-Myb. *Cell* **131,** 146–59.
7. Monticelli, S., Ansel, K. M., Xiao, C., Socci, N. D., Krichevsky, A. M., Thai, T. H., Rajewsky, N., Marks, D. S., Sander, C., Rajewsky, K., Rao, A., and Kosik, K. S. (2005) MicroRNA profiling of the murine hematopoietic system. *Genome Biol* **6,** R71.
8. Landgraf, P., Rusu, M., Sheridan, R., Sewer, A., Iovino, N., Aravin, A., Pfeffer, S., Rice, A., Kamphorst, A. O., Landthaler, M., Lin, C., Socci, N. D., Hermida, L., Fulci, V., Chiaretti, S., Foa, R., Schliwka, J., Fuchs, U., Novosel, A., Muller, R. U., Schermer, B., Bissels, U., Inman, J., Phan, Q., Chien, M., Weir, D. B., Choksi, R., De Vita, G., Frezzetti, D., Trompeter, H. I., Hornung, V., Teng, G., Hartmann, G., Palkovits, M., Di Lauro, R., Wernet, P., Macino, G., Rogler, C. E., Nagle, J. W., Ju, J., Papavasiliou, F. N., Benzing, T., Lichter, P., Tam, W., Brownstein, M. J., Bosio, A., Borkhardt, A., Russo, J. J., Sander, C., Zavolan, M., and Tuschl, T. (2007) A mammalian microRNA expression atlas based on small RNA library sequencing. *Cell* **129,** 1401–14.
9. Chen, C. Z., Li, L., Lodish, H. F., and Bartel, D. P. (2004) MicroRNAs modulate hematopoietic lineage differentiation. *Science* **303,** 83–6.
10. Brown, B. D., Gentner, B., Cantore, A., Colleoni, S., Amendola, M., Zingale, A., Baccarini, A., Lazzari, G., Galli, C., and Naldini, L. (2007) Endogenous microRNA can be broadly exploited to regulate transgene expression according to tissue, lineage and differentiation state. *Nat Biotechnol* **25,** 1457–67.
11. Landthaler, M., Gaidatzis, D., Rothballer, A., Chen, P. Y., Soll, S. J., Dinic, L., Ojo, T., Hafner, M., Zavolan, M., and Tuschl, T. (2008) Molecular characterization of human Argonaute-containing ribonucleoprotein complexes and their bound target mRNAs. *RNA* **14,** 2580–96.
12. Brennecke, J., Hipfner, D. R., Stark, A., Russell, R. B., and Cohen, S. M. (2003) bantam encodes a developmentally regulated microRNA that controls cell proliferation and regulates the proapoptotic gene hid in Drosophila. *Cell* **113,** 25–36.
13. Mansfield, J. H., Harfe, B. D., Nissen, R., Obenauer, J., Srineel, J., Chaudhuri, A., Farzan-Kashani, R., Zuker, M., Pasquinelli, A. E., Ruvkun, G., Sharp, P. A., Tabin, C. J., and McManus, M. T. (2004) MicroRNA-responsive 'sensor' transgenes uncover Hox-like and other developmentally regulated patterns of vertebrate microRNA expression. *Nat Genet* **36,** 1079–83.
14. Brown, B. D., Venneri, M. A., Zingale, A., Sergi Sergi, L., and Naldini, L. (2006) Endogenous microRNA regulation suppresses transgene expression in hematopoietic lineages and enables stable gene transfer. *Nat Med* **12,** 585–91.
15. Cao, X., Pfaff, S. L., and Gage, F. H. (2007) A functional study of miR-124 in the developing neural tube. *Genes Dev* **21,** 531–6.
16. Brennecke, J., Stark, A., Russell, R. B., and Cohen, S. M. (2005) Principles of microRNA-target recognition. *PLoS Biol* **3,** e85.
17. Doench, J. G., Petersen, C. P., and Sharp, P. A. (2003) siRNAs can function as miRNAs. *Genes Dev* **17,** 438–42.
18. Taganov, K. D., Boldin, M. P., Chang, K. J., and Baltimore, D. (2006) NF-kappaB-dependent induction of microRNA miR-146, an inhibitor targeted to signaling proteins of innate immune responses. *Proc Natl Acad Sci U S A* **103,** 12481–6.
19. Giraldez, A. J., Mishima, Y., Rihel, J., Grocock, R. J., Van Dongen, S., Inoue, K., Enright, A. J., and Schier, A. F. (2006) Zebrafish MiR-430 promotes deadenylation and clearance of maternal mRNAs. *Science* **312,** 75–9.
20. O'Connell, R. M., Rao, D. S., Chaudhuri, A. A., Boldin, M. P., Taganov, K. D., Nicoll, J., Paquette, R. L., and Baltimore, D. (2008) Sustained expression of microRNA-155 in hematopoietic stem cells causes a myeloproliferative disorder. *J Exp Med* **205,** 585–94.
21. Lim, L. P., Lau, N. C., Garrett-Engele, P., Grimson, A., Schelter, J. M., Castle, J., Bartel, D. P., Linsley, P. S., and Johnson, J. M. (2005) Microarray analysis shows that some microRNAs downregulate large numbers of target mRNAs. *Nature* **433,** 769–73.
22. Selbach, M., Schwanhausser, B., Thierfelder, N., Fang, Z., Khanin, R., and Rajewsky, N. (2008) Widespread changes in protein synthesis induced by microRNAs. *Nature* **455,** 58–63.
23. Doench, J. G. and Sharp, P. A. (2004) Specificity of microRNA target selection in translational repression. *Genes Dev* **18,** 504–11.

24. Ebert, M. S., Neilson, J. R., and Sharp, P. A. (2007) MicroRNA sponges: competitive inhibitors of small RNAs in mammalian cells. *Nat Methods* **4,** 721–6.

25. Gentner, B., Schira, G., Giustacchini, A., Amendola, M., Brown, B. D., Ponzoni, M., and Naldini, L. (2009) Stable knockdown of microRNA in vivo by lentiviral vectors. *Nat Methods* **6,** 63–6.

26. Brown, B. D. and Naldini, L. (2009) Exploiting and antagonizing microRNA regulation for therapeutic and experimental applications. *Nat Rev Genet* **10,** 578–85.

27. Krek, A., Grun, D., Poy, M. N., Wolf, R., Rosenberg, L., Epstein, E. J., MacMenamin, P., da Piedade, I., Gunsalus, K. C., Stoffel, M., and Rajewsky, N. (2005) Combinatorial microRNA target predictions. *Nat Genet* **37,** 495–500.

28. Amendola, M., Venneri, M. A., Biffi, A., Vigna, E., and Naldini, L. (2005) Coordinate dual-gene transgenesis by lentiviral vectors carrying synthetic bidirectional promoters. *Nat Biotechnol* **23,** 108–16.

29. De Palma, M. and Naldini, L. (2002) Transduction of a gene expression cassette using advanced generation lentiviral vectors. *Methods Enzymol* **346,** 514–29.

30. Follenzi, A. and Naldini, L. (2002) Generation of HIV-1 derived lentiviral vectors. *Methods Enzymol* **346,** 454–65.

Part IV

Functional Analysis of miRNAs in the Immune System: Loss-of-Function

Chapter 16

Lentivirus-Mediated Antagomir Expression

Ewa Surdziel, Matthias Eder, and Michaela Scherr

Abstract

MicroRNAs (miRNAs) are small non-coding RNAs involved in post-transcriptional gene regulation via hybridisation to mRNAs. miRNA function can be inhibited by the so-called "antagomirs" – anti-sense RNA oligonucleotides complementary to individual miRNAs. Since, in principle, any miRNA can be silenced, antagomirs provide a powerful tool to investigate the function of particular miRNAs. However, conventional methods to deliver antagomirs into cells (e.g. transfection) have been shown to only transiently interfere with endogenous miRNA expression and/or function. In this section, we describe a lentivirus-based system for stable antagomir expression to generate longterm loss-of-function phenotypes for individual miRNAs. Moreover, the described strategy is also suitable for studying the function of individual miRNAs encoded within polycistronic clusters.

This chapter provides a collection of protocols to antagonize miRNA function by lentiviral antagomir expression, which can be achieved in a wide range of target cells.

1. Introduction

MicroRNAs (miRNAs) comprise an abundant class of small non-coding RNAs, which are part of an evolutionarily highly conserved intracellular mechanism to regulate gene expression in a sequence-specific manner (1). Each miRNA is believed to regulate the expression of multiple mRNA targets. Recent reports have provided compelling evidence that a range of miRNAs is also involved in the regulation of immunity. Given that miRNA-mediated RNA interference (RNAi) has important roles in many aspects of adaptive and innate immune responses, discovering the biological functions of selected miRNAs may reveal novel concepts about the regulation of the immune system (2). Functional analysis of miRNAs requires methods to generate stable gain- and loss-of-function phenotypes for individual miRNAs and subsequent identification and isolation of modified cells. Chemically modified anti-sense oligonucleotides

Silvia Monticelli (ed.), *MicroRNAs and the Immune System: Methods and Protocols*, Methods in Molecular Biology, vol. 667,
DOI 10.1007/978-1-60761-811-9_16, © Springer Science+Business Media, LLC 2010

complementary to specific miRNAs, named "antagomirs", have been shown to only transiently interfere with miRNA function in cell culture reporter assays and in mice (3–5) (Fig. 1). In contrast, alternative approaches employ retroviral/lentiviral vectors. These viruses are known to infect a wide variety of cell types, where they can integrate into the host genome. An additional advantage of using retroviral/lentiviral gene transfer is its high ability to transduce primary cells. Furthermore, lentiviral vectors can also integrate into the host genome of non-dividing cells, giving the opportunity to alter miRNA function in cells such as primary macrophages. To date, stable reduction of miRNA function can be achieved by using vector-mediated strategies based on two distinct protocols. The so-called "sponge method" for endogenous miRNA depletion using lentiviral vectors was developed in Naldini's laboratory (6, 7). This approach is based on the insertion of complementary miRNA target (miRT) sites into the 3′ untranslated region (3′ UTR) of the GFP cDNA. Consequently, GFP expression is subjected to miRNA-mediated regulation and thus serves as a sensor of the particular miRNA knock-down (6, 7). Another strategy for generating stable miRNA loss-of-function phenotypes was developed in our lab and is described in detail in the following chapter. The principle of this method is lentivirus-mediated expression of antagomirs directed against a particular miRNA. In this system, lentivirally expressed antagomirs are transcribed from a H1-promoter located within the U3 region of the Δ3′ LTR. Expression of a GFP reporter driven by a viral SFFV (spleen focus forming virus)-LTR promoter allows tracking of transduced cells. Lentivirus-mediated antagomirs can be also used to assign specific functions to individual miRNAs encoded within polycistronic clusters (8, 9).

Stable knock-down of endogenous miRNAs will possibly allow studying the function of selected miRNAs during long-term processes, such as differentiation of immune cells from haematopoietic progenitors. Additionally, recent observations demonstrate that lentivirus-mediated knock-down of miRNA can be also functional in vivo (10).

Commercially available PCR-based assays for detection of mature miRNA (e.g. miRNA-specific quantitative RT-PCR assay named miR-qRT-PCR) can be used to determine whether antagomir expression interferes with endogenous miRNA expression. It is important to note that antagomir hybridisation to miRNAs may not always change the total level of an individual miRNA but the amount of unbound miRNA which is available for binding to target mRNA (8). In addition, antagomir-mediated miRNA silencing can be evaluated by immunoblotting of proteins known to be regulated by miRNAs. Nevertheless, stable interference with endogenous miRNA expression and/or function may be accompanied by selection processes during cell culture similar to those observed for lentivirus-mediated RNAi (11).

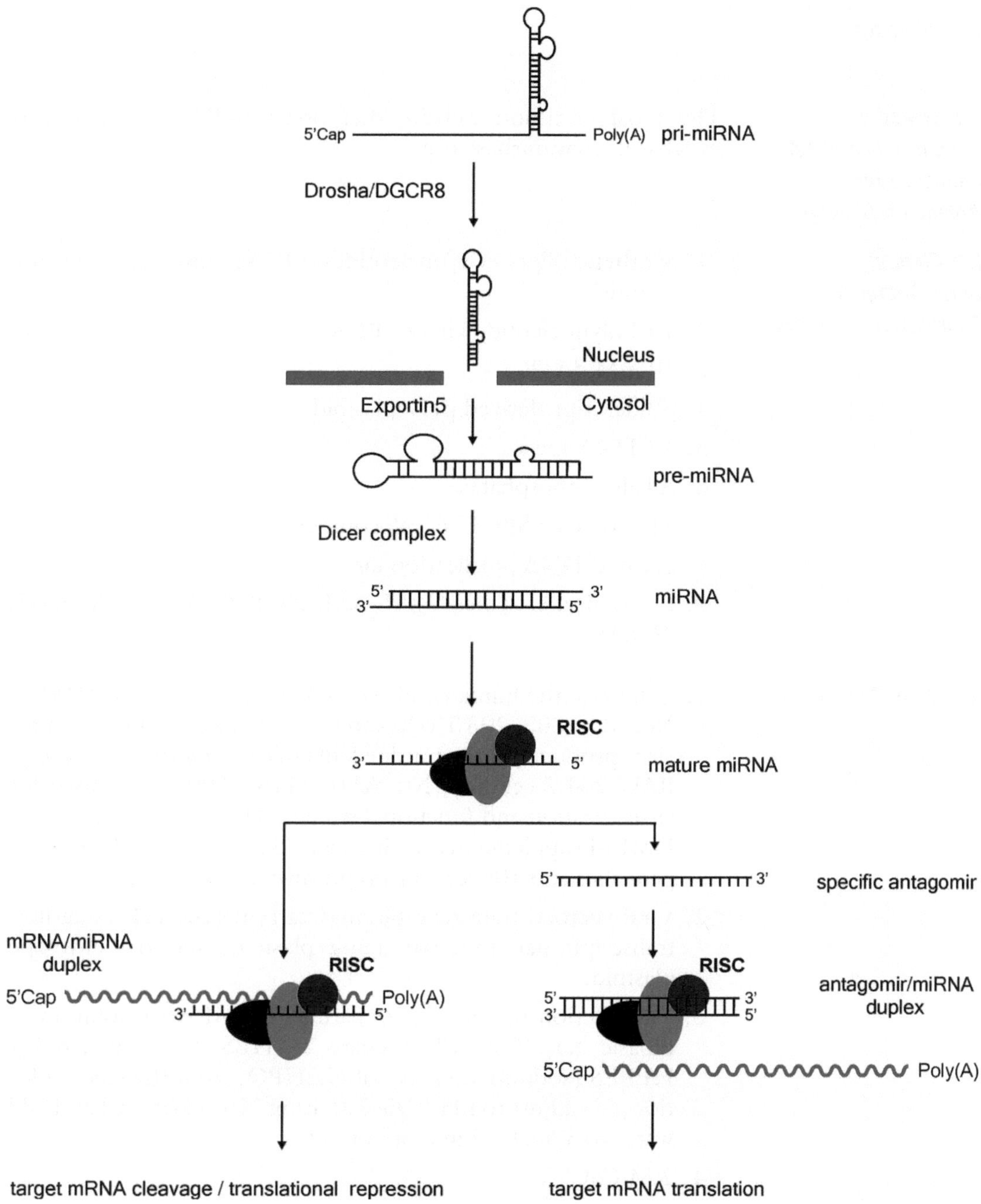

Fig. 1. Cartoon of miRNA silencing mediated by antagomirs. Transcribed pri-miRNA is cleaved by Drosha/DGCR8 within the nucleus. The resulting pre-miRNA is exported into the cytoplasm where additional processing mediated by Dicer occurs. Mature miRNAs are incorporated into the RISC (RNA-induced silencing complex). In the presence of specific antagomirs, miRNA is inhibited (by hybridisation with antagomirs) and miRNA function is also inhibited. In the absence of specific antagomirs, normal miRNA function is maintained.

2. Materials

2.1. Selection of Mature MicroRNA Sequence for Antagomir Cloning

The most common website that offers miRNA sequences is miRBase. www.mirbase.org

2.2. Cloning of H1-Antagomir Expression Cassettes

1. Synthetic oligodeoxynucleotides (ODN; sense and anti-sense strands).
2. T4 Polynucleotide kinase (PNK).
3. 10 mM dATP.
4. pBluescript-derived pH1-plasmid.
5. T4 DNA Ligase.
6. Alkaline phosphatase.
7. XL1-Blue or Stbl II *E. coli* competent bacteria.
8. Plasmid DNA purification kit.
9. Restriction enzymes: *Bgl*II, *Sal*I, *Xho*I, *Eco*RI, *SnaB*I, *Sma*I, *Hinc*II.

2.3. Virus Generation

1. Cell lines: the human embryonal kidney 293 cell line (DSMZ No. ACC 305, 293 T cells can be used as well) is preferred for virus production; the murine leukemic monocyte macrophage RAW 264.7 cell line (No. ATCC TIB-71™) can be used for virus titration and functional studies. The cells are cultured in DMEM supplemented with 10% FCS and 1% P/S (100 U/ml penicillin and 100 μg/ml streptomycin) (see Note 1).
2. Viral vectors: transgene plasmid carrying the H1-antagomir transcriptional unit, packaging plasmid, and the envelope plasmid.
3. Transfection buffer: (1) Prepare a 74 mM stock solution of dibasic Na_2HPO_4, (2) Prepare 2× HBS: 8 g NaCl, 6.5 g HEPES (sodium salt), 10 ml Na_2HPO_4 from the stock solution, (3) adjust to pH 6.95–7.0 using NaOH or HCl and add water to a final volume of 500 ml.
4. 2 M $CaCl_2$.
5. 100× protamine sulfate (400 μg/ml).
6. 0.01% (w/v) poly-l-lysine.
7. Phosphate-buffered saline (PBS; pH 7.4, Ca^{2+}- and Mg^{2+}-free).

2.4. TaqMan-Based Analysis of MicroRNA Expression (miR-qRT-PCR)

1. Trizol-based reagent for total RNA isolation.
2. Commercially available assays for specific mature miRNA detection and quantification, e.g. Applied Biosystems TaqMan® MicroRNA Assay.

2.5. Immunoblotting

1. RIPA buffer for cell lysis.
2. Separating gel 10%: 0.375 M Tris–HCl, pH 8.8, 10% Acrylamide, 0.1% SDS, 0.1% TEMED, 0.1% APS.
3. Stacking gel 5%: 0.125 M Tris–HCl, pH 6.8, 5% Acrylamide, 0.1% SDS, 0.1% TEMED, 0.1% APS.
4. SDS-Polyacrylamide Gel Electrophoresis (SDS-PAGE) running buffer: 25 mM Tris base, 250 mM glycine, 0.1% SDS.
5. Transfer buffer: 25 mM Tris base, 192 mM glycine, 20% methanol.
6. Polyvinylidene difluoride (PVDF) membrane, e.g. from Amersham.
7. Tris-buffered saline with Tween (TBST): 10 mM Tris–HCl, pH 8.0, 150 mM NaCl, 0.05% Tween 20.
8. Blocking buffer: 5% non-fat dry milk in TBST.
9. Enhanced chemiluminescent (ECL) reagents, e.g. from Amersham.
10. Stripping buffer: 0.1 M glycine, 125 mM HCl.

3. Methods

The design of specific antagomirs for the induction of particular miRNA loss-of-function phenotypes requires only the knowledge of mature miRNA sequence (approximately 22–25 nucleotides), which can be easily obtained from suitable databases, such as miRBase [www.mirbase.org]. Antagomirs can be expressed from different mammalian expression vectors. The most commonly used RNA polymerase III (Pol III) promoters are the eukaryotic H1- and U6-snRNA promoters which produce high levels of small, non-coding RNA transcripts. Chemically synthesized, self-complementary DNA oligonucleotides encompassing the sequence of the mature miRNA have to be annealed and directionally cloned into the pH1-plasmid, e.g. pBluescript-derived pH1-plasmid (*8*). Each sense oligonucleotide harbours a sequence of six thymidines as a Pol III transcription termination signal. As shown in Fig. 2, the H1-antagomir expression cassette can be inserted into the lentiviral transgene plasmid pdc-SEW (dc = double copy, S = SFFV promoter, E = EGFP, W = WPRE) within the U3 region of the Δ3′ LTR. The location in the U3 region of the Δ3′ LTR leads to duplication of the H1-cassette during reverse transcription.

Reporter gene activity allows for rapid and quantitative analysis of transduction efficiency. Since we have previously demonstrated that reporter gene activity positively correlates with the level of

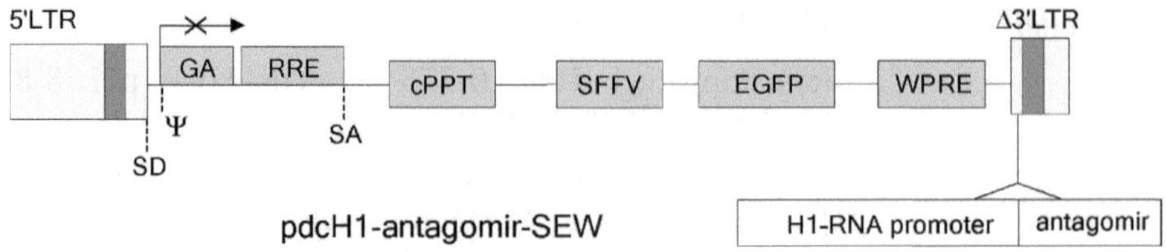

Fig. 2. Schematic representation of lentiviral transgene plasmid for antagomir expression with a Pol III expression cassette located within the U3 region of the Δ3′ LTR.

shRNA expression and consequently with the extent of target gene silencing (12), GFP fluorescence may ultimately correspond to the level of miRNA silencing upon lentiviral antagomir expression (8). Moreover, because of random lentiviral integration into the host genome, lentivirus-based antagomir transfer leads to cell populations with heterogeneous GFP expression and presumably antagomir expression. This effect can be easily monitored by flow cytometry and used to isolate cell subpopulations with different levels of miRNA reduction (by using fluorescence-activated cell sorting). Additionally, antagomir ability to knock-down selected miRNA and, in consequence, to influence miRNA natural target regulation can be validated by specific miR-qRT-PCR and reporter assay/immunoblotting, respectively (see Subheading 3.5).

3.1. Cloning of H1-Antagomir Expression Cassettes

Single-stranded ODNs (~45 nt in length) encoding (*i*) an anti-sense mature miRNA, (*ii*) a termination signal consisting of six thymidines, and (*iii*) overhang sequences from a 5′ *Bgl*II- and a 3′ *Sal*I-restriction site are phosphorylated and hybridised with the corresponding complementary single-stranded ODNs. The ODN sequences can be designed as follows: sense antagomir: 5′-GATCCC *anti-sense of mature miRNA* TTTTTTGGAAG-3′, anti-sense antagomir: 5′-TCGACTTCCAAAAAA *sense of mature miRNA* GGG-3′ (see Note 2). The resulting DNA duplex is inserted into the *Bgl*II–*Sal*I site of the dephosphorylated pH1-plasmid harbouring the H1-RNA promoter to generate pH1-antagomir. *E. coli* XL1-Blue or Stbl II competent cells are transformed with the resulting plasmid, followed by plasmid DNA purification. The proper insertion and correct sequence is confirmed by DNA restriction digestion and sequencing for each plasmid.

3.1.1. Phosphorylation and Annealing of ODNs

1. Dissolve ODNs in water to obtain a final concentration of 1 mM and take 1 μl from each ODNs (sense and anti-sense antagomir).
2. Add 1 μl 10× T4 PNK buffer.
3. Add 1 μl 10 mM ATP.
4. Add 1 μl T4 PNK (10 U/μl).
5. Add 5 μl H_2O.

6. Incubate 30–45 min at 37°C, denature at 100°C for 3 min, and slowly cool the annealed ODNs to room temperature.

3.1.2. Ligation of the Duplex into pH1-Plasmid

1. To 3 μl of the duplex (annealing reaction), add 1 μl 10× T4 ligase buffer.
2. Add 1 μl dephosphorylated plasmid pH1-plasmid (digested with *Bgl*II and *Sal*I).
3. Add 1 μl T4 DNA Ligase (400 U/μl).
4. Add 4 μl H_2O.
5. Incubate for 1 h at room temperature.
6. After transformation of XL1-Blue or Stbl II *E. coli* competent cells and plasmid preparation, the insert can be analysed by *Eco*RI/*Xho*I digestion. Positive clones are identified by inserts of ~300 bp for the pH1-antagomir plasmid.

3.2. Stable Knock-down of MicroRNA Expression by Antagomirs

To construct the double-copy variant pdcH1-antagomir-SEW, digest the plasmid pdc-SEW with *SnaB*I and dephosphorylate with alkaline phosphatase. The H1-antagomir cassette is released from pH1-antagomir by digestion with *Sma*I and *Hinc*II.

3.2.1. Lentivirus-Mediated Delivery of H1-Antagomir Expression Cassette

1. To 1 μl (~400 ng) H1-antagomir-fragment, add 1 μl 10× T4 ligase buffer.
2. Add 1 μl (100 ng) dephosphorylated plasmid pdc-SEW.
3. Add 1 μl T4 DNA Ligase (400 U/μl).
4. Add 6 μl H_2O.
5. Incubate for 1 h at room temperature.
6. After transformation of XL1-Blue or Stbl II *E. coli* competent cells and plasmid preparation, the insert can be analysed by *Pst*I digestion with positive clones identified by inserts of ~700 and ~1250 bp for the pdcH1-antagomir-SEW plasmid (see Note 3).

3.2.2. Generation of Lentiviral Vector Particles

1. 293 cells are grown in a 5% CO_2 humidified incubator at 37°C in DMEM supplemented with 10% FCS and 1% P/S.
2. Three days before transfection, plate 5×10^6 293 cells onto a poly-l-lysine (0.01% solution) coated T175 flask in 30 ml DMEM (10% FCS and 1% P/S).
3. Transfect the sub-confluent 293 cells with 40 μg of the lentiviral transgene plasmid, 30 μg packaging-, and 20 μg envelope-plasmid DNA using the calcium phosphate method (13).
4. After 16 h, wash the cells with 1× PBS (pH 7.4, Ca^{2+}- and Mg^{2+}-free) and incubate for an additional 8 h in fresh DMEM (10% FCS) medium.
5. Collect the culture supernatant containing the lentiviral particles 24–72 h after transfection.

6. Filter through a 0.45 μm pore size filter to remove cell debris and concentrate the viral particles by low-speed centrifugation (10000 × *g*, 10°C for 16 h).
7. Titrate the virus (e.g. on RAW 264.7 cells) and store the aliquots of viral particles at −80°C.
8. Use the culture medium as indicated above in Subheading 2.3.

3.2.3. Transduction and Stable Knock-down of MicroRNA in Immune Cells

1. Plate 1×10^5 RAW 264.7 cells in a 96-well plate (flat bottom) 2 h before transduction. After the indicated time, wash non-adherent cells away with 1× PBS (pH 7.4, Ca^{2+}- and Mg^{2+}-free). For transduction, supplement the remaining adherent cells with the culture medium.
2. RAW 264.7 cells are transduced twice by adding lentivirus (multiplicity of infection; MOI ~ 10) and 2 μl of protamine sulfate (final concentration 2 μg/ml) in a total volume of 200 μl.
3. Transduction is performed by overnight incubation in a 5% CO_2 humidified incubator at 37°C.
4. After transduction, wash the cells with 1× PBS (pH 7.4, Ca^{2+}- and Mg^{2+}-free) and maintain in the culture medium; analyse the transduction efficacy after 4 days.
5. Use the culture medium as indicated above in Subheading 2.3.

3.2.4. Flow Cytometry Analysis

Reporter gene activity allows for rapid and quantitative analysis of transduction efficiency. As shown in Fig. 3a, flow cytometry analysis of GFP expression in RAW 264.7 cells transduced with scrambled control (middle panel) and specific antagomir (right panel) lentiviral vectors reveals a high transduction efficiency (approximately 90%), which is maintained during cell culture (indicating stable antagomir expression).

3.3. TaqMan-Based Analysis of MicroRNA Expression

For mature miRNA expression analysis, total cellular RNA is extracted from lentivirus transduced cells and subjected to specific miR-qRT-PCR (see Note 2). As shown in Fig. 3b, RAW 264.7 macrophages transduced with specific antagomir-181b show abrogated level of mature miRNA-181b compared to the cells transduced with scrambled control (see Notes 4 and 5).

1. Isolate total cellular RNA from the transduced cells using e.g. TRIzol® reagent (Invitrogen).
2. Subject 10 ng of total cellular RNA to reverse transcription (RT) reaction in the presence of miRNA-specific stem-looped RT primer according to the manufacturer's protocol.
3. Subject the obtained cDNA to TaqMan quantification in the presence of miRNA-specific forward PCR primer, specific PCR reverse primer, and miRNA-specific TaqMan probe, as recommended by the manufacturer.

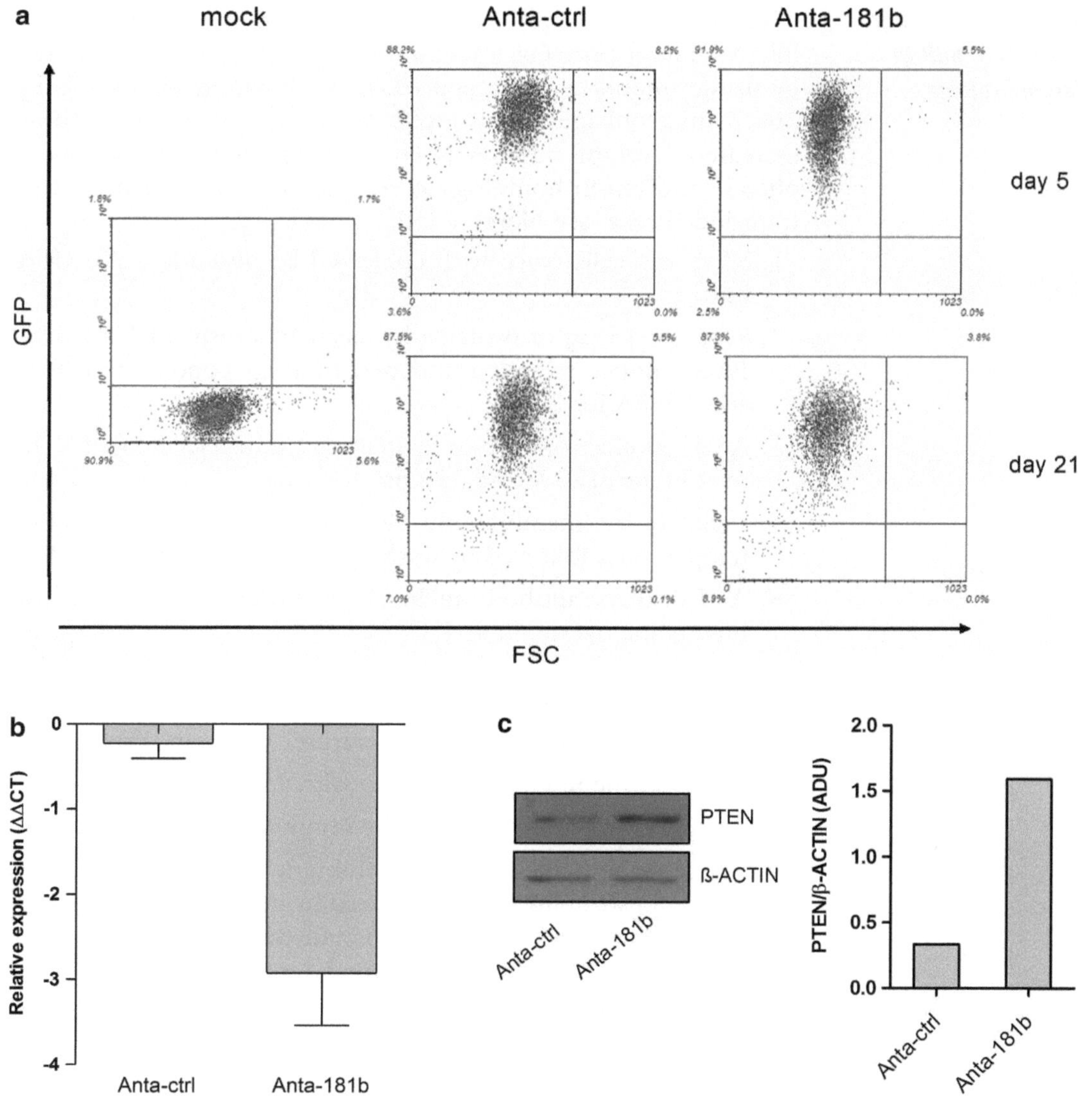

Fig. 3. Lentivirus-mediated antagomir expression. (**a**) Flow cytometry profile of RAW 264.7 macrophages transduced with scrambled control (*middle panel*) and specific antagomir-181b (*right panel*) lentiviral vectors. Note that the reporter gene fluorescence remains stable during the cell culture. (**b**) Expression level of miRNA-181b in RAW 264.7 macrophages transduced with specific antagomir-181b compared to the cells transduced with scrambled control. RNA was isolated 21 days after transduction. (**c**) Effect of miRNA-181b knock-down on its target protein PTEN in RAW 264.7 macrophages. PTEN was predicted as a miR-181b target by bioinformatics algorithms: DIANA-microT 3.0, miRDB and RNA22. PTEN protein expression level was determined by immunoblotting and densitometric analysis of band intensities (*ADU* arbitrary densitometric units). The membrane was probed with anti-PTEN antibody (1:500 dilution, Santa Cruz). Afterwards, the membrane was reprobed for β-ACTIN as a loading control (1:2000 dilution, Cell Signaling). Cell lysis was perfomed 21 days after transduction.

4. Normalisation and analysis of miRNA expression can be performed using the $2^{-\Delta\Delta CT}$ method relative to snRNA-U6 or snoRNA-202, for human or murine cells, respectively.

3.4. Immunoblotting Analysis of miRNA Target Proteins

Given that effective miRNA silencing results in upregulation of miRNA target proteins, antagomir functionality can be analysed by using immunoblotting approach. As shown in Fig. 3c, RAW 264.7 macrophages transduced with antagomir-181b show increased level of miRNA-181b target protein PTEN (phosphatase and tensin homolog) as compared to scrambled control transduced cells (see Notes 4 and 5).

1. Wash the cells twice with cold 1× PBS and add cold RIPA buffer.
2. Separate 15 μg of proteins by electrophoresis on 10% SDS-PAGE under reducing and denaturating conditions (80 V and 40 mA for 2 h).
3. After gel electrophoresis, proteins are transferred to a PVDF membrane (120 V and 250 mA for 1 h).
4. Incubate the membrane in blocking buffer for 1 h at room temperature, followed by washing three times with 1× TBST.
5. Add primary antibody in blocking buffer and incubate the membrane overnight at 4°C.
6. Wash the membrane three times with 1× TBST and incubate with horseradish peroxidase (HRP)-conjugated secondary antibody for 1 h at room temperature.
7. Wash the membrane three times with 1× TBST.
8. Use ECL system to visualise the immune complexes.
9. For reprobing, incubate the membrane at room temperature for 1 h in stripping buffer followed by intensive washing with 1× TBST; the membrane is then ready to be used as described above (starting from Subheading 3.4, **step 4**).
10. Densitometric analysis (target protein level normalised to loading control).

3.5. Detection of Lentivirus-Mediated MicroRNA Silencing

Standard techniques such as quantitative miR-qRT-PCR at the RNA level and reporter assays and immunoblotting at the protein level are used to analyse miRNA expression and function in the presence or absence of antagomirs. Phenotypic analysis of proliferation, survival, and differentiation of transduced cells can be easily monitored by several standard techniques, including trypan-blue exclusion, BrdU incorporation, apoptosis assays, or morphological and immunophenotypic analyses.

4. Notes

1. Production of high-titer lentiviral supernatants may require some training and experience (see related protocols). Make sure that the cells used for virus production are free of

Mycoplasma contamination. *Mycoplasma* is known to induce chromosomal instability and inhibit cell growth. Furthermore, *Mycoplasma* interferes with several biochemical assays, such as reverse transcription as well as proliferation assays based on thymidine incorporation. There are several commercial kits available to detect *Mycoplasma* contamination based on conventional PCR, e.g. Venor®GeM (Minerva Biolabs).

2. Mature miRNA sequences can differ between species. It is important to consider this fact for antagomir design as well as for mature miRNA detection using specific miR-qRT-PCR. On the other hand, both miRT (sponge method) and antagomirs will hybridise to similar but not identical RNA sequences limiting the specificity of miRNA silencing.
3. The use of recombination-deficient bacteria (such as *E. coli* XL1-Blue or Stbl II) is crucial for successful cloning of lentiviral plasmids.
4. Note that lentiviral gene transfer itself can affect gene expression and pathways involved in the innate immunity. Proper controls are essential to make sure that experimental results are specific.
5. The efficacy of miRNA knock-down depends on the expression of endogenous miRNA to be inhibited. In case of very high endogenous miRNA level, the induction of loss-of-function phenotypes using both lentiviral antagomir expression and the sponge technology may be difficult.

Acknowledgments

We are grateful to Maciej Cabanski (Hannover Medical School) for performing immunoblotting experiments. We also thank Michael A. Morgan (Hannover Medical School) for critical reading of the manuscript. This work was supported in part by grants of the "Deutsche Forschungsgemeinschaft" (SFB 566), H.W. & J. Hector-Stiftung.

References

1. Bartel, D. P. (2004) *Cell 116*, 281–97.
2. Lodish, H. F., Zhou, B., Liu, G., and Chen, C. Z. (2008) *Nat Rev Immunol 8*, 120–30.
3. Meister, G., Landthaler, M., Dorsett, Y., and Tuschl, T. (2004) *RNA 10*, 544–50.
4. Krutzfeldt, J., Rajewsky, N., Braich, R., Rajeev, K. G., Tuschl, T., Manoharan, M., and Stoffel, M. (2005) *Nature 438*, 685–9.
5. Krutzfeldt, J., Kuwajima, S., Braich, R., Rajeev, K. G., Pena, J., Tuschl, T., Manoharan, M., and Stoffel, M. (2007) *Nucleic Acids Res 35*, 2885–92.
6. Brown, B. D., Venneri, M. A., Zingale, A., Sergi Sergi, L., and Naldini, L. (2006) *Nat Med 12*, 585–91.
7. Brown, B. D., Gentner, B., Cantore, A., Colleoni, S., Amendola, M., Zingale, A., Baccarini, A., Lazzari, G., Galli, C., and

Naldini, L. (2007) *Nat Biotechnol 25*, 1457–67.

8. Scherr, M., Venturini, L., Battmer, K., Schaller-Schoenitz, M., Schaefer, D., Dallmann, I., Ganser, A., and Eder, M. (2007) *Nucleic Acids Res 35*, e149.
9. Venturini, L., Battmer, K., Castoldi, M., Schultheis, B., Hochhaus, A., Muckenthaler, M. U., Ganser, A., Eder, M., and Scherr, M. (2007) *Blood 109*, 4399–405.
10. Gentner, B., Schira, G., Giustacchini, A., Amendola, M., Brown, B. D., Ponzoni, M., and Naldini, L. (2009) *Nat Methods 6*, 63–6.
11. Scherr, M., and Eder, M. (2007) *Cell Cycle* 6, 444–9.
12. Scherr, M., Battmer, K., Ganser, A., and Eder, M. (2003) *Cell Cycle 2*, 251–7.
13. Graham, F. L., and van der Eb, A. J. (1973) *Virology 54*, 536–9.

Part V

miRNA Post-Transcriptional Modifications and Mechanisms of Action

Chapter 17

Solution Structure of miRNA:mRNA Complex

Mirko Cevec and Janez Plavec

Abstract

The use of contemporary nuclear magnetic resonance (NMR) methods in the studies of model systems between microRNA (miRNA) and messenger RNA (mRNA) is reviewed. We describe our studies on structural features of 33-nt RNA model construct between *let-7* miRNA and *lin-41* mRNA at the second binding site. *let-7* miRNA inhibits translation of *lin-41* gene through formation of two complexes with the target sequence within 3′ untranslated region of *lin-41* mRNA in *Caenorhabditis elegans*. The base pairing, asymmetric internal loops, and adenine bulge in both the complementary sites are important for regulation of gene expression. NMR study on the uniformly ^{13}C- and ^{15}N-labeled RNA construct has shown that RNA molecule folds into a stable structure consisting of two stem regions separated by a well-defined asymmetric internal loop. Solution-state NMR can make important contribution toward deeper understanding of assembly, folding, and structural features of miRNA:mRNA complexes.

1. Introduction

microRNAs (miRNAs) inhibit translation through formation of complexes with target sequences within 3′ untranslated regions (3′-UTR) of messenger RNAs (mRNAs). *let-7* miRNA was first discovered in the nematode *Caenorhabditis elegans*, where it silences expression of the *lin-41* gene through the miRNA–ribonucleoprotein complex (miRNP) (1). Members of *let-7* miRNA family have been isolated from many organisms including human (2). *let-7* miRNA, for example, functions as a Ras oncogene suppressor and could as such serve as a good therapeutic target for treating lung cancer (3). The interaction between *let-7* miRNA and *lin-41* mRNA in *C. elegans* involves two conserved *let-7* complementary sites (LCS1 and LCS2). Earlier studies have shown that the base pairing, asymmetric internal loops, and

Silvia Monticelli (ed.), *MicroRNAs and the Immune System: Methods and Protocols*, Methods in Molecular Biology, vol. 667, DOI 10.1007/978-1-60761-811-9_17, © Springer Science+Business Media, LLC 2010

adenine bulge in both the complementary sites are important for regulation of gene expression (4).

We studied the structural features of 33-nt RNA model construct between *let-7* miRNA and *lin-41* mRNA at the LCS2. High-resolution nuclear magnetic resonance (NMR) spectroscopy techniques require preparation of $^{13}C,^{15}N$-labeled RNA samples. The 3D structure was modeled with the use of NMR data including restraints for interatomic distances and torsion angles, and was further improved with the measurement of residual dipolar couplings (RDCs) on partially aligned RNA molecules using Pfl phages. Structural calculations utilizing simulated annealing approach in combination with the experimental restraints have shown that RNA molecule folds into a stable structure consisting of two stem regions separated by a well-defined asymmetric internal loop (5). The results of our research contribute towards deeper understanding of structural features of miRNA:mRNA complexes.

2. Materials

2.1. In Vitro Transcription with T7 RNA Polymerase

1. 1 M NaOH in ddH_2O. Filter and store at room temperature.
2. 1 M HCl in ddH_2O. Filter and store at room temperature.
3. Millex filter units.
4. RNaseZAP (Applied Biosystems/Ambion).
5. 1 M Tris–HCl in ddH_2O. Adjust pH to 8.4 at 25°C (pH 8.1 at 37°C) with NaOH or HCl. Autoclave and store at room temperature.
6. 200 mM spermidine in ddH_2O. Store at –20°C.
7. 20× Transcription buffer: 800 mM Tris–HCl, 20 mM spermidine, and 100 mM dl-dithiothreitol (DTT) in ddH_2O. Adjust pH to 8.4 at 25°C (pH 8.1 at 37°C) with NaOH or HCl. Store at –20°C.
8. 400 mg/mL poly(ethylene glycol) (PEG, average molecular weight 8,000) in ddH_2O. Store at –20°C.
9. 1 M $MgCl_2$ in ddH_2O. Autoclave and store at room temperature.
10. 1,100 U/μL T7 RNA polymerase. Store at –20°C.
11. 10× Annealing buffer: 100 mM Tris–HCl, 100 mM $MgCl_2$, target pH 8.4 at 25°C (pH 8.1 at 37°C) in ddH_2O. Autoclave and store at room temperature.
12. 100 μM template-strand DNA in ddH_2O. Store at –20°C.
13. 100 μM top-strand DNA in ddH_2O. Store at –20°C.

14. Low DNA stock (see Note 1): 2 μM template-strand DNA, 2.4 μM top-strand DNA, 1× Annealing buffer (10 mM Tris–HCl, 10 mM $MgCl_2$) in ddH_2O. Store at −20°C.
15. High DNA stock: 20 μM template strand DNA, 24 μM top strand DNA, 1× Annealing buffer (10 mM Tris–HCl, 10 mM $MgCl_2$) in ddH_2O. Store at −20°C.
16. ^{13}C,^{15}N-labeled rNTPs (see Note 2). Prepare 12 mM stock solution from 60 mM (rATP, rCTP and rUTP) and 55 mM (rGTP). Add NaOH or HCl to adjust pH to 8.4 at 25°C. Store at −20°C.

2.2. Ethanol Precipitation

1. 100 mM ethylenediaminetetraacetic acid (EDTA) in ddH_2O. Add NaOH or HCl to adjust pH to 8.1 at 25°C. Autoclave and store at room temperature.
2. 3 M NaOAc in ddH_2O. Add HCl to adjust pH to 5.2 at 25°C. Autoclave and store at room temperature.
3. Absolute ethanol.

2.3. Preparative Gel Electrophoresis

1. 10× TBE buffer: 890 mM Tris–base, 890 mM boric acid, and 20 mM EDTA in ddH_2O. Autoclave and store at room temperature.
2. 15–20% acrylamide/bis solution (19:1), 7 M urea in 1× TBE and ddH_2O.
3. *N*,*N*,*N*′,*N*′-Tetramethyl-ethylenediamine (TEMED).
4. 10% ammonium persulfate (APS) in 1× TBE. Prepare solution and separate on small aliquots. Store at −20°C.
5. Loading buffer: 8.1 M urea, 0.9 mM EDTA, 0.1% xylene cyanole (XC), and 0.1% bromophenol blue (BPB) in 1× TBE.
6. 2% dimethyldichlorosilane in octamethylcyclooctasilane (PlusOne Repel-Silane ES).
7. 2 μg/mL ethidium bromide in 1× TBE.

2.4. UV Shadowing, Electroelution and Centrifugation

1. Merck TLC plates.
2. Elutrap (Schleicher & Schuell BioScience).
3. Centricon YM-3 (nominal molecular-weight limit 3,000, Millipore).
4. 70% ethanol. Store at room temperature.
5. 0.1 M NaOH in ddH_2O. Filter and store at room temperature.
6. 5 M NaCl in ddH_2O. Autoclave and store at room temperature.
7. 1 M Na_2HPO_4 in ddH_2O. Autoclave and store at room temperature.
8. 1 M NaH_2PO_4 in ddH_2O. Autoclave and store at room temperature.

9. 100 mM sodium phosphate buffer: 100 mM Na_2HPO_4 and 100 mM NaH_2PO_4, target pH 6.8 at 25°C in ddH_2O. Autoclave and store at room temperature.
10. High salt buffer: 10 mM sodium phosphate buffer, pH 6.8, 1 M NaCl, and 7.5 mM EDTA in ddH_2O. Autoclave and store at room temperature.

2.5. NMR Sample Preparation

1. NMR buffer: 10 mM sodium phosphate buffer, pH 6.8, 20 mM NaCl in 95% H_2O, 5% ^2H_2O, or 100% ^2H_2O.
2. 50 mg/mL filamentous Pfl phage solution in 10 mM sodium phosphate buffer, pH 6.8, and 20 mM NaCl (Asla Biotech). Store at 0–5°C.

3. Methods

This contribution reviews sample preparation (6), NMR data collection, and processing (7, 8) to obtain a high-resolution structure of a 33-nt RNA model construct. In order to stabilize the secondary structure and improve the yield of RNA synthesis with the T7 RNA polymerase, two additional G:C base pairs were incorporated at the 5′-end of RNA constructs. In addition, the template strand was modified with C2′-methoxy groups on the last two residues at the 5 end to decrease the amount of shorter and longer transcripts (9).

3.1. In Vitro Transcription with T7 RNA Polymerase

1. Before running a large-scale reaction, we need to optimize reaction conditions. Optimal concentrations of rNTPs, T7 RNA polymerase and DNA template depend on template sequence. Prepare 20–60 μL reaction mixtures where you vary ingredients (see Note 3). We run 20% 8 M urea polyacrylamide analytical gels and visualize them by ethidium bromide staining. We compare the intensities of bands (Fig. 1).
2. Heat 20 μM DNA stock to 85–95°C for 2 min (to denaturate both DNA strands) and slowly cool at the end (to allow DNA duplex formation).
3. Add ingredients for reaction mixture in the following order:
   (a) ddH_2O
   (b) 1× Transcription buffer
   (c) 28 mM $MgCl_2$
   (d) 80 mg/mL PEG
   (e) 4 mM each ^{13}C,^{15}N-rNTPs
   (f) 400 nM DNA template

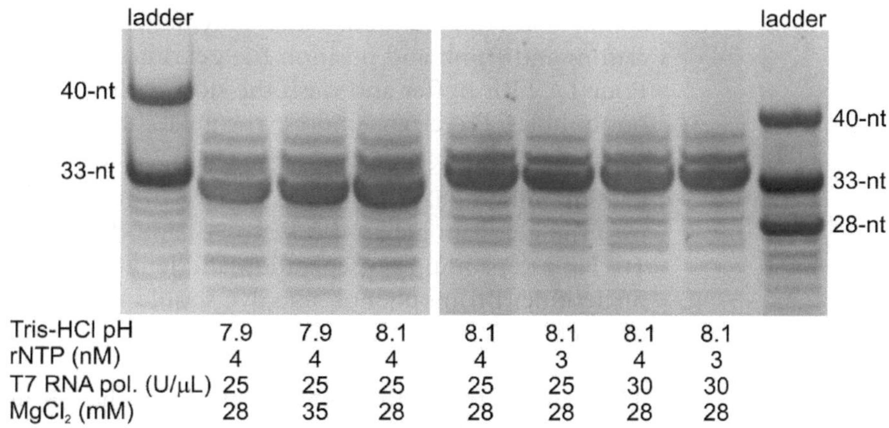

Fig. 1. Optimizing transcription yields using analytical PAGE gels.

This mixture is kept at 37°C for 15 min before adding the enzyme, which is added directly from the freezer.

(g) 25 U/µL T7 RNA polymerase

4. Incubation for 3–6 h at 37°C. After successful transcription we can observe a cloudy white precipitate due to magnesium-pyrophosphate precipitation.

3.2. Ethanol Precipitation

1. Stop the transcription reaction by adding EDTA to make it 29 mM (usually 1 mM higher than the $MgCl_2$ concentration). Then, add 1× volume of ddH_2O. Precipitate the product by adding 0.1× volume NaOAc and 2.5× volume of cold absolute ethanol. Store overnight at −20°C.
2. Balance two centrifuge bottles (see Note 4) and centrifuge for 120 min at 15,000 × *g* and 4°C. Remove ethanol and dissolve the pellet in ca. 3 mL ddH_2O. Store sample at −20°C.

3.3. PAGE

1. The target RNA molecule can be purified from abort transcripts using 6–8 denaturating preparative gels. The following description assumes a 3-mm thick gel (size 35 × 45 cm). Solutions can be scaled up or down for different gel thicknesses and sizes.
2. First clean plates, spacers, and comb with RNaseZAP, ddH_2O, and ethanol. To inhibit sticking of polyacrylamide gels to glass plates, use Repel-Silane. Then, assemble the spacers between the plates. Put the clamps on each side through the whole side length.
3. Seal the bottom with 40 mL mixture of acrylamide/bis solution, 25 µL TEMED, and 50 µL APS and wait for 30 min to polymerize; then, pour top mixture of 500 mL acrylamide/bis solution, 300 µL TEMED, and 1 mL APS, place the

comb, and wait 45 min. After polymerization remove the clamps and comb and position the gel onto the plate holder. Pour 1× TBE buffer and wash the slots with syringe to blow out bubbles. Pre-electrophorese the gel for 45 min at 400 V.

4. To prepare RNA sample, mix RNA with the same amount of loading buffer, heat the sample for 10 min at 85°C, and apply it to the gel. Run gel at 400 V for 5 h and then at 600 V for 10–15 h depending on separation and length of RNA oligonucleotide. Bromophenol blue dye should reach the bottom of a gel.

3.4. UV Shadowing, Electroelution and Centrifugation

1. The band of transcribed RNA is cut from the gel using UV shadowing and TLC silica plates. Store the gel slices at −20°C.
2. RNA is recovered from gel slices by electroelution with Elutrap. We first prepare Elutrap by cleaning all the parts with ethanol, RNaseZAP, and ddH_2O and then assemble the Elutrap. Use 1× TBE as running buffer.
3. Put the gel slices inside the electrophoresis chamber. Electro-elute for 1 h at 100 V and then for 4 h at 200 V. Reverse the polarity for approximately 20 s at 200 V in order to remove any material that may be attached to the membrane. Remove eluate from the trap using a disposable pipette and add fresh 1× TBE. Continue to electro-elute for 15 h at 200 V and at the end, reverse the polarity for 20 s at 200 V. Store the eluate.
4. Clean the Centricons with 70% ethanol and 0.1 M NaOH. Fill the sample reservoir with 2 mL ddH_2O. Put the parafilm around the top of reservoir and make holes with a needle. Place Centricons inside the centrifuge (counterbalance) and centrifuge for 90 min at 4,000 × *g* and 25°C. After each step, remove water completely. Repeat this step **4–6** times.
5. Put the electro-eluted RNA solution with pipette inside the sample reservoir. Add 1.2 mL of high-salt buffer. Counterbalance the opposite Centricons and start the centrifugation for 90 min at 4,500 × *g* and 4°C. After each step, add ca. 1.2 mL ddH_2O and save the filtrate. Repeat this step **5–7** times. At the end, the concentration of NaCl in the solution should be ca. 0.01 mM.
6. Place retentate vial over the sample reservoir, put the Centricon upside down, and transfer the concentrate into the retentate vial. Add 100 μL ddH_2O onto the membrane. Put the parafilm and make holes with a needle. Centrifuge for 10 min at 1,000 × *g* and 4°C. Repeat this step one more time.
7. Lyophilize RNA sample.

3.5. NMR Sample Preparation

1. The NMR sample is prepared by dissolving the lyophilized RNA in a NMR buffer, heated to 95°C, and snap-cooled on ice. The sample concentration is usually 1–2 mM.
2. The sample used to measure RDCs is prepared (1.0 mM in RNA) by mixing the oligonucleotide with a filamentous Pfl phage solution to a total phage concentration of 17 mg/mL.
3. Check the concentration of RNA molecule by UV spectrometer at 260 nm. Molar extinction coefficient is determined by the nearest-neighbor model.
4. UV melting of the construct is measured using a UV spectrometer equipped with a Peltier system between 5 and 95°C with a melting/annealing rate of 0.1°C/min. Sample concentration is ca. 2 μM in oligonucleotide, 10 mM sodium phosphate buffer, pH 6.8, and 20 mM NaCl.

3.6. NMR Spectroscopy

1. The following steps describe NMR experiments to investigate ^{13}C,^{15}N-labeled RNA construct. We use ^{13}C or ^{15}N decoupling during acquisition and WATERGATE pulse sequence (10) for water suppression in 95% H_2O samples. Splitting of resonances in the indirect dimensions is removed by refocusing ^{13}C and ^{15}N couplings. We record 1D ^1H NMR spectrum at 5 and 25°C for NMR sample in 95% H_2O and at 25°C for NMR sample in 100% ^2H_2O. Watson–Crick imino proton resonances are observed in the region from 12.3 to 14.5 ppm. The additional imino proton resonances are in the region from 10.5 to 11.7 ppm and originate from nonWatson–Crick base-paired residues of the asymmetric internal loop, the GAAA tetraloop and the G:U wobble base pair.
2. We establish the RNA base-pairing pattern using 2D NOESY experiments (11) (acquired on NMR sample in 95% H_2O at 5 and 25°C with mixing time of 75 and 300 ms) optimized for exchangeable imino and amino ^1H resonances (see Note 5). NOE characteristic cross-peaks of A:U base pairs are between uracil imino and adenine H2 protons, while G:C base pairs exhibit characteristic cross-peaks between guanine imino and cytosine amino protons. The NOESY spectra are used later for distance restraints calculations with cross-peaks being classified as strong (1.8–3.6 Å), medium (2.6–5.0 Å), and weak (3.5–6.5 Å).
3. 2D HNN-COSY experiments (12) allow to validate the NOESY-based assignment of base pairs and to observe non-Watson–Crick base-pairs (e.g., A:G, U:U, U:G), especially in the case where exchangeable resonances cannot be detected in NOESY experiments. The 2D HNN-COSY experiment (acquired on NMR sample in 95% H_2O at 5°C) correlates the

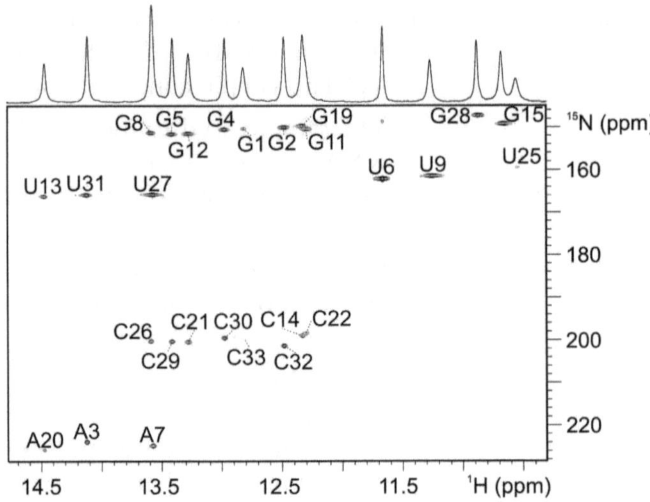

Fig. 2. 2D HNN-COSY spectrum acquired on NMR sample in 95% H_2O at 5°C.

Table 1
Chemical shift ranges in 2D ^{15}N-HSQC of 33-nt RNA molecule

	Chemical shift range (ppm)	
Atom pair	**Proton**	**Nitrogen**
Cytosine amino–N4	6.6–8.5	100–104
Guanine H1–N1	10.7–13.6	146–152
Uracil H3–N3	10.4–14.5	159–167

imino proton to adjacent *J*-correlated ^{15}N nuclei across the NH···N hydrogen bond (Fig. 2).

4. 2D ^{15}N-HSQC spectra (13) (acquired on NMR sample in 95% H_2O at 5 and 25°C) show correlations between imino or amino protons to directly bound nitrogen atoms (Table 1).
5. We use base-specific experiments for identifying the spin systems of nucleobases (NH, NH_2, H2, H5, H6, and H8). These experiments correlate exchangeable and nonexchangeable base proton resonances. We assign cytosine and uracil aromatic protons using 2D HNCCCH experiments (14) (acquired on NMR sample in 95% H_2O at 5°C) which correlate uracil imino to H6 protons or cytosine amino to H6 protons.
6. We use 2D TOCSY experiment (15) (acquired on NMR sample in 100% $2H_2O$ at 25°C) to correlate uracil and cytosine H5 to H6 protons.

7. Guanines are assigned with the use of 2D HNC-TOCSY-CH experiment (16) (acquired on NMR sample in 95% H_2O at 5 and 25°C) which correlates guanine imino protons to H8 protons.
8. We utilize 2D HCCH-TOCSY experiment (17) (acquired on NMR sample in 100% ^2H_2O at 25°C) to obtain through bond correlation between the adenine H2 and H8 protons.
9. 2D NOESY spectra (acquired on NMR sample in 100% ^2H_2O at 25°C) give information about NOE distance restraints between nonexchangeable ^1H resonances. Only resolved cross-peaks are used in the calculation of distance restraints. Upper and lower bounds are set to ±20% for mixing time (τ_m) of 75 ms, ±30% for $\tau_m = 150$ ms, and ±40% for $\tau_m = 300$ ms. NOESY spectra also give information about χ torsion angle, which is estimated from the intensity of intranucleotide H6/H8-H1′ and H6/H8-H2′ signals. Torsion angle χ is restrained to *syn* or *anti* conformation. Figure 3 shows sequential walk between H6/H8 and H2′ proton NOE cross-peaks. The sequential walk is possible because aromatic and H2′ protons are spatially close in the A-form RNA structure.
10. Further step in completing the assignment of ^1H and ^{13}C resonances of sugar moieties is performed with the help of 3D HCCH-COSY spectrum, which allows to correlate H1′ and H2′ protons by transferring magnetization through a single carbon–carbon bond, 3D HCCH-RELAY spectrum which gives additional cross-peaks to H3′ and 3D HCCH-TOCSY spectrum which gives correlation peaks between all sugar

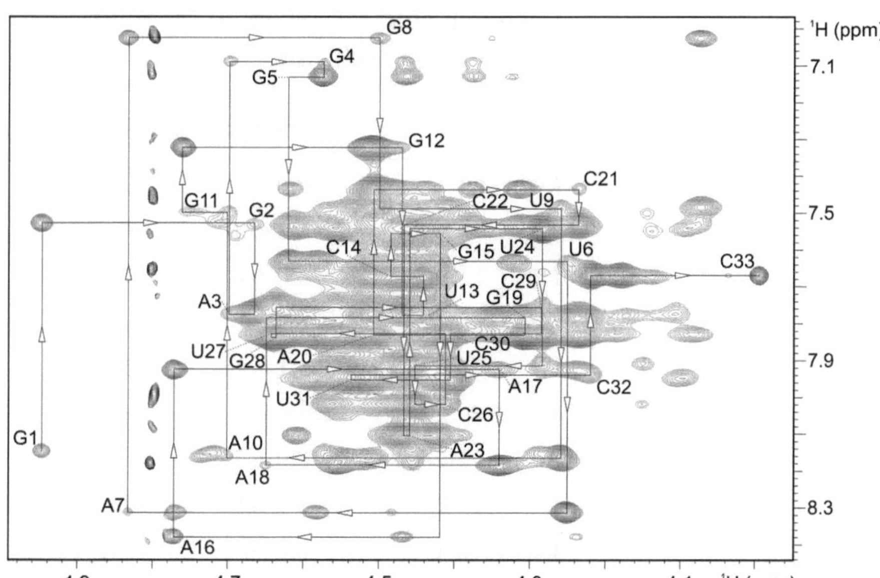

Fig. 3. The H6/H8-H2′ region of 2D NOESY spectrum ($\tau_m = 300$ ms) in 100% ^2H_2O at 25°C. Sequential connectivities are indicated by lines and arrows.

protons in the same ribose spin system (18). All the above spectra are acquired on NMR sample in 100% ^2H_2O at 25°C.

11. With the identification of nucleobase and ribose protons, we can assign all signals in 2D ^{13}C-HSQC spectrum (acquired on NMR sample in 100% ^2H_2O at 25°C), which shows correlations between aromatic or ribose protons to directly bound carbons (Table 2). In our case, due to the conformation of 33-nt RNA construct, two correlation peaks deviate from the usual range of chemical shifts. A18 H3′–C3′ exhibits ^{1}H signal at δ 5.1 ppm (^{13}C δ 72.3 ppm), and G19 H1′–C1′ exhibits ^{1}H chemical shift at δ 3.6 ppm (^{13}C δ 91.2 ppm).
12. The spin systems of nucleobases and sugar moieties are connected using 2D HCN experiment (19) (acquired on NMR sample in 100% ^2H_2O at 25°C), which correlates H1′ and H8 protons to purine N9 atoms, and H1′ and H6 to pyrimidine N1 atoms.
13. 3D NOESY-^{13}C-HSQC experiments (acquired on NMR sample in 100% ^2H_2O at 25°C with mixing time of 150 ms) help to perform the unambiguous assignment of ^{1}H–^{1}H connectivities in 2D NOESY and to obtain additional NOE distance restraints for nonexchangeable protons classified as strong (1.8–3.6 Å), medium (2.6–5.0 Å), and weak (3.5–6.5 Å). Separate experiments are recorded for aliphatic and aromatic protons.

Table 2
Chemical shift ranges in 2D ^{13}C-HSQC of 33-nt RNA molecule

	Chemical shift range (ppm)	
Atom pair	**Proton**	**Carbon**
H1′–C1′	5.3–6.1	89–93
H2′–C2′	3.9–5.0	73–76
H3′–C3′	4.0–4.8	68–75
H4′–C4′	4.1–4.6	80–84
H5′/H5″–C5′	3.9–4.7	62–68
Adenine H2–C2	7.0–8.1	151–154
Cytosine H5–C5	5.1–5.9	95–97
Uracil H5–C5	5.0–5.7	101–103
H6–C6	7.4–8.1	138–142
H8–C8	7.0–8.4	133–141

14. 2D DQF-COSY spectrum (20) (acquired on NMR sample in 100% ^2H_2O at 25°C) gives information about sugar conformation, specifically about torsion angle δ which is later restrained to N-type sugar geometry for nucleotides with absent H1′–H2′ cross-peaks. In our case, U24 nucleotide was restrained to S-type due to pronounced H1′–H2′ cross-peak.
15. 2D H(N)CO spectrum (21) (acquired on NMR sample in 95% H_2O at 5°C) gives information about two N–H···O=C hydrogen bonds in asymmetric U9:U25 base pair in the internal loop. Two hydrogen bonds involve C2 and C4 carbonyl groups as the acceptors.
16. 1D ^{31}P spectrum, 3D HCP spectrum (22) and 2D HP-COSY spectrum (acquired on NMR sample in 100% ^2H_2O at 25°C) were used to assign ^{31}P resonances, calculate coupling constants, and measure β and ε torsion angles. We restrain the β torsion angles to *trans* for absent P-H5′ and P-H5″ cross-peaks in the 2D HP-COSY spectrum. Torsion angles α and ζ are set to exclude the *trans* conformation when the range of ^{31}P resonances is narrow.
17. All the above assignment steps allow to unambiguously identify resonances belonging to residues that are unpaired within RNA construct, e.g., within some internal/terminal loops or bulges.

3.7. Residual Dipolar Couplings

1. Phages allow weak alignment of the molecules with respect to the magnetic field and to measure RDC values (only from directly coupled nuclei) (23). The quadrupole splitting of the ^2H_2O resonance was 15.2 Hz at 800 MHz.
2. We measure RDC values for ^1H–^{15}N bonds from the splitting of the cross-peaks along the ^{15}N-dimension of the 2D IPAP ^{15}N-HSQC spectra (24) (acquired on NMR sample before and after addition of phages in 90% H_2O at 25°C).
3. One-bond ^1H–^{13}C RDC values are measured for H2–C2, H6–C6, and H8–C8 bonds from 2D CE CT ^{13}C-HSQC spectrum (25) (acquired on NMR sample before and after addition of phages in 90% H_2O at 25°C).

3.8. Structure Calculation

1. The resolved NOEs are used in conjunction with heteronuclear coupling constants to perform structure calculations (26) using force-field based molecular modeling.
2. NOE cross-peak volumes are translated into distances using the $I \sim r^{-6}$ relation implemented in the Accelrys Felix 2002 program. We select the pyrimidine H5–H6 cross-peak for reference signal which is set to the reference distance of 2.45 Å.
3. NOE-derived distance restraints, torsion angle restraints, and RDCs are used in structure determination. Usually hydrogen

bond and base pair planarity restraints are applied for G:C, A:U, and G:U base pairs. No hydrogen bond and planarity restraints are used within the asymmetric internal and terminal loops.

4. Structure calculations are performed using AMBER 9 with a Wang et al. force field (27). Initial starting structures are created using 8 ps unrestrained MD at different temperatures from 300 to 2,000 K. Structures are then subjected to 60 ps of restrained simulated annealing calculations using a generalized Born implicit solvation model. The molecules are heated to 1,000 K during the first 5 ps, after which temperature is constant for 30 ps, scaled down to 100 K in the next 11 ps, and reduced to 0 K in the last 14 ps. The force constants are 35 kcal/mol/Å^2 for NOE distance, 300 kcal/mol/rad^2 for torsion angle, and 25 kcal/mol/Å^2 for base planarity restraints. The cutoff for nonbonded interactions is 20 Å. The SHAKE algorithm for hydrogen atoms is used with a tolerance of 0.0005 Å. All structures from simulated annealing are subjected to a maximum of 10,000 steps of conjugate gradient minimization.
5. A family of minimized structures with the lowest energy and the smallest NMR violations are analyzed using ptraj, suppose, and 3DNA programs.

3.9. Solution Structure

1. All structural motifs in miRNA:mRNA complexes are very important for proper functioning of *let-7* miRNA and consequent downregulation of *lin-41* gene. Procedures mentioned above helped us to determine NMR solution structure model for the 33-nt hairpin RNA molecule. A model was prepared to study a complex between the *let-7* miRNA and its second complementary site from the 3′-UTR of the *lin-41* mRNA (LCS 2). NMR data and subsequent structure calculations demonstrate that the miRNA:mRNA construct folds into a well-defined stem-loop structure and exhibits two stem regions that are separated by an asymmetric internal loop (Fig. 4).
2. The lower stem is stabilized by seven Watson–Crick base pairs and a U6:G28 wobble base pair, while the upper stem consists of four Watson–Crick base pairs. Both stems show conformational features of A-form RNA.
3. The residue U24 in the asymmetric internal loop is placed in coplanar arrangement with U9:U25 base pair. The puckering of the sugar ring of U24 is in the South conformation (C2′-endo). The torsion angles ζ in U24 and α, β, and ε in U25 adopt conformations outside the usual ranges for A-form RNA. A10:A23 base pair has hydrogen bond between the A10 amino proton and A23 N1. It is stacked above the U9:U25:U24 base triplet, which makes the asymmetric internal loop very well-defined and thermodynamically stable.

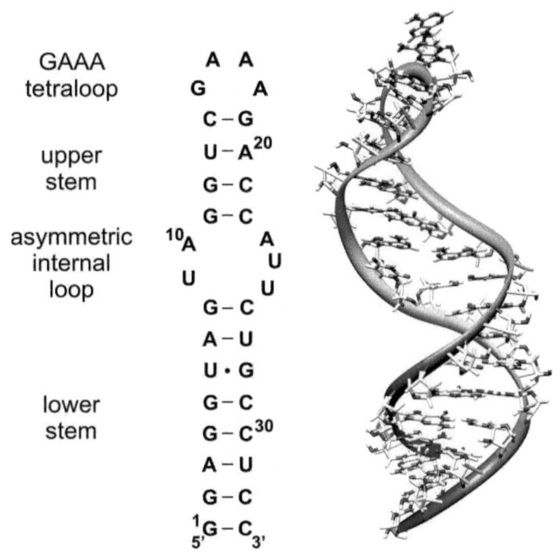

Fig. 4. Schematic representation and high-resolution model of the 33-nt RNA construct (PDB 2JXV) mimicking the complex of *let-7* miRNA with 3′-UTR of the *lin-41* mRNA (LCS2).

4. The asymmetric internal loop in our model system bends both stems in such a way that the major groove becomes wider. As a result, the lower and upper stems are not collinear. The analysis showed that their helical axes exhibited an angular bend of ~20°.
5. Residues G15 and A18 from stable GAAA tetraloop form a sheared G15:A18 mismatch. Adenines A16 and A17 are stacked on A18, which is positioned directly above G19 H1′.

4. Notes

1. We order a 1 μmol synthesis for the top strand and 1 μmol synthesis for the template strand. DNA template is prepared in 1.2× excess of top strand.

   Top strand 5′-TAATACGACTCACTATAG-3′
   Template strand 3′-ATTATGCTGAGTGATATCC…5′
2. rNTPs are purchased as lithium salts in 5 mM Tris, pH 7.5. We prepare stock solution by mixing together individual rNTPs in equimolar ratios, adjust the pH to 8.4 at 25°C with NaOH and store at –20°C. We can increase one of the rNTPs if the amount of that nucleotide in the sequence is bigger. For example, in 33-nt RNA molecule there are 10 guanines, 7 uracils, 8 adenines, and 8 cytosines. The prepared stock solution was 13 mM for guanine and 12 mM for all the other rNTPs.

3. We need to optimize transcription conditions for better yield. We can optimize Tris–HCl pH from 7.9 to 8.2 at 37°C. It is possible to raise the concentration of each rNTP to 4 mM. The $MgCl_2$ concentration required is dependent on the total rNTP concentration. Optimal is a ratio rNTP:$MgCl_2$ = 1:1.75. The enzyme concentration should be carefully varied from 15 to 45 U/μL to ensure that the optimum has been found; we used 25 U/μL. Additional amount of DNA strand is not inhibitory. Optimal DNA strand concentrations are between 50 and 400 nM; we used 400 nM DNA strand. We found out that PEG improves reaction yields.
4. We prepare two centrifuge bottles by washing them with ethanol, water, RNaseZAP, and ddH_2O; then, we autoclave them.
5. NOESY distance restraints from exchangeable protons are valuable to establish spatial relations of sequential nucleotides as well as connectivities across the asymmetric internal loop.

Acknowledgements

We would like to thank the Ministry of Higher Education, Science and Technology and the Slovenian Research Agency (grant numbers P1-0242 and Z1-2138) for their financial support.

References

1. Reinhart B. J., Slack F. J., Basson M., Pasquinelli A. E., Bettinger J. C., Rougvie A. E., Horvitz H. R. and Ruvkun G. (2000) The 21-nucleotide *let-7* RNA regulates developmental timing in *Caenorhabditis elegans*. *Nature* **403,** 901–906.
2. Pasquinelli A. E., Reinhart B. J., Slack F., Martindale M. Q., Kuroda M. I., Maller B., Hayward D. C., Ball E. E., Degnan B., Muller P., Spring J., Srinivasan A., Fishman M., Finnerty J., Corbo J., Levine M., Leahy P., Davidson E. and Ruvkun G. (2000) Conservation of the sequence and temporal expression of *let-7* heterochronic regulatory RNA. *Nature* **408,** 86–89.
3. Johnson C. D., Esquela-Kerscher A., Stefani G., Byrom M., Kelnar K., Ovcharenko D., Wilson M., Wang X., Shelton J., Shingara J., Chin L., Brown D. and Slack F. J. (2007) The *let-7* microRNA represses cell proliferation pathways in human cells. *Cancer Res.* **67,** 7713–7722.
4. Vella M. C., Reinert K. and Slack F. J. (2004) Architecture of a validated microRNA::target interaction. *Chem. Biol.* **11,** 1619–1623.
5. Cevec M., Thibaudeau C. and Plavec J. (2008) Solution structure of a *let-7* miRNA:*lin-41* mRNA complex from *C. elegans*. *Nucleic Acids Res.* **36,** 2330–2337.
6. Milligan J. F. and Uhlenbeck O. C. (1989) Synthesis of small RNAs using T7 RNA polymerase. *Methods Enzymol.* **180,** 51–62.
7. Varani G., Aboul-ela F. and Allain F. H.-T. (1996) NMR investigation of RNA structure. *Prog. Nucl. Magn. Reson. Spectrosc.* **29,** 51–127.
8. Furtig B., Richter C., Wohnert J. and Schwalbe H. (2003) NMR spectroscopy of RNA. *ChemBioChem* **4,** 936–962.
9. Kao C., Zheng M. and Rudisser S. (1999) A simple and efficient method to reduce nontemplated nucleotide addition at the 3 terminus of RNAs transcribed by T7 RNA polymerase. *RNA* **5,** 1268–1272.

10. Piotto M., Saudek V. and Sklenar V. (1992) Gradient-tailored excitation for single-quantum NMR spectroscopy of aqueous solutions. *J. Biomol. NMR* **2,** 661–665.
11. Kumar A., Ernst R. R. and Wuthrich K. (1980) A two-dimensional nuclear Overhauser enhancement (2D NOE) experiment for the elucidation of complete proton-proton cross-relaxation networks in biological macromolecules. *Biochem. Biophys. Res. Commun.* **95,** 1–6.
12. Dingley A. J. and Grzesiek S. (1998) Direct observation of hydrogen bonds in nucleic acid base pairs by internucleotide $^2J_{NN}$ couplings. *J. Am. Chem. Soc.* **120,** 8293–8297.
13. Kay L. E., Keifer P. and Saarinen T. (1992) Pure absorption gradient enhanced heteronuclear single quantum correlation spectroscopy with improved sensitivity. *J. Am. Chem. Soc.* **114,** 10663–10665.
14. Simorre J. P., Zimmermann G. R., Pardi A., Farmer II B. T. and Mueller L. (1995) Triple resonance HNCCCH experiments for correlating exchangeable and nonexchangeable cytidine and uridine base protons in RNA. *J. Biomol. NMR* **6,** 427–432.
15. Bax A. and Davis D. G. (1985) MLEV-17-based two-dimensional homonuclear magnetization transfer spectroscopy. *J. Magn. Reson.* **65,** 355–360.
16. Simorre J. P., Zimmermann G. R., Mueller L. and Pardi A. (1996) Correlation of the guanosine exchangeable and nonexchangeable base protons in ^{13}C-/^{15}N-labeled RNA with an HNC-TOCSY-CH experiment. *J. Biomol. NMR* **7,** 153–156.
17. Marino J. P., Prestegard J. H. and Crothers D. M. (1994) Correlation of adenine H2/H8 resonances in uniformly ^{13}C labeled RNAs by 2D HCCH-TOCSY: a new tool for ^{1}H assignment. *J. Am. Chem. Soc.* **116,** 2205–2206.
18. Pardi A. and Nikonowicz E. P. (1992) Simple procedure for resonance assignment of the sugar protons in ^{13}C-labeled RNAs. *J. Am. Chem. Soc.* **114,** 9202–9203.
19. Riek R., Pervushin K., Fernandez C., Kainosho M. and Wuthrich K. (2001) [^{13}C,^{13}C]- and [^{13}C,^{1}H]-TROSY in a triple resonance experiment for ribose-base and intrabase correlations in nucleic acids. *J. Am. Chem. Soc.* **123,** 658–664.
20. Rance M., Sorensen O. W., Bodenhausen G., Wagner G., Ernst R. R. and Wuthrich K. (1983) Improved spectral resolution in COSY ^{1}H NMR spectra of proteins via double quantum filtering. *Biochem. Biophys. Res. Commun.* **117,** 479–485.
21. Muhandiram D. R. and Kay L. E. (1994) Gradient-enhanced triple-resonance three-dimensional NMR experiments with improved sensitivity. *J. Magn. Reson. B* **103,** 203–216.
22. Marino J. P., Schwalbe H., Anklin C., Bermel W., Crothers D. M. and Griesinger C. (1994) A three-dimensional triple-resonance ^{1}H,^{13}C,^{31}P experiment: sequential through-bond correlation of ribose protons and intervening phosphorus along the RNA oligonucleotide backbone. *J. Am. Chem. Soc.* **116,** 6472–6473.
23. Hansen M. R., Hanson P. and Pardi A. (2000) Filamentous bacteriophage for aligning RNA, DNA, and proteins for measurement of nuclear magnetic resonance dipolar coupling interactions. *Methods Enzymol.* **317,** 220–240.
24. Ottiger M., Delaglio F. and Bax A. (1998) Measurement of *J* and dipolar couplings from simplified two-dimensional NMR spectra. *J. Magn. Reson.* **131,** 373–378.
25. Davis A. L., Keeler J., Laue E. D. and Moskau D. (1992) Experiments for recording pure-absorption heteronuclear correlation spectra using pulsed field gradients. *J. Magn. Reson.* **98,** 207–216.
26. Mackerell A. D. (2004) Empirical force fields for biological macromolecules: overview and issues. *J. Comput. Chem.* **25,** 1584–1604.
27. Cornell W. D., Cieplak P., Bayly C. I., Gould I. R., Merz K. M., Ferguson D. M., Spellmeyer D. C., Fox T., Caldwell J. W. and Kollman P. A. (1995) A second generation force field for the simulation of proteins, nucleic acids, and organic molecules. *J. Am. Chem. Soc.* **117,** 5179–5197.

Chapter 18

MiRNA Editing

Dylan E. Dupuis and Stefan Maas

Abstract

RNA editing by A-to-I modification is a widespread mechanism in complex organisms that leads to the posttranscriptional alteration of protein coding as well as noncoding sequences. MiRNA transcripts have been recognized as a major target for RNA editing enzymes, and single-nucleotide changes through editing can impact the biogenesis of mature miRNAs, as well as the target specificity of the regulatory RNA. Bona fide A-to-I RNA editing events are validated experimentally through parallel analysis of genomic DNA and transcribed sequences of miRNA genes isolated from the same specimen through gene-specific amplification and sequencing of endogenous transcripts.

1. Introduction

A-to-I RNA editing is a posttranscriptional modification resulting in the enzymatic modification of an adenosine-to-inosine nucleotide in RNA. It affects RNAs with partially double-stranded RNA folds and is catalyzed by the adenosine deaminase acting on RNA (ADAR) family of enzymes (1–4). Editing by ADARs can be very site specific, as seen in cases where a single nucleotide within a protein-coding sequence is altered. This modification can then in turn lead to a single amino acid substitution in the protein product since inosine is interpreted as guanosine by the translational machinery (1–4). Apart from coding sequences, A-to-I RNA editing can modify RNA splice sites (5, 6) and noncoding RNAs, including miRNA sequences. In fact, since the initial report of miRNA editing in 2004 (7), miRNA transcripts are today considered as a major target of ADARs. It has been shown that modifications caused by editing can influence both the biogenesis and function of mature miRNAs (8–12). Editing can interfere with processing by both Drosha

Silvia Monticelli (ed.), *MicroRNAs and the Immune System: Methods and Protocols*, Methods in Molecular Biology, vol. 667,
DOI 10.1007/978-1-60761-811-9_18,

and Dicer (9, 12). However, there are several miRNAs identified in which A-to-I RNA editing leads to an increase in mature miRNA expression (9). The variation in how A-to-I RNA editing regulates miRNA processing likely depends on the number of edited sites as well as the location of those sites within the miRNA precursor.

A-to-I RNA editing also has the ability to regulate miRNA targeting (9, 10) when modifications occur within the miRNA seed sequence or at other locations important for target recognition. Through such modifications, editing can not only reduce regulation of the primary target but also can redirect the miRNA to a new target altogether.

A 2008 survey of 209 human pri-miRNA transcripts concluded that an estimated 16% of pri-miRNAs are targeted by A-to-I RNA editing (9). This study also revealed a strong bias for editing to occur at the adenosine within UAG trinucleotides. Such editing events comprise about 50% of all editing events identified in pri-miRNAs. Additionally, mature miRNAs have also been investigated directly for evidence of A-to-I RNA editing (10). Due to their small size, these investigations require RNA size selection and isolation of the small RNA fraction followed by poly-A tailing, adapter ligation, and cloning of the sequences. The development of high-throughput sequence technology has led to deep sequencing analysis of mature miRNAs, which also can be used to detect edited variants of wild-type miRNA sequences (13). The methods for experimental determination of RNA editing in miRNAs described here include techniques to analyze pri-miRNA transcripts using human miRNA22 as an example, which was the first miRNA sequence reported to undergo A-to-I editing (7).

2. Materials

2.1. Cell Culture

1. Dulbecco's Modified Eagle's Medium (DMEM) supplemented with 10% fetal bovine serum (FBS) and 1× antimycotic, antibiotic (final concentration 100 IU penicillin, 100 μg/ml streptomycin, and 0.25 μg/ml amphotericin B).
2. Solution of trypsin (0.25%) and ethylenediamine tetraacetic acid (EDTA) (1 mM).

2.2. RNA Isolation

1. 1× PBS.
2. Trizol solution (Invitrogen, Carlsbad, CA): This reagent contains phenol and is therefore very hazardous. Toxic in contact with skin and if swallowed, causes burns. Vapors should not

be inhaled. It is recommended to perform the pipetting of the solution under a chemical fume hood.

3. Chloroform.
4. Isopropyl alcohol.
5. Ethanol 70%.
6. DNAse I and 10× DNAse I buffer (NEB, Ipswich, MA).

2.3. Reverse Transcription and PCR

1. Superscript reverse transcriptase II (Invitrogen, Carlsbad, CA) with 5× buffer.
2. 20 mM dNTP mix.
3. RNAsin (Promega Biosciences, Madison, WI).
4. 0.1 M DTT.
5. N6 random oligonucleotides (Promega Biosciences, Madison, WI).
6. Taq DNA polymerase with 10× buffer and 50 mM $MgCl_2$ solution.

2.4. Purification and Sequencing

1. Phenol:chloroform:isoamylalcohol (25:24:1).
2. Chloroform:isoamylalcohol (24:1).
3. Sodium acetate 3 M, pH 5.2.
4. Ethanol 100 and 70%.
5. Agarose.
6. DNA loading buffer.
7. Ethidium bromide.
8. QIAEX II gel extraction kit (Qiagen, Hilden, Germany).

2.5. Subcloning of PCR Products and Sequencing

1. pBluescript II plasmid vector (Stratagene, La Jolla, CA).
2. Kpn I (10 U/μl) and Eco RI (20 U/μl) restriction enzymes plus reaction buffers.
3. T4 DNA ligase plus 10× T4 DNA ligase buffer.
4. DH5α Z-competent *Escherichia coli* cells.
5. SOB medium.
6. LB agar plates with 100 μg/ml ampicillin and 30 μg/ml X-Gal (from 40 mg/ml solution in dimethylformamide).
7. LB medium with 100 μg/ml ampicillin.
8. DNA miniprep spin isolation kit (Qiagen, Hilden, Germany).

2.6. ADAR Overexpression Analysis

1. ADAR1 and ADAR2 mammalian expression constructs (such as described in (14)).
2. SuperFect transfection reagent (Qiagen, Hilden, Germany).

2.7. Analysis of Genomic DNA from the Same Specimen

1. Lysis buffer: 10 mM Tris–HCl pH 7.5, 10 mM EDTA, 10 mM NaCl, 0.5% (w/v) SDS.
2. Proteinase K (Fisher Scientific, Pittsburgh, PA) in distilled water, 10 mg/ml stock solution, subject to "self-digestion" for 30 min at 55°C before each use to activate the catalytic domains. Store at −20°C.
3. RNAse A (EMD Chemicals, Gibbstown, NJ), 10 mg/ml in 10 mM Tris–HCl pH 7.5, 1 mM EDTA, 50% glycerol. Store at room temperature.

3. Methods

The RNA editing analysis of any target requires the selection of the appropriate specimen. In case of miRNAs, due to their often highly selective expression, it is important to establish if a particular cell type or tissue does express detectable levels of the miRNA of interest. As a result of various deep sequencing and miRNA-specific expression studies, it is possible using existing databases and the literature to determine the expression status of a given miRNA (at least in several mammalian species, *Drosophila*, and *C. elegans*).

3.1. Cell Culture

Cervix carcinoma HeLa cells are cultivated using standard procedures and grown at 37°C, 5% CO_2 until confluent. HeLa cells are known to express functional ADAR enzymes. For editing analysis, the amount of cells obtained from a confluent well of a 6-well plate is sufficient (see Note 1).

3.2. RNA Isolation

1. The cells (see Note 2) are harvested with 0.8 ml of Trizol reagent for a single well of a 6-well plate by pipetting the reagent onto the cells, tilting the plate and repeated pipetting of the solution, and rinsing the well with the fluid until all the cells have dislodged and are dissolved in the Trizol. The solution is then transferred to a 1.7-ml microcentrifuge tube.
2. Following the manufacturer's protocol for isolation of RNA using Trizol, incubate at room temperature for 5 min, followed by the addition of 160-µl chloroform and centrifugation at 12,000 × *g* for 15 min at 4–8°C. The mixture separates into a lower red, phenol–chloroform phase, an interphase, and a colorless upper aqueous phase containing the RNA.
3. The supernatant is transferred into a new tube (see Note 3) and the extraction step can be repeated if desired (see Note 4).
4. For RNA precipitation, 0.4-ml isopropyl alcohol is added to the supernatant and mixed. Incubate samples at room

temperature for 10 min and centrifuge at no more than 12,000 × *g* for 10 min at 4–8°C.

5. The supernatant is removed then the RNA pellet is washed once with 0.8 ml 70% ethanol. Mix by vortex and centrifuge at 7,500 × *g* for 5 min at 4–8°C.
6. Remove all supernatant and air-dry the pellet for 5–10 min at room temperature. Resuspend the RNA in 20-μl DEPC-treated water. Now the RNA is ready for reverse transcription and PCR (see Note 5).

3.3. Reverse Transcription and PCR

Unless there is a specific base position within a given miRNA sequence that is to be analyzed, the aim is to evaluate the occurrence of editing within the complete pre-miRNA sequence of ca. 75–125 nucleotides plus flanking regions of the pri-miRNA. To this end, it is desired to reverse transcribe most of the pri-miRNA transcripts. This is best achieved by using random primers for reverse transcription, in particular, as sometimes the beginning and end of the respective miRNA gene are not well characterized. However, alternatively, a miRNA-specific reverse primer for reverse transcription can be used to reduce the complexity of the resulting cDNA sample and to enhance the efficient cDNA synthesis of low copy transcripts. Many miRNA transcripts are subject to splicing. This allows for the placement of the PCR primers for amplification of the miRNA cDNA on different exons, which ensures the amplification of cDNA vs. any DNA contaminations in the sample (see Note 5). In general, for primer design any conventional primer selection software can be used. Aim for an amplicon size of between 200 and 500 bp as the efficiency of amplification and the yields for isolation and purification of the amplicons are optimal within this range. Figure 1a shows the human miRNA22 gene structure with the position of amplification primers relative to the position of the exons and introns of this miRNA gene and flanking the exon that harbors the pre-miRNA22 sequence.

1. 50% (10 μl) of the RNA prepared in Subheading 3.2 is combined with 1 μl of random primers (400–500 ng) and brought to a total of 18.5 μl with DEPC-treated water. The mixture is incubated for 10 min at 70°C and followed by placing the tubes on ice.
2. During the incubation, a master mix for reverse transcription is prepared on ice with (for each reverse transcription reaction) 6 μl 5× RT buffer, 1.5 μl 0.1 M DTT, 1 μl RNasin, and 3 μl 20 mM dNTPs. 11.5 μl of this mix is pipetted to the RNA/primer sample, mixed by vortexing, and spun down.
3. At this point, 10–20% of the total volume can be removed into a new tube to serve as a mock reverse transcriptional control (see Note 6).

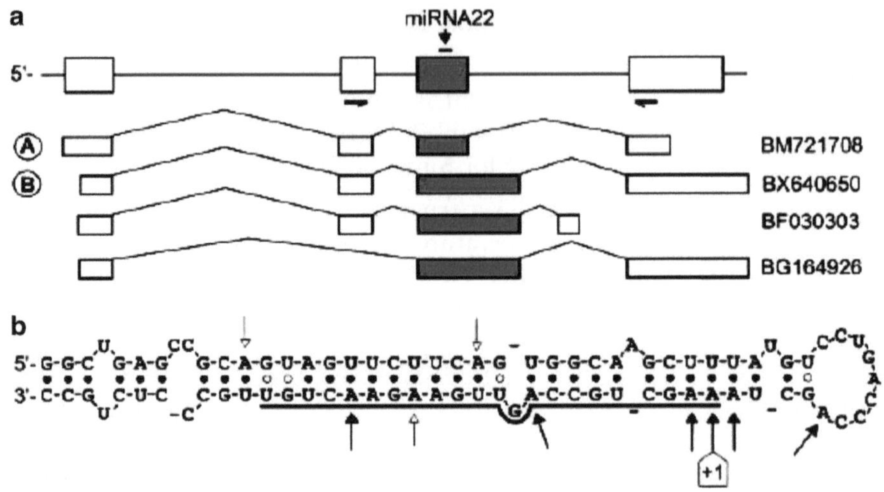

Fig. 1. A-to-I RNA editing analysis of miRNA22. (**a**) The exon/intron structure of the human miRNA22 gene as deduced from expressed sequences with GenBank accession numbers. Exons are shown as *boxes*, introns as *lines*. The location of the mature miRNA22 sequence and the positions of the oligonucleotide primers used for editing analysis of two different splice variants A and B are indicated. (**b**) Predicted RNA secondary structure of pre-miRNA22 with the mature miRNA sequence *underlined*. Edited positions in human and/or mouse tissues (*filled arrowheads*) and additional sites found only in ADAR1 overexpressing cell lines (*open arrowheads*) are indicated (reproduced from ref. *7* with permission from Cold Spring Harbor Laboratory Press).

4. The tube is then prewarmed to 42°C, and reverse transcription is initiated by adding 0.5 μl of Superscript reverse transcriptase II.
5. Reactions are incubated for 1 h at 42°C, followed by heating the cDNA samples to 95°C for 5 min to inactivate the reverse transcriptase. Now the cDNA is ready for the PCR reaction.
6. For a total reaction volume of 100 μl, 10 μl 10× PCR buffer, 5 μl 50 mM $MgCl_2$, 4 μl of each 10 μM concentrated oligonucleotide primer, 2 μl 20 mM dNTP mix, 1.2 μl template cDNA, and 0.4 μl Taq DNA polymerase are combined on ice, mixed by vortexing, and transferred to a thin-walled PCR tube.
7. A PCR thermocycler with heated lid is programmed with the following cycle conditions (see Note 7): (a) 3 min at 94°C, (b) 30 s at 94°C, 30 s at 55°C, 30 s at 72°C, (c) 10 min at 72°C, and (d) hold at 4°C. Step b is repeated 35 times, steps a, c, and d only once.
8. The PCR is analyzed for productive amplification of the expected size by running 10% of the reaction out on a 2% agarose gel followed by ethidium bromide staining and UV detection of DNA bands (see Note 8).

3.4. Purification and Sequencing

Upon successful amplification of the miRNA-specific cDNA fragment, the amplicon is prepared for sequencing by phenol–chloroform extraction, precipitation, and gel purification.

One extraction with a phenol/chloroform/isoamylalcohol mixture is followed by another extraction with chloroform/isoamylalcohol, and the aqueous supernatant is subjected to precipitation with sodium acetate plus ethanol. This purification step is most efficient with an initial sample volume of at least 100 μl. It is suggested that volumes below 100 μl be adjusted to 100 μl using distilled water.

1. A volume of phenol/chloroform/isoamylalcohol mixture is added to an equal volume of sample. Mix by vortex, then centrifuge at 13,000 × *g* for 5 min.
2. The aqueous phase is transferred to a new microcentrifuge tube, and a volume of chloroform/isoamylalcohol mixture is added in volume equal to that of the sample. Mix by vortex then centrifuge at 13,000 × *g* for 5 min.
3. The aqueous phase is transferred to a new microcentrifuge tube, and the DNA is precipitated by adding a volume of 3 M sodium acetate equal to 10% of the volume of the initial PCR product. Add 100% ethanol equal to 250% volume of the initial PCR product. Mix by vortex then centrifuge at 13,000 × *g* for 30 min.
4. The supernatant is removed, and the DNA pellet is washed once with 500 μl of 70% ethanol. This is then centrifuged at 13,000 × *g* for 5 min.
5. The supernatant is removed, and the DNA pellet is air-dried for 5 min at room temperature or until all residual ethanol has evaporated.
6. The DNA pellet is resuspended in 20 μl of distilled water. To this solution, 2 μl of 10× DNA sample buffer is added, then the mixture is loaded onto a 2% agarose gel, and run at 6 V/cm for about 1 h (until the unincorporated primers are well separated from the amplicon band).
7. The DNA band is excised from the gel with a scalpel, and the DNA is extracted from the agarose using QIAEX II gel extraction kit according to the manufacturer's instructions. The DNA is eluted in 50 μl of Tris/EDTA buffer (Elution buffer).
8. 10% of the eluted DNA is run out on a 2% agarose gel to evaluate purity and concentration as judged by comparison to DNA size marker bands. For good quality sequencing results, a concentration of at least 30 ng/μl DNA should be present. The DNA is then subjected to dideoxy sequencing using standard protocols, and one of the two PCR primers that were used for initial amplification is used for the sequencing reaction (see Note 9).

3.5. Subcloning of PCR Products and Sequencing

If the overall editing levels within the target miRNA are smaller than about 20% and in general to obtain more accurate quantitative data on the editing extent at each editing site, the PCR products are subcloned into pBluescript vector and then individual recombinant clones are isolated and sequenced (see Note 10). An additional advantage of this process is that it allows for the detection of positive or negative coupling between editing sites within the same target RNA.

1. PCR is performed as described above using the initial PCR product as a template in a re-PCR with oligonucleotide primers that have 5′-extensions with incorporated restriction sites. The 5′-sequence 5′-GACGAGTGGTACC-3′ (introducing a Kpn I restriction site) is added to the upstream primer, while the sequence 5′-GGAATTC-3′ is added to the downstream primer (introducing an Eco RI restriction site).
2. Purify the amplicons by phenol/chloroform extraction and ethanol precipitated as described above.
3. Purified amplicons are digested by Kpn I for 3 h at 37°C in a total volume of 100 μl.
4. Restriction digest is purified by phenol/chloroform extraction and ethanol precipitation, then DNA is resuspended in distilled water, and digested with Eco RI for 3 h under the same conditions.
5. Purify the DNA as described above through phenol/chloroform extraction and precipitation followed by gel purification.
6. pBluescript vector is treated like the PCR amplicons and successively digested with Kpn I and Eco RI, followed by gel purification.
7. The digested and purified amplicons are ligated into the vector and transformed into *E. coli* Z-competent DH5α cells. Transformed bacteria is plated on LB/ampicillin/X-Gal agar plates
8. Ampicillin-resistant colonies of white color (indicating a recombinant clone) are picked and grown out overnight in 4-ml liquid LB medium containing ampicillin.
9. Plasmid DNAs from individual cultures are isolated using a DNA miniprep kit (see Note 10), and the obtained plasmids are subjected to DNA sequencing using standard T7 primer, which will yield the sense cDNA sequence as a readout.

Figure 1b depicts human pre-miRNA22 indicating which adenosines were found to undergo RNA editing.

3.6. ADAR Overexpression Analysis

Once in vivo RNA editing within a miRNA transcript has been established through the methods described above, an ADAR overexpression experiment in human cells that endogenously

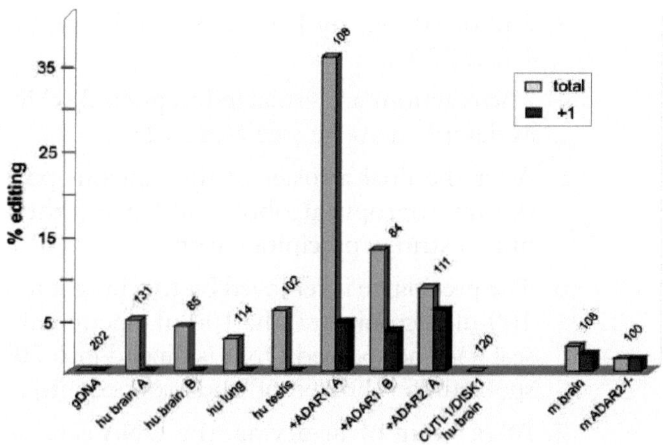

Fig. 2. Editing levels of miRNA22 precursor molecules in various human tissues, human cell lines, wild-type mouse brain, and brains of ADAR2 knock-out mice. A PCR product derived from the human miRNA22 genomic region (gDNA), as well as the reverse transcribed and amplified coding sequences from human CUTL1 (CCAAT displacement proteinlike) and DISK1 (disrupted in Schizophrenia 1) genes, were analyzed as negative controls. The number of individually sequenced clones is indicated above each column. In addition to the total extent of editing (percent of molecules edited at one or more of the 17 adenosines within the pre-miRNA), the results for the +1 position of miRNA22 are shown because they point toward a pronounced site selectivity of ADAR2 vs. ADAR1 (reproduced from ref. *7* with permission from Cold Spring Harbor Laboratory Press).

express the miRNA under investigation can provide further evidence that indeed the observed base modifications are mediated specifically by ADARs. Furthermore, it can also reveal if editing at the detected sites may be preferentially mediated by either ADAR1 or ADAR2.

1. For the purpose of analyzing human miRNA22, a mammalian expression construct for ADAR1 or ADAR2 is transfected through standard methods (such as transfection with SuperFect reagent) into human HeLa cells (see Note 11), which endogenously express miRNA 22.
2. 24–36 h after transfection, the cells are harvested using Trizol solution and RNA editing status in pri-miRNA22 is analyzed as described above.

Figure 2 shows results obtained for human miRNA22 editing in human tissues, as well as human cell lines, mouse tissues, and ADAR1 and ADAR2 overexpressing human cells.

3.7. Analysis of Genomic DNA from the Same Specimen

1. Genomic DNA of the same specimen is isolated using standard procedures. The cells from one well of a 6-well plate are washed twice with 1× PBS and harvested with 500 μl lysis buffer.
2. The suspension is transferred to microcentrifuge tubes, and 10 μl of a 10 mg/ml Proteinase K solution is added. The suspension is then incubated overnight at 55°C while inverting.

3. 3 μl of 10 mg/ml RNAse A is added and then incubated for 1 h at 37°C.
4. The reactions are subjected to phenol/chloroform extraction as described above (see Note 12).
5. After the final transfer of the aqueous phase to a new tube, 0.9-ml isopropyl alcohol is added and the tubes are inverted until a stringy precipitate forms.
6. The precipitate is removed by touching it to the sealed end of a 100-μl micropipette (the 100-μl pipette is flamed at one end to seal it). The spooled DNA is dipped into 70% ethanol, and the spooled tip is broken off and dropped into a microfuge tube.
7. After 5 min of air-drying, the DNA is resuspended in 100-μl distilled water. The genomic DNA is now ready for PCR.

The analysis of RNA editing through PCR, purification, and sequencing is analogous to that for cDNA, except that the gDNA is the template in the PCR and primers that are designed to amplify the genomic region of the gene are used.

3.8. Error Analysis

The theoretical background of A/G discrepancies resulting from errors during reverse transcription and PCR can be calculated as $P = a \cdot c + b \cdot c \cdot d = 3.4 \times 10^{-5} \times 17 + 0.8 \times 10^{-5} \times 17 \times 24 = 0.4 \times 10^{-2}$, with a being the error rate of Superscript reverse transcriptase (3.4×10^{-5}; (15)), b the error rate of Taq DNA polymerase (0.8×10^{-5}; (16)), c the number of adenosines analyzed, and d the number of template doublings during PCR (estimated for 30 cycles of amplification). In case of the human miRNA22 analysis, one can therefore expect 0.4 base changes affecting adenosine in 100 sequences, corresponding to 1 base change due to mutation in 250 sequences. Because changes of A to C and A to T are also possible, this error rate is likely an overestimation as the analysis only detects A-to-G changes. The results from analysis of genomic DNA isolated from human brain is in line with this value, as within 200 sequenced clones not a single A/G change was detected (7). As additional controls, RT-PCR and sequencing of coding regions from human CUTL1 (BC025422) and DISC1 (AK025293) RNAs were performed yielding the same result as for the genomic DNA.

4. Notes

1. Essentially, a single cell is sufficient to amplify a cDNA target, such as a pri-miRNA precursor, but practically, the use of ca. 10,000 cells from the well of a 6-well plate yields sufficient

RNA to ensure that even miRNAs of low expression level can be detected and allows for repetition of the experiment to optimize the amplification protocol, if needed.

2. Alternatively, tissue specimen or other cell lines may be used as starting material depending on the miRNA to be analyzed and the species to be investigated. The main difference to the RNA isolation protocol between cells and tissue sample is that the tissue is placed into 1-ml Trizol reagent per 100-mg tissue and homogenized by douncing.
3. When transferring the supernatant, avoid any material from the interphase and the lower organic phase. It is recommended to rather leave a few percent of the supernatant behind than to risk contaminating the RNA phase with protein or DNA from the other phases.
4. If the starting material is high in proteins, fat, or polysaccharides (such as brain tissue), it is recommended to perform an additional step of phenol–chloroform extraction. To this end, add one volume of phenol:chloroform:isoamylalcohol reagent (25:24:1 ratio) to the solution, mix by shaking vigorously, and centrifuge at 12,000 × *g* for 15 min at 4–8°C. Then proceed with the protocol as described.
5. After preparation of total RNA from cells or tissues using Trizol, there will likely be traces of genomic DNA present (or traces of plasmid DNA if the cells were transfected with plasmid DNA). These DNA contaminations are of no concern for the subsequent steps of the protocol if the target that is being analyzed is a spliced RNA and if the PCR primers that are used span at least one intron. This means that it is possible to distinguish after amplification, the product of the spliced cDNA sequences from any genomic sequences that are amplified with the same primers. In addition, the genomic fragments are not amplified under the cycling conditions used for the spliced cDNA, because introns in mammalian species are often very long. In cases where the to be analyzed, miRNA sequence lacks introns or the amplification strategy does not allow for the primers to be located on separate exons, it is critical to eliminate the traces of DNA from the RNA isolate before continuing with RT-PCR. This is accomplished through DNAse digestion of the sample using DNAse I in 1× DNAse I buffer for 1 h, phenol–chloroform extraction and precipitation of the RNA and resuspension in DEPC-treated water. This whole procedure should be repeated at least three times before the RNA sample can be tested for the absence of DNA traces. This is done by using the RNA (without reverse transcription) as a template in a PCR using the same primers that will be used for the cDNA. Any detectable amplification product of the expected size indicates contamination, and additional rounds of DNAse treatment need to be performed.

6. The mock reverse transcription reaction is critical in cases where the RNA has previously been treated with DNAse to remove any genomic or plasmid DNA from the RNA preparation. When the amplification products obtained from the pri-miRNA transcripts cannot be distinguished from products originating from DNA templates, then the parallel PCR on the mock samples will serve as a control that no DNA contamination persists.
7. The cycling parameters need to be optimized for each template to be amplified for optimal yield. The described settings usually work to amplify most sequences, but especially high G/C content and extremely low expression level may require special conditions, buffers, polymerases for amplification, or a second reamplification step using the first PCR product as a template.
8. In case of weak or missing amplification of target sequences, the PCR conditions can be optimized to allow amplification or second-step PCR can be performed with the same or nested primers to boost yield.
9. The conclusions that can be drawn from the direct sequencing of PCR products strongly depend on the data quality. DNA purity, sequence primer specificity, and target sequence environment all influence the resolution and signal-to-noise ratio for sequencing. Usually, there is a small level of noise visible in the electropherogram. Since editing is detected through the evaluation of double peaks of A and G signals at the editing site, distinguishing what constitutes bona fide editing signal vs. background noise is critical. Especially in cases of low editing frequency (<20%), it is often necessary to proceed with Subheading 3.5 in order to clearly establish the existence of cDNAs that carry a G at the position in question. If the sequence data is of good quality and moderate to high editing extent revealed, then the approximate percentage of editing at the site can be calculated by comparing the relative peak heights of the A and G signals.
10. The total number of clones that should be analyzed in each case depends on the editing level at the modification sites. To obtain statistically significant data, the number of independent clones that need to be sequenced increases with decreasing editing extent.
11. To control for variation in transfection efficiencies and inter-assay variation, triplicates of transfections should be performed using a 6-well plate format.
12. During the phenol/chloroform purification, mix only by shaking, but do not vortex to minimize shearing of chromosomal DNA.

Acknowledgments

This work was supported, in part, by R15 NS057739 to SM.

References

1. Bass, B. L. (2002) RNA editing by adenosine deaminases that act on RNA, *Annu Rev Biochem* **71**, 817–846.
2. Gommans, W. M., Dupuis, D. E., McCane, J. E., Tatalias, N. E., and Maas, S. (2008) Diversifying exon code through A-to-I RNA editing, in *DNA RNA Editing* (Smith, H., Ed.), pp. 3–30, Wiley & Sons, Inc., New York.
3. Hoopengardner, B. (2006) Adenosine-to-inosine RNA editing: perspectives and predictions, *Mini Rev Med Chem* **6**, 1213–1216.
4. Maydanovych, O. and Beal, P. A. (2006) Breaking the central dogma by RNA editing, *Chem Rev* **106**, 3397–3411.
5. Athanasiadis, A., Rich, A., and Maas, S. (2004) Widespread A-to-I RNA editing of Alu-containing mRNAs in the human transcriptome, *PLoS Biol* **2**, e391.
6. Lev-Maor, G., Sorek, R., Levanon, E. Y., Paz, N., Eisenberg, E., and Ast, G. (2007) RNA-editing-mediated exon evolution, *Genome Biol* **8**, R29.
7. Luciano, D. J., Mirsky, H., Vendetti, N. J., and Maas, S. (2004) RNA editing of a miRNA precursor, *RNA* **10**, 1174–1177.
8. Blow, M. J., Grocock, R. J., van Dongen, S., Enright, A. J., Dicks, E., Futreal, P. A., Wooster, R., and Stratton, M. R. (2006) RNA editing of human microRNAs, *Genome Biol* **7**, R27.
9. Kawahara, Y., Megraw, M., Kreider, E., Iizasa, H., Valente, L., Hatzigeorgiou, A. G., and Nishikura, K. (2008) Frequency and fate of microRNA editing in human brain, *Nucleic Acids Res* **36**, 5270–5280.
10. Kawahara, Y., Zinshteyn, B., Sethupathy, P., Iizasa, H., Hatzigeorgiou, A. G., and Nishikura, K. (2007) Redirection of silencing targets by adenosine-to-inosine editing of miRNAs, *Science* **315**, 1137–1140.
11. Yang, W., Chendrimada, T. P., Wang, Q., Higuchi, M., Seeburg, P. H., Shiekhattar, R., and Nishikura, K. (2006) Modulation of microRNA processing and expression through RNA editing by ADAR deaminases, *Nat Struct Mol Biol* **13**, 13–21.
12. Kawahara, Y., Zinshteyn, B., Chendrimada, T. P., Shiekhattar, R., and Nishikura, K. (2007) RNA editing of the microRNA-151 precursor blocks cleavage by the Dicer-TRBP complex, *EMBO Rep* **8**, 763–769.
13. Landgraf, P., Rusu, M., Sheridan, R., Sewer, A., Iovino, N., Aravin, A., Pfeffer, S., Rice, A., Kamphorst, A. O., Landthaler, M., Lin, C., Socci, N. D., Hermida, L., Fulci, V., Chiaretti, S., Foa, R., Schliwka, J., Fuchs, U., Novosel, A., Muller, R. U., Schermer, B., Bissels, U., Inman, J., Phan, Q., Chien, M., Weir, D. B., Choksi, R., De Vita, G., Frezzetti, D., Trompeter, H. I., Hornung, V., Teng, G., Hartmann, G., Palkovits, M., Di Lauro, R., Wernet, P., Macino, G., Rogler, C. E., Nagle, J. W., Ju, J., Papavasiliou, F. N., Benzing, T., Lichter, P., Tam, W., Brownstein, M. J., Bosio, A., Borkhardt, A., Russo, J. J., Sander, C., Zavolan, M., and Tuschl, T. (2007) A mammalian microRNA expression atlas based on small RNA library sequencing, *Cell* **129**, 1401–1414.
14. Gommans, W. M. and Maas, S. (2008) Characterization of ADAR1-mediated modulation of gene expression, *Biochem Biophys Res Commun* **377**, 170–175.
15. Potter, J., Zheng, W., and Lee, J. (2003) Thermal stability and cDNA synthesis capability of SuperScript reverse transcriptase, *Focus* **25**, 19–24.
16. Cline, J., Braman, J. C., and Hogrefe, H. H. (1996) PCR fidelity of pfu DNA polymerase and other thermostable DNA polymerases, *Nucleic Acids Res* **24**, 3546–3551.

Part VI

Bioinformatic Analysis and Target Prediction

Chapter 19

Computational Prediction of MicroRNA Targets

Xiaowei Wang

Abstract

One critical step in miRNA functional studies is to identify the gene targets that are directly regulated by miRNAs. In this chapter, we describe a computational algorithm and an online database, miRDB, for miRNA target prediction. In miRDB, flexible Web search interface has been developed for the retrieval of target prediction results generated by the newly developed computational algorithm. In addition, a wiki editing interface has been established to allow anyone with Internet access to make contributions on miRNA functional annotation. All data stored in miRDB are freely accessible at http://www.mirdb.org.

1. Introduction

As of 2010, over 700 human miRNAs have been identified. Despite the relatively small number of miRNAs, both computational and experimental studies have shown that thousands of human protein-coding genes are regulated by miRNAs (1–3). Thus, miRNAs are considered to be master regulators of many important biological processes, including the regulation of the immune system.

Because of their critical roles in the regulation of gene expression, the functional characterization of miRNAs has become one of the most active research fields in biology in recent years. Accordingly, there has been an exponential growth for the number of PubMed publications on miRNA research. There were only about 100 miRNA papers published in 2003, in contrast to the over 1,500 miRNA papers published in 2008. At present, experimental identification of miRNA targets is difficult, and miRNA researchers rely primarily on computational tools to initially identify the targets of interest (4). However, one major issue in this research field is that the available computational

Silvia Monticelli (ed.), *MicroRNAs and the Immune System: Methods and Protocols*, Methods in Molecular Biology, vol. 667,
DOI 10.1007/978-1-60761-811-9_19, © Springer Science+Business Media, LLC 2010

tools are insufficient for the accurate prediction of miRNA targets. Although multiple computational approaches have been proposed recently, this remains a major challenge for bioinformatists because of the very limited sequence complementarity between miRNAs and their targets, as well as the scarcity of experimentally validated gene targets to guide bioinformatics design (4).

Recent studies have identified useful features that could be applied to miRNA target prediction. For example, the miRNA 5′-end, known as the "seed region," usually shows perfect Watson–Crick complementarity to the target binding site in the transcript 3′-untranslated region (UTR). This is by far the most effective feature for target prediction and has been included in most target prediction algorithms. Unfortunately, the seed match feature alone is insufficient to identify miRNA targets because the seed sequence is very short and a large number of nontarget transcripts also contain seed complementary sequences. Thus, a combination of multiple features is required to build a prediction model. Recent studies have also shown the importance of the evolutionary conservation of the seed complementary sequence in the target binding site. Both experimental and computational analyses indicate that many miRNA target sites are evolutionarily conserved. Thus, this feature can be used to significantly reduce the false positive rate of target prediction. It has also been proposed that incorporating the secondary structure of the target site is helpful to identify biologically important targets as the accessibility of the target site is an important requirement for miRNA binding (4).

One promising strategy for target prediction is to use machine learning approaches. Machine learning algorithms, such as support vector machines (SVMs, see Note 1), attempt to extract relevant information from data automatically using computational and statistical methods. Machine learning has been applied to many diverse fields including biological research, but has not been widely applied to miRNA target prediction. One major obstacle is the lack of high-quality training data for building robust prediction models. There is only a limited number of validated miRNA targets reported in the literature (5). In addition, most of these reported targets were validated because they were predicted miRNA targets by existing bioinformatics algorithms. As a result, the validation data are biased toward these algorithms and less useful for developing new target prediction algorithms.

In this chapter, we describe a new bioinformatics algorithm and a database for miRNA target prediction. These computational tools have been described in detail in our recent publications (6, 7). Genome-wide miRNA target prediction results are available from the online database, miRDB, which is freely accessible at http://www.mirdb.org.

2. Methods

2.1. A Machine Learning Algorithm for miRNA Target Prediction

In this study, we used microarray data to improve the accuracy of bioinformatic target prediction. We began by analyzing a public microarray transcriptional profiling dataset for miRNA functional studies (8). Based on this profiling analysis, we developed a machine learning algorithm, MirTarget2, by combining many heterogeneous prediction features in the algorithm training process (6). Comparative data analysis on independent experimental data indicates that MirTarget2 has superior performance over previously published algorithms (6).

2.1.1. Preparation of the Training Data

A public microarray dataset was used as the training data in our target prediction analysis (8). The downloaded microarray dataset is by far the largest of its kind for miRNA functional studies. In the public study, multiple miRNAs were individually overexpressed, and the global effects on gene expression were measured by microarrays. In this way, miRNA functions were characterized by globally analyzing miRNA-downregulated genes. More interesting to us, this microarray study has also made available a large experimental dataset that could potentially be used to improve bioinformatics target prediction. In our computational analysis, downregulated and unchanged genes due to miRNA overexpression were identified and their 3′-UTR sequences were retrieved from the NCBI databases. By comparing downregulated genes and unchanged genes directly, we were able to identify many useful predictive features for target prediction as described in detail below.

2.1.2. Selection of Training Features for Target Prediction

A critical step in computational modeling for building predictive classifiers is to identify key characteristics, called "training features," which can be used as the basis for separating targets from nontargets. In our study, 131 training features relevant to miRNA target prediction were selected by analyzing 1,471 transcript sequences from downregulated or unchanged genes. A typical miRNA target site has perfect complementarity to the miRNA seed sequence. There are four major types of seed sequences: positions 1–8 (defined as *seed 8* in our study), positions 1–7 (as *seed 7a*), positions 2–8 (as *seed 7b*), and positions 2–7 (as *seed 6*). Although all seed types are useful for target prediction, our computational analysis indicated that seed 7b is the most important seed type for prediction. Thus, all the selected training sequences are required to contain seed 7b matching sites. The 131 selected training features were from five major categories as described below:

1. *Seed conservation*. The seed-pairing site in a target 3′-UTR is often conserved across multiple species. This is a main selection filter in almost all existing target prediction algorithms.

Usually, a candidate site is rejected if the site is not conserved across multiple species. In our training process, seed conservation was also considered, but not as a requirement. In this way, we were able to predict both conserved and nonconserved miRNA target binding sites. Transcript 3′-UTR sequences from human gene orthologs in mouse, rat, dog, and chicken were analyzed to identify miRNA seed matches, and the level of seed conservation was recorded as a training feature.

2. *Seed type*. A seed 7b site is also a site for seed 8 if the terminal base is a match. Therefore, terminal base match was recorded as a training feature in our analysis to represent seed 8 sites. The presence of seed 7a is also relevant to miRNA target identification, and thus, the presence of the seed 7a site in a 3′-UTR was recorded as another training feature. In this way, in addition to seed 7b, seed 8 and seed 7a were also considered for data modeling.
3. *Base composition*. Local 3′-UTR regions surrounding the candidate miRNA binding sites were analyzed for their base composition. Compared to unchanged genes, the sites in the downregulated genes had a significantly lower GC content in general. All four base counts were significantly different between candidate sites in the downregulated and unchanged genes, with C as the most underrepresented base in the downregulated gene sites. In addition to the four mononucleotide counts, the frequencies of all 16 dinucleotides were determined and recorded as training features. Base composition at individual positions of the target site was also analyzed. Many of the position-specific base counts were statistically significant, reflecting the overall site requirement for low GC content. However, there were also multiple interesting novel observations that may be related to specific functional requirements. For example, nucleotide C was significantly absent at positions immediately upstream of the miRNA seed binding site in the downregulated genes when compared with the unchanged genes. The absence of C cannot be explained by the low GC content requirement since there was no significant difference in nucleotide G count at the same positions. A typical miRNA/target binding duplex has a loop or bulge structure in this region, and the absence of C might be related to this requirement. Another example is nucleotide A count at positions immediately downstream of the miRNA seed binding site. Although there was no difference in nucleotide T count at these positions, the A count was significantly higher in candidate sites from the downregulated genes. These position-specific nucleotide counts were recorded as SVM training features.

4. *Secondary structure*. A target site is not likely to be functional if it is not accessible to miRNA binding. RNA secondary structure prediction is a challenging task, and in general, the prediction accuracy decreases dramatically as the sequence length increases. In our study, a short length of 25 nucleotides on each side of the seed binding site was included in the structural analysis. Local secondary structure of a candidate site was calculated with RNAfold (9). The propensity for secondary structure formation was measured by the Gibbs free energy change (ΔG) and recorded as a training feature. Besides the overall accessibility of a candidate site, the base-pairing potential of individual nucleotides was also evaluated and significant positions were considered to capture potential position-specific structural effects.

   The secondary structure of the miRNA/target hybridization duplex was calculated to determine the level of nucleotide pairing potential at each position. Nucleotides 13–17 in a miRNA were significantly more likely to match perfectly to candidate sites in the downregulated genes than to those in the unchanged genes. On the other hand, position 10 was more unstructured in the downregulated genes. A typical miRNA binding duplex has a bulge/loop following the seed binding region, which likely results in an exposed base at position 10. These significant base positions were combined to build a training feature to evaluate the overall position-specific base pairing of the binding duplex.

5. *Location in 3′-UTR*. Previous studies suggest that miRNA targeting is related to the target site location as a site in the middle of a long 3′-UTR is less likely to be functional (10, 11). In our analysis, candidate sites from the downregulated genes and unchanged genes were examined to determine whether they were at least 600 or 900 nucleotides away from both ends of the UTRs. In this way, two training features were recorded (target site location >600 or >900 bases).

2.1.3. Construction of Target Prediction Model

Machine learning algorithms are powerful tools for combining training features to achieve optimal predictive accuracy. A machine learning algorithm, which we named MirTarget2, was developed by integrating the sequence training features described above. MirTarget2 was developed based on an SVM framework in which all 131 training features were combined. In this way, nonlinear interactions among these features can be captured and used for model improvement. In addition, MirTarget2 was able to integrate features that were heterogeneous in nature, and both numerical and categorical features were combined and analyzed within a common computational framework.

A score was calculated for each target candidate by the prediction model, MirTarget2. The MirTarget2 score distributions for the downregulated and unchanged genes were compared to evaluate the predictive power of the scoring system (Fig. 1). The score distribution for the unchanged genes was significantly different from that for the downregulated genes. On average, the scores for the unchanged genes were much lower, with a major peak below 20. About 90% of the unchanged genes were correctly classified by calculating the area to the left of the score 50. In contrast, the downregulated genes had a more spread-out score distribution, reflecting the fact that about 50% of the genes had scores higher than 50. Thus, a threshold score 50 was chosen for the maximal separation of the downregulated and unchanged genes.

2.1.4. Evaluation of Algorithm Performance with Independent Data

The performance of MirTarget2 was independently evaluated with our recently published miR-124a time-course microarray data (12). In this microarray experiment, a human miRNA, miR-124a was overexpressed in HepG2 cells, and changes in global expression profiles were evaluated by microarrays at multiple time points. The miR-124a dataset had not been used for model training and thus was used here as independent validation data for model testing. MirTarget2 was compared to three other widely used algorithms, TargetScan (11), PicTar (13), and miRanda (14). In our analysis, the algorithm performance was compared by evaluating the overall prediction performance for identifying miRNA-downregulated genes. Genome-wide target prediction was performed using different algorithms for all the genes

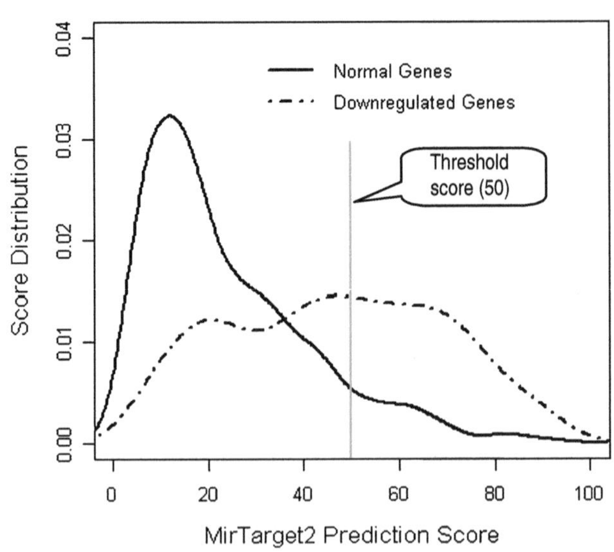

Fig. 1. Target prediction score distributions for the downregulated and unchanged genes. A threshold score of 50 was chosen for the maximal separation of the unchanged and downregulated genes.

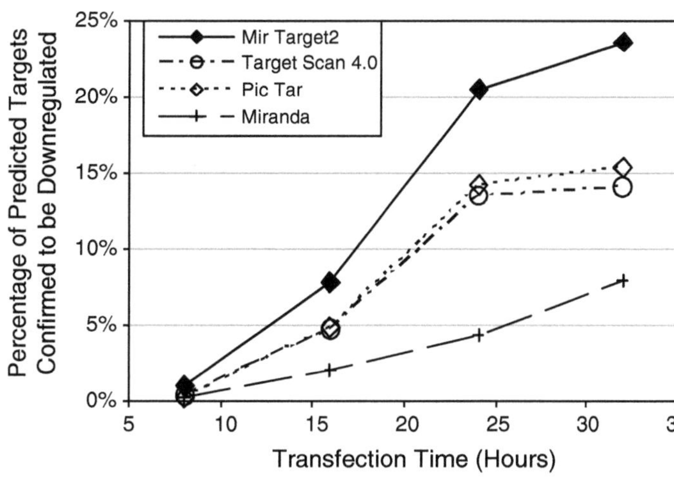

Fig. 2. Performance comparison of four target prediction algorithms using an independent microarray dataset. Four algorithms were compared, MirTarget2, TargetScan, PicTar and miRanda. Gene expression profiles were analyzed at 8, 16, 24 and 32 h after miR-124a overexpression. The figure shows the percentage of predicted mR-124a targets by different algorithms that were confirmed to be downregulated in the microarray experiment.

represented on the microarrays with detectable expression levels. Among these algorithms, MirTarget2 was the most selective one at predicting downregulated genes (Fig. 2). Among all predicted miR-124a targets by MirTarget2, 24% of them were confirmed to be downregulated at 32 h by microarrays. In contrast, the percentages of confirmed predicted targets were much lower from other published algorithms (8–15%). Thus, MirTarget2 had significantly improved performance over prior algorithms.

2.2. miRDB: an Online Database for miRNA Target Prediction

2.2.1. Presentation of Computationally Predicted miRNA Targets

As described in the previous section, we have developed a new computational algorithm for miRNA target prediction (6). To help other miRNA researchers to take advantage of this new algorithm, genome-wide target prediction was performed, and the predicted targets were imported into an online database, miRDB (7). miRDB stores predicted gene targets for miRNAs from five species: human, mouse, rat, dog, and chicken. The detailed statistics is listed in Table 1. As of version 3.0, miRDB contains 2,295 miRNAs targeting 58,953 unique genes. All predicted targets are freely accessible from miRDB using the Web search interface at http://www.mirdb.org. Alternatively, all computational prediction results can be batch downloaded for both the current and previous miRDB versions.

A Web query interface was established to retrieve target prediction results by miRNA name, target GenBank accession, NCBI Gene ID, or gene symbol (Fig. 3a, see Notes 2 and 3). The search

Table 1
miRDB target prediction statistics (version 3.0)

Species	miRNA	Gene target	Unique gene target
Human	703	236,543	16,856
Mouse	570	176,627	17,803
Rat	291	51,836	10,246
Dog	290	29,653	5,427
Chicken	441	64,456	8,621
Total	2,295	559,115	58,953

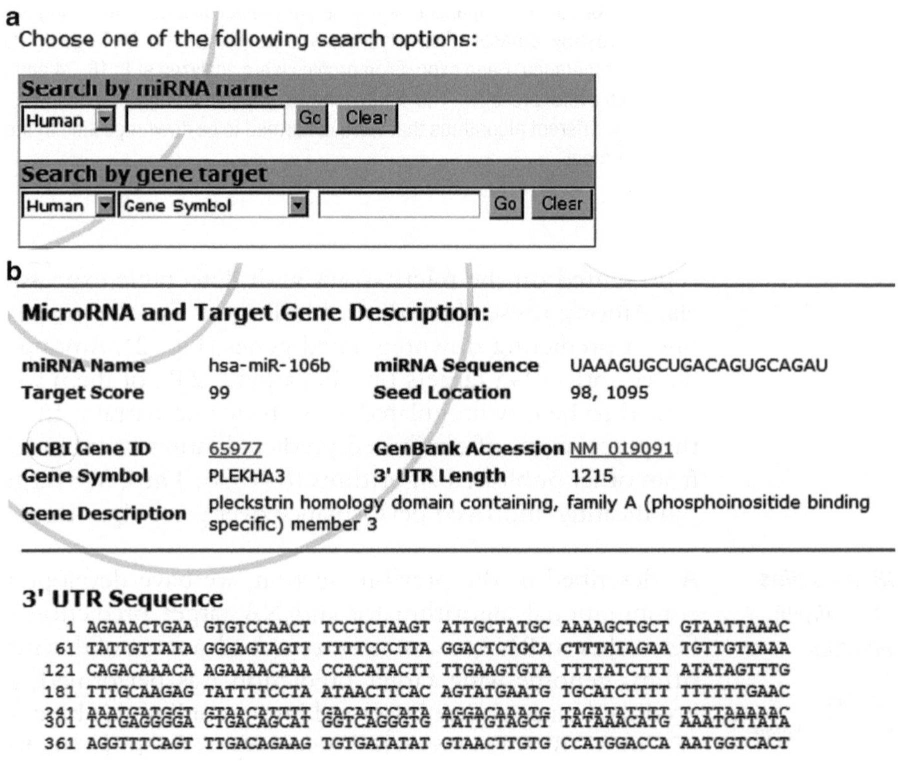

Fig. 3. miRNA target search with the standard query interface in miRDB. (**a**) A screenshot of the Web search interface. (**b**) A screenshot of retrieved target prediction data.

result is sorted by target prediction score, which was calculated by the prediction algorithm. The target score represents the confidence level for target prediction (see Note 4). A screen shot for target search is presented in Fig. 3b. The search result page contains information for both the miRNA and the gene target. In addition, the target seed binding sites in the 3′-UTR are also highlighted.

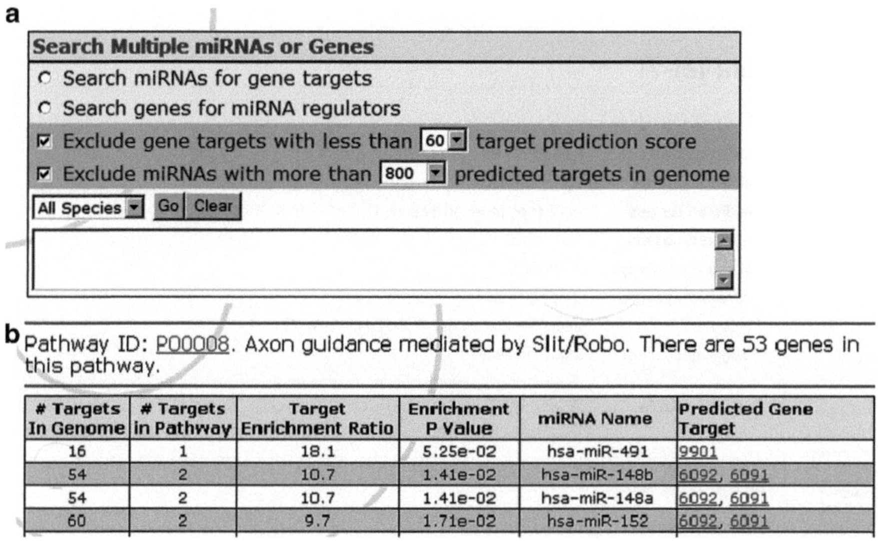

# Targets In Genome	# Targets in Pathway	Target Enrichment Ratio	Enrichment P Value	miRNA Name	Predicted Gene Target
16	1	18.1	5.25e-02	hsa-miR-491	9901
54	2	10.7	1.41e-02	hsa-miR-148b	6092, 6091
54	2	10.7	1.41e-02	hsa-miR-148a	6092, 6091
60	2	9.7	1.71e-02	hsa-miR-152	6092, 6091

Fig. 4. Advanced target search for multiple miRNAs or targets. (**a**) A screenshot of the advance Web search interface. (**b**) A screenshot of retrieved pathway target data.

The simple search interface described above is designed for the analysis of one miRNA or gene target at a time. If a user is interested in analyzing multiple miRNAs or gene targets together, then the target mining search interface should be used (Fig. 4). For example, a user could use this advanced search interface to determine whether a group of related genes in the same biological pathway are targeted by any miRNA (see Note 5). To add more flexibility in target mining, search filters are also available for the exclusion of less interesting miRNAs or gene targets (see Note 6). Besides the query interface for user-provided lists of genes or miRNAs, miRDB also presents target prediction data for precompiled pathways imported from PANTHER (15). Potential miRNA target enrichment in specific pathways was evaluated by identifying miRNAs that were significantly associated with the pathways using the hypergeometric test. In this way, potential links between miRNAs and biological pathways may be discovered.

2.2.2. A miRNA Functional Annotation Catalog

One popular strategy to present functional miRNA data is to organize the annotation data by miRNA precursors. While useful to present miRNA gene information in the genome, this data presentation strategy also creates major challenges for the annotation of miRNA functions (see Note 7). For example, mature miRNA hsa-let-7f has two precursors in the genome, and thus, there would be two separate annotation pages describing hsa-let-7f functions. As a result, database redundancy is inevitable. To address this issue, miRDB adopts a new strategy by focusing on mature miRNAs, which are the carriers of miRNA functions. Functional annotations for one mature miRNA are organized and presented in a single Web

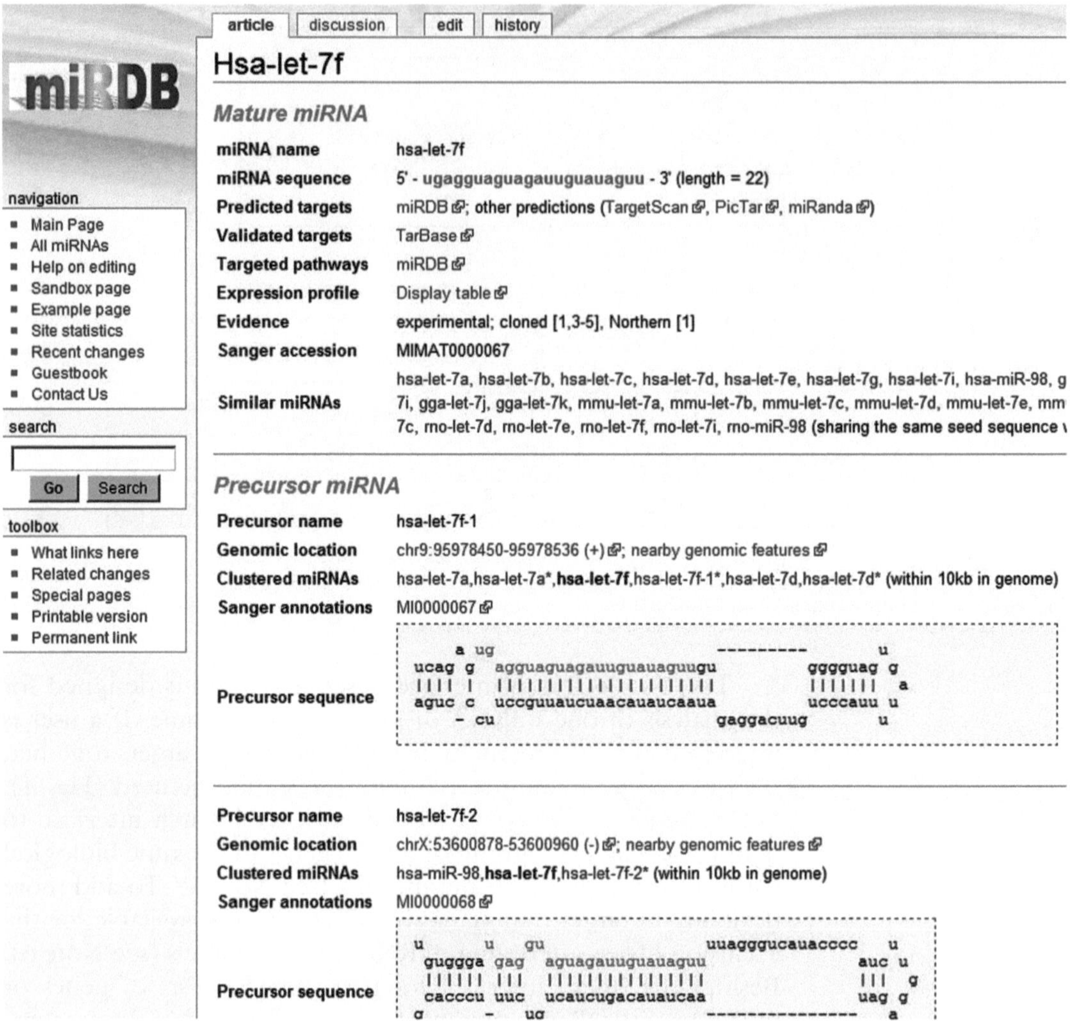

Fig. 5. A screenshot of the miRNA functional annotation page. miRNA hsa-let-7f is presented here as an example.

page. In this way, miRDB provides a centralized view of the functional annotations for individual miRNAs.

A screenshot of a miRNA functional annotation Web page is presented in Fig. 5. The official miRNA names and sequence data were imported from Sanger miRBase (14). In addition, each miRNA annotation page contains dynamic Web links to predicted gene targets and pathway targets stored in miRDB, as well as experimentally validated targets from TarBase (5). The tissue expression profile of a miRNA is presented based on data from recent profiling studies (16). As demonstrated by previous studies, miRNAs sharing the same seed sequence usually target similar sets of genes (2, 8). Thus, these related miRNAs are considered to have similar functions and presented as part of the functional annotations. miRNA precursor information, including precursor name, sequence, and genomic location, is also presented. The secondary structure of the precursor was calculated with RNAfold (9) and then presented in the annotation Web page.

2.2.3. The Wiki Interface of miRDB for User-Provided Annotations

A typical wiki Web server allows anyone with Internet access to make contributions by editing the Web page. Although widely successful in many Web-based projects (one famous example is Wikipedia), the wiki model has been relatively unexplored by the biological research community. As a new attempt for data annotation, we established a wiki interface for miRDB using the MediaWiki package, which is widely used to build wiki applications including Wikipedia. All miRNA annotation pages in miRDB can be edited by anyone via a Web browser. A History tab is associated with each miRNA page for version control of the annotation data, so that undesired changes can be easily rolled back. The wiki functional annotation pages and computational target prediction pages in miRDB are cross-referenced to each other via dynamic Web links to provide an integrated Web-based environment for miRNA functional studies.

3. Notes

1. SVMs are universal constructive machine learning procedures based on statistical learning theory. SVM has been applied in many diverse applications such as pattern recognition, computational biology, and image analysis. The basic concept is that by maximizing the separation between the two classes in a nonlinear mathematically determined feature space, SVM not only reduces the training error but more importantly also achieves better generalization on unseen data.
2. There are two ways to search miRDB for predicted miRNA targets: (a) *Search by miRNA names.* Partial names are allowed. If there is more than one match, all the matched miRNAs will be returned and you may choose from one of those miRNAs to view their predicted targets. If there is only one match, the target prediction result will be presented directly. The partial name search can be useful if you need to do a general search. For example, by typing in "hsa," you will retrieve all human miRNAs with predicted targets; (b) *Search by gene target information.* There are three options to do target search: GenBank Accession, NCBI Gene ID, or Gene Symbol. You have to enter the exact ID or symbol, and no partial match is allowed. In this way, a single gene record will be retrieved if it is predicted to be a miRNA target.

3. Because of the sequence redundancy in GenBank, each gene is usually represented by more than one GenBank record. miRDB uses the NCBI Gene index files to map multiple sequence records to the same gene record. As a result, a different GenBank accession number other than the originally submitted one may be presented. However, both accessions represent the same gene.
4. All the predicted targets have target prediction scores between 50 and 100. These scores are assigned by the prediction tool, MirTarget2. The higher the score, the more confidence we have in this prediction. That is why the search result is ordered by prediction score. In our experience, a predicted target with prediction score >80 is most likely to be real. If the score is below 60, you need to be cautious, and it is recommended to have other independent supporting evidence as well.
5. The Target Mining page provides advanced search options for miRNAs or their gene targets. First, you need to click on one of the radio buttons to choose either miRNA search or gene target search. When searching for miRNA targets, full mature miRNA names are required; when searching for miRNAs, you may provide either NCBI gene IDs or official gene symbols. If symbols are used in the search, you also need to specify the species. Please use spaces or commas to separate the entries.
6. There are two optional check boxes for the exclusion of miRNAs with too many predicted targets or targets with low scores. You may adjust the threshold values to tailor for your needs. The default recommendation is to include targets with scores >60 and miRNAs with <800 targets.
7. Most miRNA functional studies are focused on mature miRNAs since they are the carriers of miRNA functions. For example, most miRNA microarray profiling and real-time PCR assays are designed to detect the expression of mature miRNAs. Thus, it is logical to focus primarily on mature miRNAs when functional annotations are presented.

References

1. Lim LP, Lau NC, Garrett-Engele P, et al. (2005) Microarray analysis shows that some microRNAs downregulate large numbers of target mRNAs. *Nature* **433**:769–73.
2. Lewis BP, Burge CB, Bartel DP. (2005) Conserved seed pairing, often flanked by adenosines, indicates that thousands of human genes are microRNA targets. *Cell* **120**:15–20.
3. Miranda KC, Huynh T, Tay Y, et al. (2006) A pattern-based method for the identification of microRNA binding sites and their corresponding heteroduplexes. *Cell* **126**:1203–17.
4. Rajewsky N. (2006) MicroRNA target predictions in animals. *Nat Genet* **38** Suppl:S8–13.
5. Sethupathy P, Corda B, Hatzigeorgiou AG. (2006) TarBase: a comprehensive database of experimentally supported animal microRNA targets. *RNA* **12**:192–7.
6. Wang X, El Naqa IM. (2008) Prediction of both conserved and nonconserved microRNA targets in animals. *Bioinformatics* **24**:325–32.

7. Wang X. (2008) miRDB: a microRNA target prediction and functional annotation database with a wiki interface. *RNA* **14**:1012–7.
8. Linsley PS, Schelter J, Burchard J, et al. (2007) Transcripts targeted by the microRNA-16 family cooperatively regulate cell cycle progression. *Mol Cell Biol* **27**:2240–52.
9. Hofacker IL. (2003) Vienna RNA secondary structure server. *Nucleic Acids Res* **31**:3429–31.
10. Gaidatzis D, van Nimwegen E, Hausser J, Zavolan M. (2007) Inference of miRNA targets using evolutionary conservation and pathway analysis. *BMC Bioinformatics* **8**:69.
11. Grimson A, Farh KK, Johnston WK, Garrett-Engele P, Lim LP, Bartel DP. (2007) MicroRNA targeting specificity in mammals: determinants beyond seed pairing. *Mol Cell* **27**:91–105.
12. Wang X, Wang X. (2006) Systematic identification of microRNA functions by combining target prediction and expression profiling. *Nucleic Acids Res* **34**:1646–52.
13. Krek A, Grun D, Poy MN, et al. (2005) Combinatorial microRNA target predictions. *Nat Genet* **37**:495–500.
14. Griffiths-Jones S, Grocock RJ, van Dongen S, Bateman A, Enright AJ. (2006) miRBase: microRNA sequences, targets and gene nomenclature. *Nucleic Acids Res* **34**:D140–4.
15. Mi H, Lazareva-Ulitsky B, Loo R, et al. (2005) The PANTHER database of protein families, subfamilies, functions and pathways. *Nucleic Acids Res* **33**:D284–8.
16. Liang Y, Ridzon D, Wong L, Chen C. (2007) Characterization of microRNA expression profiles in normal human tissues. *BMC Genomics* **8**:166.

Chapter 20

Large-Scale Integration of MicroRNA and Gene Expression Data for Identification of Enriched MicroRNA–mRNA Associations in Biological Systems

Preethi H. Gunaratne, Chad J. Creighton, Michael Watson, and Jayantha B. Tennakoon

Abstract

The discovery of microRNAs (miRNAs) revealed a hidden layer of gene regulation that is able to integrate multiple genes into biologically meaningful networks. A number of computational prediction programs have been developed to identify putative miRNA targets. Collectively, the miRNAs that have been discovered so far have the potential to target over 60% of genes in our genome. A minimum of six consecutive nucleotides in the 5′-seed (nucleotides 2–8) in the miRNA must bind through complimentary base pairing to the 3′-untranslated (3′-UTRs) of target genes. Given the small sequence match required, a given miRNA has the potential to target hundreds of genes and a given mRNA can have 0–50 miRNA binding sites. The low-throughput nature of the query design (gene by gene or miRNA by miRNA) and a fairly high rate of false positives and negatives uncovered by the limited number of functional studies remain as the major limitations. Programs that integrate genome-wide gene and miRNA expression data determined by microarray and/or next-generation sequencing (NGS) technologies with the publicly available target prediction algorithms are extremely valuable on two fronts. First, they allow the investigator to fully capitalize on all the data generated to reveal new genes and pathways underlying the biological process under study. Second, these programs allow the investigator to lift a small network of genes they are currently following into a larger network through the integrative properties of miRNAs. In this chapter, we discuss the latest methodologies for determining genome-wide miRNA and gene expression changes and three programs (Sigterms, CORNA, and MMIA) that allow the investigator to generate short lists of enriched miRNA:target mRNA candidates for large-scale miRNA:target mRNA validation. These efforts are essential for determining false positive and negative rates of existing algorithms and refining our knowledge on the rules of miRNA–mRNA relationships.

1. Introduction

MicroRNAs (miRNAs) are small ~22 nucleotide noncoding RNAs that have been predicted to target >60% of the genes in our genome to mediate posttranscription gene silencing (1, 2). The

Silvia Monticelli (ed.), *MicroRNAs and the Immune System: Methods and Protocols*, Methods in Molecular Biology, vol. 667, DOI 10.1007/978-1-60761-811-9_20, © Springer Science+Business Media, LLC 2010

key determinants for miRNA–mRNA target associations lie in the 5′-seed region (nucleotides 2–8) in miRNA and the 3′-untranslated region (3′-UTR) of mRNA targets (2). The miRNA–mRNA target association is catalyzed mainly by the action of Argonaute (Ago) family of proteins in the RNA-induced silencing complex (RISC) (3). Base pairing of at least six consecutive nucleotides within the 5′-seed of the miRNA with the target site on the mRNA is reported to be required at a minimum. However, binding can occur through the entire length of the miRNA. miRNA–mRNA duplexes that form with perfect or near perfect complementarity have been shown to result in mRNA cleavage between nucleotides 10 and 11 (4) of the miRNA resulting ultimately in mRNA cleavage and decay (4, 5). By contrast, when binding occurs through imperfect complementarity, the mRNA target is generally kept intact and silencing occurs through translational repression (6).

With the advent of microarray and next-generation sequencing (NGS) technologies in the postgenome era, it is now possible to determine genome-wide miRNA–mRNA associations that are significant to specific cellular contexts or systems such as the immune system. A number of target prediction algorithms, which are primarily based on searches for matches between miRNA seed sequences and 3′-UTRs of genes, have been developed and freely available (7). Such programs offer users the possibility of quickly searching for potential targets on a miRNA by miRNA basis or potential miRNAs on a gene-by-gene basis. However, these approaches are too cumbersome and do not offer optimal solutions to integrate the glut of microarray (gene and miRNA expression) and sequencing (mRNA-seq and miRNA-seq) data that is becoming available on a daily basis. More recently, several groups have written programs and software packages to address this issue and offer solutions for the large-scale three-way integration of gene expression data, miRNA expression data and miRNA–mRNA target predictions (8). These programs offer the users the possibility of reaping the full benefit of these genome-wide studies. It is becoming increasingly clear that miRNAs are very different from the traditional transcriptional repressors that we are familiar with. Overexpression and loss-of-function studies suggest that most miRNAs have only a limited influence on their target genes (approximately two- to ten-fold repression) on its own. It appears that the main role of miRNAs is to fine-tune gene expression by coordinately downregulating multiple genes within and across pathways to integrate them into meaningful networks in relation to specific cellular states. The question then is what is the impact of global shifts in miRNA profiles on the transcriptome and proteome of a given cellular state. Furthermore, when aiming to assess the role of a given miRNA in relation to a specific biological process, it is essential to consider its impact on all of its targets. Consequently, programs that integrate expression data with target prediction data are vital to understand the role of miRNAs in the immune system. In this chapter, we examine in detail three programs that allow the large-scale integration of genome-wide expression and miRNA target prediction data.

2. Materials

2.1. Gene Expression Data

2.1.1. Microarrays

While classical northern blotting and quantitative real-time PCR continue as techniques used for gene expression studies of single or small sets of genes over the past two decades, high-throughput microarray-based techniques have been increasingly applied in this field to measure several thousands of genes at a time. Microarray technology was first described by Schena et al. in 1995 (9). Over the years, DNA chip based technologies have widely demonstrated the power of this high-throughput parallel synthesis based method. Microarray DNA chips contain thousands of probes arranged on a regular pattern. Microarrays produce quantitative gene expression data based on relative dye intensities corresponding to DNA hybridized to probes immobilized on chips (10). A typical microarray-based experiment consists of preparing a DNA chip based on target DNAs, generating a hybridization solution containing a mixture of fluorescently labeled cDNAs, incubating fluorescently labeled cDNAs with DNA chip followed by data detection based on laser technologies, and finally computer assisted statistical testing and data analysis. To disseminate data analyzed by researchers for public use, microarray data can be stored in NCBI microarray data repository Gene Expression Omnibus (GEO) (http://www.ncbi.nlm.nih.gov/geo) (11) using a standardized framework, termed microarray markup language (MAML).

MAML employs a standard format to describe microarray experiment details, which include experimental design, array design, samples, hybridization procedures and parameters, images, quantitation, and controls.

Several commercial producers have introduced microarrays with different features. The microarrays available in the current market differ from one another in terms of the technologies utilized for fabrication and their probe design architecture. Some of the popularly known commercial manufacturers are given below:

Affymetrix GeneChip (http://www.affymetrix.com). Affymetrix was one of the first microarrays to appear in the market (12). Unlike in the case of traditional microarrays where cloning libraries are used for probe design, Affymetrix employs an in silico light directed synthesizing technology to produce probes on a glass chip (10).

Bypassing management of clone libraries and ability to synthesize highly ordered DNA oligomers in silico are the two distinct advantages of the Affymetrix design.

Agilent (http://www.agilent.com) employs an inkjet-based method to print whole cDNA or oligos on chips (13). Chips produced by Agilent offer 60-mer probes compared to the 25-mer probes offered by Affymetrix (10).

Nimblegen (http://www.nimblegen.com/) (14) uses a digital light processor to synthesize microarrays, apart from their use in transcriptome analysis. NimbleGen chips containing specific sequences are used to capture large genomic fragments, which can be subject to further analysis using Nimblegens GS FLX sequencing system (10).

CombiMatrix (http://www.combimatrix.com) offers custom arrays generated by a powerful computer-directed semiconductor microelectrode based on chip synthesis method, which can be programmed to generate a given array of oligonucleotides on chips (15). Signal detection can be carried out by either laser scanning or electrochemical methods (10).

Illumina bead array (http://www.illumina.com) (16) conventional microarrays are manufactured by spotting oligonucleotides on two-dimensional substrates (17). On the contrary, Illumina bead based arrays are produced by means of random assembly of bead pools on a patterned substrate (17). Illumina's technology offers higher oligo densities on their chips and thus higher throughputs by virtue of the intrinsic size of the beads and patterned substrates compared to conventional chips.

While array-based technologies and applications continue to grow, a plethora of information would be available for researchers through GEO in future. This would be a very valuable tool to facilitate cross-reference samples, identify signatures associated with disease, personalize medicine, and most importantly provide a global view of all biological processes through a platform for systematic in depth analysis of DNA and RNA variation.

2.2. miRNA Expression Data

2.2.1. MicroRNA Microarrays

The overall approach of miRNA profiling through microarrays remains similar to the approach employed in microarrays for gene expression profiling. Mature miRNAs are isolated and purified from tissue or cell samples using classical Trizol-based isolation or commercially available kits. The purified fragment of RNA is enriched and labeled. Array probes are designed by using locked nucleic acid (LNA) or chemically modified oligos and spotted on microarrays. Hybridization is then carried out and signal intensities measured using a laser scanner. Finally, quantification and data analysis is carried out using computer software. Unlike in the case of mRNA arrays designing arrays for miRNAs is challenging in that arrays must be designed to discriminate between the mature miRNAs and their precursors, miRNA microarrays should be capable of detecting subtle differences of even a single-base difference of mature sequences (18). Short sequence length of 18–25 nt of mature sequences and wide range of melting temperatures (T_m) of mature miRNAs are significant problems in miRNA microarray design (19). In spite of the challenges, several miRNA microarrays have been designed and are currently available commercially. Synthetic oligonucleotides or cDNA fragments are used in miRNA microarray probe design. More recently, synthetic oligonucleotides with chemical modifications providing high molecular affinities facilitating hybridization have been employed. AT-rich probes are known to show lesser hybridization affinity compared to GC-rich probes (20). Higher degrees of sensitivity can be achieved by introduction of A/T analogs, which enhance overall duplex stability (21). Substitution of A and T with 2^0-O-methyl-2,6-diaminopurineand2^0-O-methyl-5-methyluridine, respectively, has shown two- to threefold increases in relative hybridization (22). LNAs first described by Wengel and coworkers in 1998 are a novel class of conformationally restricted oligonucleotide analogs, which show high thermal stabilities toward complimentary RNA and DNA (23). Chemically engineered LNAs have nucleotide analogs containing a bridging methylene group between C4′ and O2′ of the ribose ring (24). High thermal stabilities of LNAs bound to complimentary nucleic acid facilitates the design of short probes with excellent mismatch discrimination. Some of the commercially produced miRNA microarrays are discussed next.

2.2.1.1. Agilent miRNA Microarray (http://www.home.agilent.com)

Agilent miRNA microarrays are produced using unique chemically unmodified probes. Chemically unmodified oligos are immobilized on an array platform by means of a short stilt, and to the 5′ end of the anchored oligo a G residue is included and an extended hairpin attached, the 3′ end of the sample miRNAs are labeled by means of a Cy molecule attached to a C residue. When sample is introduced, hybridization takes place and the 5′ G residue of the probe complimentary to the 3′ Cy labeled C residue binds resulting fluorescence. The hairpin functions as a bridge connecting the 5′ end of the anchored oligo and the 3′ end of the hybridized miRNA. Agilent claims that the inclusion of the G residue to 5′ end of the probe increases stability of binding to target miRNA and the hairpin destabilizes probe hybridization to larger nontarget RNAs and hence provides a higher degree of specificity. Agilent's G44071A human miRNA microarray platform uses sequences from Sanger miRNA database (miRBase) version 12 and is capable of detecting unique 866 human and 89 viral miRNAs. Agilent also produces several arrays in the G44 series for human mouse and rat miRNAs, which use different versions of the Sanger database ranging from version 9.1 to 12.0 as the reference source for sequences. In Agilent miRNA arrays, 40–60 mer unmodified oligonucleotides are directly synthesized on the array by Agilent's proprietary SurePrint inkjet technology. A unique feature of Agilent's technology is the use of end labeling instead of conventional polymerase based methods where sample nucleotide damage within the substrate has been an issue. End labeling is insensitive to nucleotide damage and is particularly advantageous when testing preserved or chemically treated samples. Agilent's platform requires only small input amounts in the 100 ng range of total RNA due to the high-yield end labeling method. As the labeling method does not require size fractionation or amplification, undesired bias introduced from these two steps is eliminated (25).

2.2.1.2. Exiqon LNA Microarrays (http://www.exiqon.com)

Exiqon uses melting temperature (T_m) matched LNA probes in their miRNA microarray design. Exiqon's miRNA microarrays are marketed under the name miRCURY LNA™. In addition to probes for miRBase sequences, which the Exiqon system uses as a reference for their microarrays, Exiqon arrays contain probes called mirPLUS™ capture probes, which target proprietary miRNAs that have been defined by Exiqon company through cloning and sequencing of human normal and diseased tissues. Through these proprietary sequence probes, scientists would be able to gain unique information about miRNAs, which have not been defined elsewhere. As of August 2009 in the Exiqon Web site, a typical miRCURY LNA™ was listed as being capable of capturing 854 mature human miRNAs, 80 mature viral miRNAs, and 428 mature Exiqon-defined human mirPLUS™ miRNAs (26).

2.2.1.3. Invitrogen (http://www.invitrogen.com)

Invitrogen offers the NCode™ Human miRNA Microarray Kit V3 and NCode™ Multi-Species miRNA Microarray Kit V2 as integrated miRNA profiling systems, which include reagents for RNA isolation labeling and array hybridization. As of the date of writing this chapter (30 August 2009), it was listed in the Invitrogen Web site that the Human miRNA Microarray Kit V3 contains probe sequences targeting nearly all of the known human miRNAs in the Sanger miRBase as well as probe sequences for 373 novel putative miRNAs. The Multi-Species version was listed as having probes for the Sanger miRBase Sequence Database, Release 9.0, for human, mouse, rat, *Drosophila melanogaster*, *Caenorhabditis elegans*, and Zebrafish. Each NCode™ microarray slide comes fully blocked and ready to use. In case where starting material has concentrations <500 ng total RNA or equivalent cells/tissue, Invitrogen provides a miRNA amplification kit called the NCode™ miRNA amplification system. Once the total RNA is extracted and ready for hybridization, labeling can be carried out using an NCode™. Rapid miRNA labeling system, which is based on a poly-A tailing reaction on RNA molecules followed by ligation of dye labeled Alexa Flour™ DNA polymer by means of an oligoDT bridge. Invitrogen offers the choices of employing either preprinted or self-printed microarrays using NCode™ Human or multispecies microarray probes for experiments. Analysis of results can be performed by means of NCode™ profiler software. Invitrogen also provides a range of reagents under the NCode™ name for verification and further analysis of results by qPCR (27).

2.2.1.4. LC Sciences (http://www.lcsciences.com)

With the LC Sciences µParaFlo microfluidic miRNA Microarray chips assays can be performed with a minimum of 5 µg total RNA (28). The mirVana Isolation Kit (Ambion) is recommended. The small RNA (<300 nt) fraction is size fractionated with YM-100 Microcon Centrifugal Filter Device (Millipore) and 3′-extended with a poly-A tail by poly-A polymerase. An oligonucleotide tag is ligated to the poly-A tail for subsequent fluorescent dye staining. This platform allows dual labeling using Cy5 and Cy3 tags to label two RNA samples to be compared in dual-sample experiments. Hybridization is performed overnight on a µParaFlo microfluidic chip using a microcirculation pump (Atactic Technologies). On the microfluidic chip, each detection probe consists of a chemically modified nucleotide "coding" segment complementary to target miRNA (from miRBase, http://microrna.sanger.ac.uk/sequences/) or other RNA (control or customer defined sequences) and a spacer segment of polyethylene glycol to extend the "coding" segment away from the substrate surface. The detection probes are synthesized in situ with photogenerated reagent (PGR) chemistry on a Digital Light Projector (Texas Instruments) based synthesis system (29). Flexible DNA chip synthesis is gated by deprotection using solution photogenerated acids. The hybridization melting temperatures are balanced by adjusting length and chemical modifications of the detection probes (29). Hybridization is carried out in 100 µL 6× SSPE buffer (0.90 M NaCl, 60 mM Na_2HPO_4, 6 mM EDTA, pH 6.8) containing 25% formamide at 34°C followed by a stringent wash at 52°C. Hybridization images are collected with a laser scanner (GenePix 4000B, Molecular Device) and signal intensity values extracted using ArrayPro image processing software (MediaCybernetics). Data analysis is carried out by first subtracting the background and then normalizing with a cyclic LOWESS filter (locally weighted regression). For two-color experiments, the ratio of two sets of detected signals ($\log_2$ transformed and balanced) and *p*-values of the *t*-test are calculated; a *p*-value of less than 0.01 is used to select significantly differentially detected signal. Data classification is accomplished by hierarchical clustering based on average linkage and Euclidean distance metric, and visualized with TIGR's Multiple Experimental Viewer (MeV) (30).

Quantile normalization on the channel values is used to normalize two-color data within each chip to make single channel values within and between arrays more comparable and to improve the multiarray data analysis. The single channel normalized values are used in subsequent data analysis. Construction of a dendrogram on the single channel values, both before and after normalization, is recommended to examine the effect of normalization on the treatment differences.

2.2.2. mRNA-seq: Next-Generation Sequencing

Completion of the human reference genome by the international human genome sequencing consortium and US-based Celera genomics was a cornerstone of human scientific endeavor. This achievement clearly paved way for a new exciting era of scientific research. The human genome sequencing project commenced in the year 1990; by 2000 a draft version of the human genome was made available and a completed version was released in the year 2003. During the human genome sequencing project era, the two widely used technologies were the original enzymatic dideoxy sequencing method pioneered by Fred Sanger and colleagues (31) and the Maxam and Gilbert method, which was described during the same year (32). The chemical degradation based Maxam and Gilbert method was particularly used in cases that were not easily resolved by the popular Sanger technique (33). As the human genome project progressed, the need for fast automated sequencers became imminent and companies with commercial interests were quick to step in to make improvements to the Sanger-based technique. In spite of the advances made in the Sanger technique through introduction of automated capillary sequencers, particularly the sample preparation steps, which involved cloning of sequences into bacterial artificial chromosomes (BACs) or yeast artificial chromosomes (YACs) and artifacts related to sample preparation remained obstacles of making Sanger-based sequencing a completely automatable high-throughput method. In view of this fact, several companies came up with novel sequencing technologies, which had massively parallel high-throughput capabilities enabling genome-scale analysis in a relatively short period of time. These sequencing technologies are termed NGS technologies. As of today, three platforms, namely Roche Applied Science 454 platform, the Illumina platform, and Applied Biosystems ABI SOLiD system are widely used in research laboratories. More recently, the Helicos single-molecule sequencing device, HeliScope was released to the market. A brief description of the 454, Illumina and SOLiD systems are given in the following paragraphs.

2.2.2.1. The 454 GenomeSequencer FLX Instrument (Roche Applied Science) (http://www.454.com/)

The 454 FLX pyrosequencer, which was released in 2004, was the first to be introduced to the market as an NGS (34). In pyrosequencing, each time a nucleotide gets incorporated to the nucleotide chain through a polymerizing reaction, pyrophosphate is released, and the released pyrophosphate leads to a series of downstream events, which results in the production of firefly luciferase (35). In the 454 system, DNA fragments are ligated with special adapters. One of the adapters facilitates binding of the DNA molecule to a bead. Beads containing single DNA fragments are subject to emulsion PCR and followed by a denaturation step. Initial amplification of sample DNA is necessary to generate sufficient signal strength in the sequence by synthesis step, which is subsequently carried out on beads containing copies of a given fragment immobilized on an optical fiber chip. In the 454 setup, each bead with its amplified fragment is individually addressable by a CCD camera at the fluorescence detection stage. In the sequence by synthesis stage, polymerase enzyme, primers, and a given labeled nucleotide of known identity are provided to each bead at a time, and the resultant fluorescence due to the pyrosequencing reaction is measured via the optical fibers equipped to a smart camera. By introducing labeled nucleotides of a given kind at each subsequent cycle of the polymerizing reaction, the nucleotides being incorporated to the growing fragment in each cycle can be detected by fluorescence measurement, and the sequence of each fragment can be decoded and assembled using sophisticated computer software. The 454 system is capable of detecting sequences in the 400–500 bp range and generates around 100 MB of data in a single run. A newer improved version of the 454 FLX called Titanium would provide a data output of around 500 MB. High costs of operation and generally low reading accuracy in homopolar stretches have been cited as drawbacks of the 454 system (33).

2.2.2.2. The Illumina (Solexa) Genome Analyzer (http://www.illumina.com/)

The Solexa sequencers were first introduced to the market in the year 2006 (36) and Illumina acquired Solexa in the year 2007 (33). The Solexa system is based on sequencing by synthesis method, which uses a technology called "Reversible termination". The basic workflow of the Illumina platform involves five main stages. The initial step involves randomly fragmenting DNA and ligating adaptors to random fragments. The second step involves attaching DNA to a special glass slide and is followed by a third step, where solid-phase bridge amplification is carried out using unlabelled nucleotides. The fourth step involves denaturing amplified double-stranded DNA on the slide, and finally the fifth step involves carrying out a PCR using labeled nucleotides and photographing.

Unlike in the case of the 454 instrument where a single variety of nucleotide is incorporated in each cycle of the fluorescence generating polymerizing step, the Illumina instrument introduces all four labeled nucleotides to the polymerizing reaction at once. However, due to a chemical modification of the nucleotides, each time a nucleotide gets incorporated into the growing DNA chain termination of polymerization occurs. At this stage, a smart CCD camera photographs fluorescence signals resulting from nucleotides, which got incorporated to each individually addressable amplified cluster of DNA fragments, which are generated at the bridge amplification stage. Once photographing of all clusters is completed, termination is reversed and another set of nucleotides are introduced, and once incorporation takes place, the reaction is terminated and clusters are photographed. Eventually all photographic data are analyzed and the sequences are assembled using computer software. The sequence read length achieved by this technology is around 35 bp, and an advantage of this system is its ability to generate huge amounts of data in a single run. The Illumina GA2 sequencers released in 2008 had the ability to generate around 1.5 GB of data in a single read setup and around 3.0 GB of data using a paired run. The ability of the instrument to generate massive amounts of data having short sequence lengths has made this instrument particularly well suited for small RNA based research, which generally does not demand long sequence reads. With various modifications in sample preparation and the use of different reagents, the Illumina platform can be used in a versatile fashion for ChipSeq and Bisulfite sequencing experiments as well.

2.2.2.3. The Applied Biosystems ABI SOLiD System (http://www3.appliedbiosystems.com/)

In contrast to the polymerase reactions used in 454 and Illumina methods, the Applied Biosystems SOLiD technology uses a ligation-based reaction to incorporate fluorescent-labeled nucleotides in the sequencing step (37). However, the Solid system shares similarities with 454 and Illumina as it utilizes an adapter ligated library and emulsion PCR on magnetic beads at the sample preparation stages. The overall work flow of the solid system can be summarized as follows. Initially, an emulsion PCR step is carried out on adapter ligated DNA fragments anchored to magnetic beads to provide sufficient fluorescence intensities during the detection step. The magnetic beads containing the amplified fragments are then transferred to a flow cell slide where a ligation reaction is carried out. The ligation reaction uses a primer, which attaches to the 5 prime end of the adaptor that immobilizes DNA fragments on the magnetic bead. DNA ligase and specific 8 mers whose fourth and fifth bases are specifically encoded with attached fluorescent labels are introduced to the reaction. Fluorescent detection is followed after each extending ligation step. After ligation and detection, a regeneration step in which the 8 mers including the fluorescent labels are removed is carried out and a primer corresponding to a single base displacement (n–1) from the 3′ end of the adapter attaching the DNA fragment is introduced, and the ligation cycle is followed while the two encoded bases are read. Similar cycles are carried out starting with primers, which correspond to *n*–2, *n*–3, *n*–4, and *n*–5. In each cycle, the encoded two bases are interrogated and data stored. Finally, when all rounds of ligation have been completed, a computer builds the sequence by decoding the stored data as two base pair calls. A distinct advantage of this system is the use of two base pair encoding. As a result of two base pair encoding, it is possible to discriminate between base calling errors, true polymorphisms and single base deletions of the sequence by alignment against a high quality reference. The sequence length in the solid systems is defined in between 25 and 35 by the user. A sequencing run in a SOLiD system can yield 2–4 GB of DNA sequence data (35).

Information regarding the HeliScope instrument is available at http://www.helicosbio.com/ (38). There are also several other companies, which are in the process of manufacturing single-molecule based powerful sequencers employing *state-of-the-art* technologies. The following links provide information regarding these systems, which are either in the developmental phase or are ready to step into the market: VisiGen Biotechnologies (http://visigenbio.com/) (39), Pacific Biosciences (http://www.pacificbiosciences.com/index.php) (40), Sequenom (http://www.sequenom.com) (41), Oxford Nanopore Technologies, UK (http://www.nanoporetech.com/) (42), BioNanomatrix (http://bionanomatrix.com/) (43), and Complete Genomics company (http://www.completegenomics.com/) (44).

2.2.2.4. Small RNA Sequencing

The small RNA fraction is prepared for Illumina sequencing by the ligation of 5′ and 3′ RNA adapters according to Illumina's small RNA protocol, which can be found in the link http://www.illumina.com/downloads/rnaDGESmallRNA_Datasheet.pdf (45). Illumina's small RNA adaptors are ligated to the 5′ and 3′ ends of size selected <30 nt RNA. Adapter-modified DNA fragments will be enriched by PCR and further gel purified prior to sequencing. Small RNA sequencing for each sample is then performed using the Illumina Genome Analyzer (GA-2) according to the manufacturer's small RNA protocol. Typically, this protocol results in over 5–10 million small RNA sequence reads per sample per lane.

2.2.2.5. Bioinformatics Platform for Analyzing Small RNA Sequence Reads

A number of high-throughput computational pipeline have been developed for analyzing small RNA sequence reads generated by NGS technologies including Illumina sequencing (46). Our pipeline is described in (46, 47). For each sample, all unique sequence reads with a minimum read count of 10 are aligned to a reference set of miRNAs. The reference set is adaptable and currently consists of the 678 human and 472 mouse mature miRNA sequences found in the miRNA database (miRBase version 11.0) plus 227 miRNA predictions from Berezikov et al. (48). It has been observed that the flexibility of DICER processing of the precursor miRNA produces a variety of sequence fragments, which may be active (49). To account for this, we perform a local Smith–Waterman alignment of each unique sequence read against each of the mature miRNAs in the reference, allowing for a 3-base overhang on the 5′ end and a 6-base overhang on the 3′ end. The alignments are scored such that a matching or overhanging base counts as two points and mismatches as –1. Each unique sequence read, which achieves a per-base alignment score of 2 (i.e., a perfect match) is associated with each mature miRNA for which it achieved that score. The read counts of all redundantly aligning reads are equally apportioned to all mature miRNAs to which they align.

2.2.2.6. Identification of Novel MicroRNAs

Each specimen is expected to generate multiple sequences that are not sufficiently similar to any known human miRNA. For this purpose, a number of algorithms have been developed to evaluate the likelihood that the unique sequence that does not align with a known miRNA is a putative novel miRNA. Our novel miRNA discovery pipeline is described in Creighton et al. (8, 47). First, all small RNA sequences that do not align with known miRNA precursors are mapped to the reference genome sequence of the species the small RNA is derived from (i.e., human, mouse, etc.). Each exact sequence match is fetched along with 100 bases flanking either side. These ~220-bp sequences are then tested for miRNA-like hairpin structure. The ~220-bp putative precursor sequences are evaluated with the Vienna package (www.tbi.univie.ac.at/RNA/) (50). Each of the unique sequences that map to a larger hairpin structures is tested for the Ambros criteria, which states that "authentic" miRNA sequences must map to one arm of a single-loop hairpin with a minimum free energy less than –25 kcal/mol (51, 52). Hairpins with overly large or unbalanced loops and unique sequences that map to the loop of the hairpin are rejected: After folding the read plus flanking sequence, the sequence is trimmed down to include only the plausible precursor and then folded again to ensure that the precursor was not artificially stabilized by neighboring sequence. Sequences appropriately placed in miRNA-like hairpins are considered to be "putative mature miRNAs" (pmms). Strong conservation of the mature miRNA, significant (but possibly weaker) conservation of the hairpin arm opposite the mature miRNA, and little or no conservation of the hairpin loop are considered a positive sign. Poorly conserved sequences are also considered since not all known miRNAs are conserved. If both the mature miRNA sequence and the miRNA-star sequence are found among the sequences, this candidate is considered a definitive confirmed novel miRNA. If there is a substantial difference in abundance, the more abundant form is defined to be the mature miRNA and the less abundant form the miRNA-star sequence.

2.3. miRNA Target Prediction Programs

miRNA:mRNA target predictions for a number of different species are now available in public Web sites. We recommend the PicTar algorithm (http://pictar.bio.nyu.edu) (53), which uses predictions from Krek et al. (54); TargetScan algorithm (http://www.targetscan.org) (55), which uses predictions from Lewis et al. (56); and the miRanda algorithm (http://www.microrna.org) (57). The Sigterms software currently uses all three algorithms, and CORNA software is adapted for miRanda predictions (58).

Currently available algorithms are diverse, both in approach and in performance and all have room for improvement (7). A comparative description of some of the better known algorithms and their features are given below.

2.3.1. TargetScan (http://www.targetscan.org/)

TargetScan provides target predictions for mammalian/vertebrates offering predictions with site conservation consideration as well as without site conservation consideration (55). In predicting targets, the algorithm takes into account parameters such as stringent seed pairing, site number and factors influencing site accessibility. In the mode where site conservation is taken into account, there is an option to rank by preferential conservation instead of site context (7).

2.3.2. PicTar (http://pictar.mdc-berlin.de/)

PicTar provides target predictions for a wider variety of clades including mammalian/vertebrate, fly, and worm (53). The factors taken into consideration in this algorithm are stringent seed pairing for at least one of the sites of the miRNA, site number, and overall pairing stability (59). PicTar takes into consideration site conservation for all cases and does not offer a feature where target predictions can be done without taking conservation into account (7).

2.3.3. miRanda (http://www.microrna.org)

The miRanda algorithm is capable of making miRNA target predictions for mammal/vertebrate, fly, worm as well as additional species (56). In its criteria for target prediction, the algorithm takes into account site number, pairing to most of the miRNA, and moderately stringent seed paring (60).

2.3.4. PITA (http://genie.weizmann.ac.il/pubs/mir07/mir07_prediction.html)

The PITA algorithm is capable of predicting miRNA–mRNA targets for mammalian/vertebrate, fly, and worm clades with site conservation consideration as well as without site conservation consideration (61). In its model for target predictions, PITA uses predicted site accessibility and stability as well as moderately stringent base paring and the number of sites (62).

3. Methods

Methods and software for integrating gene expression results with miRNA expression can help to maximally assess the role of miRNAs as integrators of genes into biologically meaningful networks. This is based on the fact that a given miRNA typically has predicted target sites in the 3′-UTRs of hundreds of genes and a given mRNA has multiple binding sites for several different miRNAs. In addition, genes that belong to specific pathways or networks are coordinately regulated. For all these reasons, it is essential that miRNA–mRNA association analyses are dealt with in the context of genome-wide changes in transcripts. The ultimate aim is to determine predicted miRNA–mRNA pairs that are correlated in expression in the context of a specific experiment. These could be the genes which are significantly differentially expressed when comparing two different biological states or genes that remain correlated in a treatment time course.

Current insight suggests that miRNAs exert their biologic effects by posttranscriptionally targeting gene expression; it follows that low expression of a given miRNA in a given system should conceivably cause a concomitant reversal of expression patterns for in silico predicted gene targets. Given this, we could define a miRNA–mRNA *functional* pair as consisting of a miRNA being predicted to interact with a given mRNA, where the two are also anticorrelated with each other in terms of expression. Public gene targeting prediction databases usually provide Web interface, where the user can look up predicted miRNA–mRNA functional pairs for a specific miRNA or gene of interest. In cases where the number of genes of interest (e.g., a set of genes arising from an expression profiling experiment) is in the hundreds, a gene-by-gene approach to looking up miRNA–mRNA pairs becomes impractical. Below we describe public software tools designed to make the task of integrating lists of genes and miRNAs easier.

3.1. CORNA (http://corna.sf.net)

CORNA (63) is an open-source package for the free statistical software R (http://www.r-project.org) (64) and allows scientists to analyze gene lists in the context of miRNA target predictions. In particular, when a list of genes and a list of miRNA target predictions are given, CORNA will carry out enrichment analysis to determine whether the gene list is enriched for particular miRNA targets more than that can be expected by chance. For example, the input gene list can come from a significant gene list from a microarray experiment or a biological pathway. Further methods within CORNA exist to test for significant associations between miRNAs, pathways, and gene ontology (GO) terms and to display quantitative data associated with miRNA targets. CORNA employs three complementary statistical methods for enrichments analysis of relationships within lists of genes: the HyperGeometric test, Fisher's exact test, and the χ^2-test. Central to the flow of information through CORNA is the gene list, from which the user may test for significant miRNA target associations. The user may also start with a miRNA, find genes that are targeted by that miRNA, and then test that gene list for enrichment of KEGG pathways or GO terms. The user may also plot quantitative data associated with the targets of a particular miRNA. CORNA exclusively uses R vectors and data frames and includes functions for reading miRNA target data directly from miRBase (65) and microRNA.org (60). There are also helper functions to read gene and GO term data using biomaRt (66); microarray data directly from GEO (67); and pathway data directly from KEGG (68). A comprehensive tutorial exists at http://corna.sf.net.

3.2. Sigterms (http://sigterms.sourceforge.net)

Like CORNA, the Sigterms package allows the user to obtain miRNA–mRNA relationships for an entire set of genes (69). While CORNA runs with R, Sigterms consists of a set of Excel macros. The user enters a set of selected genes into an Excel "Annotation" workbook, which represents the entire set of genes on the gene profiling platform. The Annotation workbook can contain miRNA target predictions from one of the three commonly used algorithms (TargetScan, PicTar, and miRanda), as well GO annotation or other pathway information. Annotation workbooks for a given gene array platform representing human or mouse genes can be found at http://sigterms.sourceforge.net.

The user-provided list of genes is first entered into a Microsoft Excel document. The software will then look up the genes in the Annotation workbook to retrieve all miRNA–mRNA pairs for the given algorithm. For each miRNA, Sigterms computes an enrichment statistic that determines if the set of genes that are differentially expressed in the context of an experiment have binding sites more than expected by chance for that particular miRNA. Sigterms outputs the entire set of miRNA–mRNA pairs into an Excel worksheet; the user can then filter this worksheet for the *miRNAs* of interest (e.g., those miRNAs that are anticorrelated in expression with the genes). For computing the one-sided Fisher's exact tests for enrichment of a set of targets for a particular miRNA within the set of genes, the reference gene set determined by the complete probe set on a given array is used. To account for multiple testing of miRNAs, Monte Carlo simulation testing is performed using a 100 randomly generated gene sets. For a given gene set and a given target prediction database, the number of miRNAs having a nominal significant p-value ($p < 0.05$) for target enrichment is computed for each of the 100 random tests. To calculate FDR, the average number of miRNA associations less than or equal to the given nominal p-value for the 100 random tests is used. The ultimate goal is to identify predicted targets within the gene set, that are enriched or overrepresented, which could help to implicate roles for specific miRNAs and miRNA-regulated genes in the system under study.

3.3. MMIA (http://129.79.233.81/~MMIA/mmia_main.html)

MMIA (which stands for "MicroRNA and mRNA integrated analysis") is a Web-based application meant to provide a "one-stop" combined analysis of the miRNA/mRNA input data for various pathway-associated gene sets (70). The user inputs mRNA expression data as a tab-delimited text file along with either a miRNA expression data table or a list of top expressed miRNAs. Given the user-defined statistical cutoff values, MMIA defines the differentially expressed genes and miRNAs from the data. Using miRNA prediction algorithms (TargetScan, PITA, and PicTar), MMIA then matches the upregulated or overexpressed genes with the downregulated or underexpressed miRNAs, and vice versa. MMIA can also generate heat maps of the data and search mRNA–miRNA pairs for pathway-related gene set enrichment. The MMIA software offers a convenient way for users to upload and analyze their data, though less flexible in how the analysis is carried out, as compared to CORNA or Sigterms.

Programs such as CORNA, Sigterms, and MMIA provide investigators without substantial bioinformatics support means by which they could make optimal use of their gene and miRNA expression data. The aim is to generate a list of miRNA–mRNA associations that are significantly correlated in the experiment of interest. The goal is to provide short lists of miRNA–mRNA pairs to be validated by direct biochemical assays, which establish that the miRNA–mRNA pair occurs in a duplex and coimmunoprecipitates in Argonaute complexes (71) and functional assays that demonstrate that the 3′-UTR of the mRNA is responsive to the cognate miRNA in luciferase or GFP reporter systems (72).

Acknowledgments

PHG and JBT are supported by a 1 R01 HL095382-01 grant. The authors would like to thank Gayani Rajapakse, Ana Hernandez, and Rajib Ghosh at University of Houston, Department of Biology and Biochemistry for their assistance in preparing this manuscript.

References

1. Freidman, R.C., Farh, K.K., Burge, C.B., and Bartel, D. (2009) Most mammalian mRNAs are conserved targets of microRNAs. *Genome Res* **19**, 92–105.
2. Bartel, D.P. (2004) MicroRNAs: genomics, biogenesis, mechanisms, and function. *Cell* **116**(2), 281–97.
3. Meister, G., Landthaler, M., Patkaniowska, A., Dorsett, Y., Teng, G., and Tuschl, T. (2004) Human Argonaute 2 mediates RNA cleavage targeted by miRNAs and siRNAs. *Mol Cell* **15**, 185–97.
4. Elbashir, S.M., Martinez, J., Patkaniowska, A., Lendeckel, W., and Tuschl, T. (2001) Functional anatomy of siRNAs for mediating efficient RNAi in *Drosophila melanogaster* embryo lysate. *EMBO* **20**(23), 6877–88.
5. Song, J.J., Smith, S.K., Hannon, G.J., and Joshua-Tor, L. (2004). Crystal structure of Argonaute and its implications for RISC slicer activity. *Science* **305**, 1434–7.
6. Olsen, P. H. and Ambros, V. (1999). The lin-4 regulatory RNA controls developmental timing in *Caenorhabditis elegans* by blocking LIN-14 protein synthesis after the initiation of translation. *Dev Biol* **216**, 671–80.
7. Bartel, D.P. (2009) MicroRNAs: target recognition and regulatory functions. *Cell* **136**(2), 215–33. Review.
8. Creighton, C.J., Reid, J.G., and Gunaratne, P.H. (2009) Expression profiling of microRNAs by deep sequencing. *Brief Bioinform* **10**(5), 490–97.
9. Schena, M., Shalon, D., Davis, R.W., and Brown, P.O. (1995) Quantitative monitoring of gene expression patterns with a complementary DNA microarray. *Science* **270**, 467–70.
10. Pariset, L., Chillemi, G., Bongiorni, S., Spica, V.R., and Valentini, A. (2009) Microarrays and high-throughput transcriptomic analysis in species with incomplete availability of genomic sequences. *N Biotechnol* **25**(5), 272–9.
11. NCBI microarray data repository Gene Expression Omnibus (Geo), Accessed on August 26, 2009 at http://www.ncbi.nlm.nih.gov/geo/.
12. Affymetrix GeneChip, Accessed on August 27, 2009 at http://www.affymetrix.com.
13. Agilent chip, Accessed on August 31, 2007 at http://www.agilent.com.
14. Nimblegen, Accessed on August 28, 2009 at http://www.nimblegen.com/.
15. CombiMatrix, Accessed on August 28, 2009 at http://www.combimatrix.com.
16. Illumina bead array, Accessed on August 27, 2009 at http://www.illumina.com.
17. Fan, J.B., Oliphant, A., Shen, R. et al. (2003) Highly parallel SNP genotyping. *Cold Spring Harb Symp Quant Biol* **68**, 69–78.
18. Shingara, J., Keiger, K., Shelton, J. et al. (2005) An optimized isolation and labeling platform for accurate microRNA expression profiling. *RNA* **11**, 1461–70.
19. Yin, J.Q., Zhao, R.C., and Morris, K.V. (2008) Profiling microRNA expression with microarrays. *Trends Biotechnol* **26**(2), 70–6.
20. Lockhart, D.J., Brown, E.L., Wong, G.G., Chee, M.S., and Gingeras, T.R. (1996) Expression monitoring by hybridization to high-density oligonucleotide arrays. *Nat Biotechnol* **14**, 1675–80.
21. Prosnyak, M.I., Veselovskaya, S.I., Myasnikov, V.A. et al. (1994) Substitution of 2-aminoadenine and 5-methylcytosine for adenine and cytosine in hybridization probes increases the sensitivity of DNA fingerprinting. *Genomics* **21**, 490–94.
22. Rampal, J.B., ed. (2001) DNA arrays: methods and protocols. In *Methods in Molecular Biology*, Vol. 170. Humana Press, Totowa.
23. Kumar, P., Singh, S.K., Koshkin, A.A., Rajwanshi, V.K., Meldgaard, M., and Wengel, J. (1998) The first analogues of LNA (locked nucleic acids): phosphorothioate-LNA and 2′-thio-LNA. *Bioorg Med Chem Lett* **8**(16), 2219–22.
24. Arora, A., Kaur, H., Wenger, J., and Maiti, S. (2008) Effect of locked nucleic acid (LNA) modification on hybridization kinetics of DNA duplex. *Nucleic Acids Symp Ser* **52**, 417–18.
25. Agilent human, mouse, and rat miRNA microarrays product note. Agilent Technologies, Accessed on August 27, 2009 at http://www.home.agilent.com.
26. Exiqon LNA microarrays, Accessed on August 29, 2009 at http://www.exiqon.com.
27. Invitrogen, Accessed on August 28, 2009 at http://www.invitrogen.com.
28. LC Sciences, Accessed on August 30, 2009 at http://www.lcsciences.com.
29. Gao, X., Le Proust, E., Zhang, H. et al. (2001) Flexible DNA chip synthesis gated by deprotection using solution photogenerated acids. *Nucleic Acids Res* **29**, 4744–50.

30. The institute for genomic research, Accessed on August 29, 2004 at http://www.tigr.org/.
31. Sanger, F., NIcklen, S., and Coulson, S. (1977) DNA sequencing with chain-terminating inhibitors. *Proc Natl Acad Sci U S A* **74**, 5463–67.
32. Maxam, A.M. and Gilbert, W. (1977) A new method for sequencing DNA. *Proc Natl Acad Sci U S A* **74**, 560–4.
33. Ansorge, W.J. (2009) Next-generation DNA sequencing techniques. *N Biotechnol* **25**(4), 195–203. Review.
34. The 454 genome sequencer FLX instrument (Roche Applied Science), Accessed on August 28, 2009 at http://www.454.com/.
35. Mardis, E.R. (2008) Next-generation DNA sequencing. *Annu Rev Genomics Hum Genet* **8**, 387–402.
36. The Illumina (Solexa) Genome Analyzer, Accessed on August 30, 2009 at http://www.illumina.com/.
37. The Applied Biosystems ABI SOLiD system, Accessed on August 30, 2009 at http://www3.appliedbiosystems.com/.
38. Helicos Biosciences Corporation, Accessed on August 28, 2009 at http://www.helicosbio.com/.
39. Visigen Biotechnologies Inc, Accessed on August 30, 2009 at http://visigenbio.com/.
40. Pacific Biosciences, Accessed on August 28, 2009 at http://www.pacificbiosciences.com/index.php.
41. Sequenom Inc, Accessed on August 28, 2009 at http://www.sequenom.com.
42. Oxford Nanopore Technologies, UK, Accessed on August 28, 2009 at http://www.nanoporetech.com/.
43. BioNanomatrix, Accessed on August 28, 2009 at http://bionanomatrix.com/.
44. Complete Genomics company, Accessed on August 28, 2009 at http://www.completegenomics.com/.
45. Illumina Inc, Accessed on August 28, 2009 at http://www.illumina.com/downloads/rnaDGESmallRNA_Datasheet.pdf.
46. Reid, J.G., Nagaraja, A.K., Lynn, F.C. et al. (2008) Mouse let-7 miRNA populations exhibit RNA editing that is constrained in the 5′-seed/cleavage/anchor regions and stabilize predicted mmu-let-7a:mRNA duplexes. *Genome Res* **18**(10), 1571–81.
47. Creighton, C.J., Nagaraja, A.K., Hanash, S.M., Matzuk, M.M., and Gunaratne, P.H. (2008) A bioinformatics tool for linking gene expression profiling results with public databases of microRNA target predictions. *RNA* **14**(11), 2290–6.
48. Berezikov, E., Plasterk, R.H.A., and Cuppen, E. (2002) GENOTRACE: cDNA-based local GENOme assembly from TRACE archives. *Bioinformatics* **18**(10), 1396–97.
49. Zamore, P. and Du, T. (2005) microPrimer: the biogenesis and function of microRNA. *Development* **132**, 4645–52.
50. Vienna package, Accessed on August 29, 2009 at http://www.tbi.univie.ac.at/RNA/.
51. Ambros, V., Bartel, B., Bartel, D.P. et al. (2003) A uniform system for microRNA annotation. *RNA* **9**(3), 277–9.
52. Mathews, D.H., Sabina, J., Zuker, M., and Turner, D.H. (1999) Expanded sequence dependence of thermodynamic parameters improves prediction of RNA secondary structure. *J Mol Biol* **288**, 911–40.
53. PicTar algorithm, Accessed on August 27, 2009 at http://pictar.bio.nyu.edu.
54. Krek, A., Grun, D., Poy, M.N. et al. (2005) Combinatorial microRNA target predictions. *Nat Genet* **37**, 495–500.
55. TargetScan algorithm, Accessed on August 29, 2009 at http://www.targetscan.org.
56. Lewis, B.P., Burge, C.B., and Bartel, D.P. (2005) Conserved seed pairing, often flanked by adenosines, indicates that thousands of human genes are microRNA targets. *Cell* **120**(1), 15–20.
57. miRanda algorithm, Accessed on August 28, 2009 at http://www.microrna.org.
58. John, B., Enright, A.J., Aravin, A., Tuschl, T., Sander, C., and Marks, D.S. (2004) microRNA target detection. *PLoS Biol* **2**(11), 363.
59. Lall, S., Grun, D., Krek, A. et al. (2006). A genome-wide map of conserved microRNA targets in *C. elegans*. *Curr Biol* **16**, 460–71.
60. Betel, D., Wilson, M., Gabow, A., Marks, D.S., and Sander, C. (2008) The microRNA.org resource: targets and expression. *Nucleic Acids Res* **36**, 149–53.
61. The PITA algorithm, Accessed on August 30, 2009 at http://genie.weizmann.ac.il/pubs/mir07/mir07_prediction.html.
62. Kertesz, M., Iovino, N., Unnerstall, U., Gaul, U., and Segal, E. (2007). The role of site accessibility in microRNA target recognition. *Nat Genet* **39**, 1278–84.

63. Wu, X. and Watson, M. (2009) CORNA: testing gene lists for regulation by microRNAs. *Bioinformatics* **25**(6), 832–3.
64. The R project for statistical computing, Accessed on August, 27, 2009 at http://www.r-project.org.
65. Griffiths-Jones, S., Saini, H.K., Dongen, S.V., and Enright, A.J. (2006) miRBase: tools for micro RNA genomics. *Nucleic Acid Res* **36**, 154–8.
66. Durinck, S., Morean, Y., Kasprzyk, A. et al. (2005) BioMart and Bioconductor: a powerful link between biological databases and microarray data analysis. *Bioinformatics* **21**(16), 3439–40.
67. Barrett, T., Suzek, T.C., Troup, D.B. et al. (2008) NCBI GEO: mining millions of expression profiles – database and tools. *Nucleic Acids Res* **33**, 562–6.
68. Kanehisa, M., Araki, M., Goto, S. et al. (2008) KEGG for linking genomes to life and the environment. *Nucleic Acids Res* **36**, 480–4.
69. Sigterms, Accessed on August 28, 2009 at http://sigterms.sourceforge.net.
70. miRNA and mRNA Integrated Analysis (MMIA), Accessed on August 28, 2009 at http://129.79.233.81/~MMIA/mmia_main.html.
71. Karginov, F.V., Conaco, C., Xuan, Z. et al. (2007) A biochemical approach to identifying microRNA targets. *Proc Natl Acad Sci U S A* **104**(49), 19291–6.
72. Ebert, M.S., Neilson, J.R., and Sharp, P.A. (2007) MicroRNA sponges: competitive inhibitors of small RNAs in mammalian cells. *Nat Methods* **4**(9), 721–6.

Part VII

miRNA and Viruses

Chapter 21

Identification and Validation of the Cellular Targets of Virus-Encoded MicroRNAs

Kin-Hang Kok, Ting Lei, and Dong-Yan Jin

Abstract

Since the identification of the first virus-encoded microRNA (miRNA) in Epstein–Barr virus (EBV)-infected B cells in 2004, viral miRNAs have been found in different groups of herpesviruses. Viral miRNAs play an important role in regulating both viral and cellular gene expression. Identification and characterization of the cellular targets of viral miRNAs will not only advance our understanding of virus–cell interaction but might also reveal new strategies for the developments of antivirals. Our demonstration of the targeting of p53 upregulated modulator of apoptosis (PUMA) by an EBV-encoded viral miRNA provides one mechanism by which a viral miRNA facilitates viral replication by promoting cell survival. Using EBV miRNAs as an example, in this chapter, we detail the experimental procedures that can be used to identify and validate cellular targets of viral miRNAs.

Abbreviations

BART	BamA rightward transcript
CMV	Cytomegalovirus
EBV	Epstein–Barr virus
HSV-1	Herpes simplex virus 1
HSV-2	Herpes simplex virus 2
KSHV	Kaposi's sarcoma-associated herpesvirus
NPC	Nasopharyngeal carcinoma
PUMA	p53-upregulated modulator of apoptosis
SV40	Simian virus 40
UTR	Untranslated region

Silvia Monticelli (ed.), *MicroRNAs and the Immune System: Methods and Protocols*, Methods in Molecular Biology, vol. 667, DOI 10.1007/978-1-60761-811-9_21, © Springer Science+Business Media, LLC 2010

1. Introduction

Herpesviruses have evolved different microRNA (miRNAs) to facilitate their persistent infection of host cells (1–5). For example, Epstein–Barr virus (EBV) expresses more than 20 miRNAs and, some of them are highly abundant in both B cells and epithelial cells latently infected with EBV (5). As one of the most successful human pathogens, EBV has developed different strategies to subvert cellular control of immune response and apoptosis. It is, therefore, not surprising that the abundantly expressed EBV-encoded miRNAs might target different cellular transcripts that encode proapoptotic and immunomodulatory proteins (4, 6).

Both viral and cellular miRNAs utilize the RNA silencing machinery of the host cell to suppress gene expression by either translational repression or more rarely mRNA cleavage. The recognition of target mRNA requires Watson–Crick base pairing between the miRNA and 3′UTR of the transcript. One of the methods to identify cellular targets of viral miRNA is based on the search for sequence complementarity between viral miRNA and the 3′UTR of expressed transcripts. Below, we describe how we perform bioinformatic analysis and then experimentally validate cellular targets of miR-BART5, an EBV-encoded miRNA (see Note 1). Before searching for miRNA targets, it is critical to confirm the expression of miR-BART5 in the host cells (Subheading 3.1). We then carry out bioinformatic analysis to short-list a number of candidate genes that might be targeted by this viral miRNA (Subheading 3.2). The shortlisted gene targets are further validated in cultured cells using dual luciferase assay (see Note 1) (Subheading 3.3). Finally, after confirming the expression of miR-BART5 and its gene target [p53-upregulated modulator of apoptosis (PUMA)] in EBV-infected cells as well as patient samples, functional analyses should be performed to shed light on the biological significance of miR-BART5 targeting of PUMA.

2. Materials

1. Trizol.
2. 5 × RNA loading dye.
3. 10 × TBE.
4. 2 × SSC.
5. 2 × SSC, 0.5% SDS.
6. Zeta-Probe GT membrane (Bio-Rad).

7. ULTRAhyb-Oligo hybridization buffer (Ambion).
8. 10 × T4 kinase buffer.
9. T4 polynucleotide kinase.
10. [γ-^{32}P] ATP (10 mCi/ml, 5,000 Ci/mmol).
11. G-50/G-25 Sephadex column (Amersham).
12. 12% denaturing acrylamide gel [8 M Urea, 12% acrylamide (acrylamide:bis-acrylamide = 19:1) in 1 × TBE buffer].
13. pmirGLO vector (Promega).
14. Dual luciferase assay (Promega).
15. Genomic clone for 3′UTR cloning (imaGenes).

3. Methods

3.1. Detection of Viral miRNA in Virus-Infected Cells

The following protocol is for northern blotting of miR-BART5 in a nasopharyngeal carcinoma cell line C666-1, which consistently harbors EBV (7). C666-1 cells are used because the expression of BART miRNAs is particularly abundant in EBV-infected epithelial cells.

3.1.1. Sample Preparation

1. C666-1 cells are grown in 10-cm tissue culture plates until confluence (around 1 × 10^7 cells). Cells are then washed with 1× PBS twice. 1 ml of Trizol (Invitrogen) is added to extract total RNA (see Note 2).
2. Cells are lysed with Trizol for 5 min at room temperature (see Note 3) and then transferred into a 1.5-ml Eppendorf tube.
3. Add 0.2 ml chloroform and mix thoroughly by 1-min vortexing.
4. The mixture is then centrifuged at 12,000 × *g* for 15 min at 4°C.
5. Carefully remove the tube from centrifuge and transfer 0.5 ml of the upper colorless aqueous portion (see Note 4) of the lysate into a new Eppendorf tube.
6. Add 0.5 ml isopropan-2-ol into the aqueous portion and incubate at 4°C for 10 min. Precipitated RNA is then centrifuged at 12,000 × *g* for 10 min at 4°C.
7. The white pellet (~2 mm diameter) is washed with 1 ml of ice-chilled 70% ethanol. Cell pellet is air-dried (see Note 5) and resuspended in 20 μL DEPC-treated ddH$_2$O. Resuspended RNA must be stored at −80°C.
8. 20 μg of RNA is then denatured with 5× loading dye at 95°C for 2 min.

3.1.2. Probe Preparation

1. DNA oligonucleotide (perfectly complementary to the sequence of mature miRNA) is adjusted to 10 pmol/μL.
2. Prepare the following reaction mix (50 μL) and incubate at 37°C for 1 h.

Oligonucleotide (10 pmol/μL)	1 μL
10× T4 kinase buffer	5 μL
T4 polynucleotide kinase	1 μL
[γ-^{32}P]ATP (10 mCi/ml, 5,000 Ci/mmol)	5 μL
H_2O	38 μL

3. Reaction mix is purified by passing through G-50 (if the probe is longer than 20 nucleotides) or G-25 column (if the probe is shorter than 20 nucleotides) and stored at 4°C.

3.1.3. Northern Blotting

1. Northern blotting is performed using Hoefer miniVE unit. 12% denaturing acrylamide gel is prerun at 10 mA for 15 min in 1× TBE buffer.
2. 20 μg of denatured RNA sample is loaded and run at 150 V constantly for 2 h.
3. Gel is electroblotted in 0.5× TBE using Bio-Rad Zeta-Probe membrane (8×10 cm) at 30 V constantly for 1.5 h (see Note 6).
4. Membrane is UV cross-linked at 1,200×100 μJ/cm^3 for 100 s.
5. Prehybridize the membrane in 8 ml (1 ml per 10 cm^3) of ULTRAhyb-Oligo buffer at 42°C for 30 min.
6. Add 10 μL of purified radiolabeled DNA probe to the ULTRAhyb-Oligo buffer and incubate at 42°C overnight.
7. Wash the membrane twice with 2×SSC, 0.5% SDS at 42°C for 30 min (see Note 7).
8. Hybridized radiolabeled probe is detected by PhosphorImager.

3.2. Bioinformatic Search for Candidate Target Genes

In the following protocol, we describe the use of online database and software, as well as the selection criteria of the predicted target gene.

1. Fetch the mature miRNA sequence of miR-BART5 (MI0003727) from miRBase (http://microrna.sanger.ac.uk/) (8) and save in FASTA format.
2. Fetch all sequences of human 3′UTR from Ensembl (http://www.ensembl.org/biomart) using window-based BioMart generic data management system. Select the most updated database (Ensembl 56) and the right dataset (*Homo sapiens*

genes GRCH37). Choose sequences of 3′UTR only under "Attributes," export all the results, and save in FASTA format.

3. Run Miranda (9) using miR-BART5 as input 1 and 3′UTR as input 2, and select the top 40 candidates with the lowest minimal free energy (mfe) (see Note 8).
4. Further, select 10 candidates out of the 40 based on the following criteria (10):
   (a) Seed sequence (5′end of the miRNA that perfectly matches to the target mRNA) must be perfectly matched (at least six nucleotides, nt) with the sequence of the potential target, the more matches, the better.
   (b) Target sites that are close to the stop codon (approximately 15 nt) might have a hindrance effect and should not be selected.
   (c) Multiple target sites in one candidate gene's 3′UTR might be cooperative in gene silencing.
   (d) AU-rich sequences, instead of GC rich, near the target sites might facilitate miRNA recognition.
5. After selection of candidate genes, they can be searched for target sites of human miRNAs using TargetScanHuman (http://www.targetscan.org) (11). This provides a list of miRNAs (either conserved or not) which potentially target your input gene. In addition, it also provides the degree of sequence conservation and the alignment against other species.

3.3. Design of Luciferase Reporters and the Assay

Dual luciferase assay is a highly sensitive and well-controlled method to measure the activity of luciferase reporter protein overexpressed in cells. Proposed target sequence can be placed at the 3′UTR of the luciferase gene to mimic the real miRNA target site in the candidate mRNA. In our design, two types of luciferase reporter are used for target validation. One is the sensor of miR-BART5 and its mutant. The other is the luciferase reporter, which contains two tandem copies of the potential target sequence.

3.3.1. Design of miR-BART5 Luciferase Sensor and Its Mutant

1. Two tandem copies of sequence perfectly complementary to miR-BART5 are inserted into 3′end of firefly luciferase gene of pmirGLO vector (see Note 9). A spacer (an EcoRI site, GAATTC) is added between the two copies to facilitate effective mRNA cleavage induced by miR-BART5 (see Note 10).
2. The insert can be made by annealing the sense-strand oligonucleotide and the antisense-strand oligonucleotide. The annealed oligonucleotides are then inserted into the pmirGLO vector by classical cloning method.

3. The mutant can be made by the same strategy except that two nucleotides within the seed sequence are mutated. This mutant sensor should not be repressed by miR-BART-5.
4. Transfect the cells in 24-well plate format and harvest the cells for dual luciferase assay at 36 h posttransfection.
5. The level of repression should be calculated as follows:

[firefly luc (sensor)/Renilla luc (sensor)]/[firefly luc (mutant)/ Renilla luc (mutant)).

3.3.2. Construction of Candidate Gene Luciferase Reporter and Its Mutant

1. Using an approach similar to Subheading 3.3.1, the potential target sequence of the 3′UTR of the candidate gene is inserted into pmirGLO reporter. Three more nucleotides flanking the potential target sequence should be added to eliminate the possibility of false negative.
2. If more than one target site are found in one candidate gene, more reporters are needed to confirm the accessibility of each potential site.
3. After the validation of the target sites (see Note 11), full length 3′UTR is amplified from genomic clone to replace the 3′UTR of firefly luciferase gene in the pmirGLO vector.
4. The mutant reporter is then made by mutating two nucleotides in the target site (corresponding to the seed sequence of the miR-BART5), within the full length luciferase reporter.
5. The level of repression of the candidate gene reporter can be compared with that of the sensor (Subheading 3.3.1).

4. Notes

1. The sequence of most miRNA targets is not perfectly complementary to that of miRNA (12). However, the degree and pattern of matching are not conserved in all known miRNA:mRNA pairs. The difficulty to identify miRNA targets is ascribed to the lack of reliable bioinformatic tools. Thus, experimental validation is most important.
2. In this method, total RNA is extracted. Although alternative method can be used to preferentially obtain small RNAs of <200 bp, in our hands, no significant difference in miRNA detection was observed using the two protocols.
3. Cells are lysed in the presence of Trizol. Remember to pipette up and down to reduce viscosity of the cell lysis (dissociation

of nucleoprotein complex) so that the yield of RNA can be significantly increased.

4. It is important not to collect anything from the interphase (the middle thin milky layer) and the red lower phase (the phenol–chloroform portion).
5. RNA pellet should not be overdried. The best time to rehydrate the pellet is when it turns from white to colorless.
6. The small pore size of the positively charged Zeta-Probe GT membrane is good for small RNA retention and cross-linking.
7. Background signal can be reduced by additional washing with 2× SSC (supplemented with 2 μg/ml RNase A) at a 5-min interval.
8. The length of miRNA is around 20–25 nt. mfe is calculated based on the number of nucleotides which are perfect matches (G:C, A:U) or mismatches (G:U) between miRNA and the potential 3′UTR target. More matching should have lower mfe (e.g., mfe of miR-BART5 against PUMA 3′UTR is around −26), and thus, higher mfe (−19 or higher) is relatively less desirable.
9. pmirGLO vector is composed of both firefly and Renilla luciferase gene driven by PGK and SV40 promoter, respectively. Because firefly luciferase gene is driven by a relatively weak promoter, miRNA target sites inserted 3′ to this gene might be more sensitive to the repressive effect of miRNA. Renilla luciferase gene included in the same vector help eliminate context-dependent nonspecific effect during transient cotransfection.
10. Generally speaking, the target site, which is perfectly complementary to the sequence of the mature miRNA, will trigger mRNA cleavage (13). The inhibition (as determined by luciferase activity) triggered by the cognate miRNA is relatively stronger than that induced by an imperfectly matched miRNA.
11. Most experimentally validated target sites are imperfectly matched to the sequence of miRNA. The use of the miR-BART5 sensor is to provide the reference for the functionality and abundance of the miRNA. Normally, the repression of the sensor is more than 80%. Since the level of repression is calculated by the wild-type reporter (firefly luc/Renilla luc) normalized by the mutant reporter (firefly luc/Renilla luc), the repression level of the candidate gene luciferase reporter accurately reflects the effect of miRNA on the target site inserted to the 3′UTR.

References

1. Ghosh, Z., Mallick, B., and Chakrabarti, J. (2009) Cellular versus viral microRNAs in host-virus interaction. *Nucleic Acids Res* **37**, 1035–48.
2. Pfeffer, S., Zavolan, M., Grässer, F.A., Chien, M., Russo, J.J., Ju, J., John, B., Enright, A.J., Marks, D., Sander, C., and Tuschl, T. (2004) Identification of virus-encoded microRNAs. *Science* **304**, 734–6.
3. Cullen, B.R. (2009) Viral and cellular messenger RNA targets of viral microRNAs. *Nature* **457**, 421–5.
4. Choy, E.Y., Siu, K.L., Kok, K.H., Lung, R.W., Tsang, C.M., To, K.F., Kwong, D.L., Tsao, S.W., and Jin, D.Y. (2008) An Epstein-Barr virus-encoded microRNA targets PUMA to promote host cell survival. *J Exp Med* **27**, 2551–60.
5. Cai, X., Schäfer, A., Lu, S., Bilello, J.P., Desrosiers, R.C., Edwards, R., Raab-Traub, N., and Cullen, B.R. (2006) Epstein-Barr virus microRNAs are evolutionarily conserved and differentially expressed. *PLoS Pathog* **2**, e23.
6. Xia, T., O'Hara, A., Araujo, I., Barreto, J., Carvalho, E., Sapucaia, J.B., Ramos, J.C., Luz, E., Pedroso, C., Manrique, M., Toomey, N.L., Brites, C., Dittmer D.P., and Harrington, W.J. Jr. (2008) EBV microRNAs in primary lymphomas and targeting of CXCL-11 by ebv-mir-BHRF1-3. *Cancer Res* **68**, 1436–42.
7. Cheung, S.T., Huang, D.P., Hui, A.B.Y., Lo, K.W., Ko, C.W., Tsang, Y.S., Wong, N., Whitney, B.M., and Lee, J.C.K. (1999) Nasopharyngeal carcinoma cell line (C666-1) consistently harbouring Epstein-Barr virus. *Int J Cancer* **83**, 121–6.
8. Griffiths-Jones, S., Grocock, R.J., van Dongen, S., Bateman, A., and Enright, A.J. (2006) miRBase: microRNA sequences, targets and gene nomenclature. *Nucleic Acids Res* **34**, D140–4.
9. Betel, D., Wilson, M., Gabow, A., Marks, D.S., and Sander, C. (2008) The microRNA.org resource: targets and expression. *Nucleic Acids Res* **36**, D149–53.
10. Grimson, A., Farh, K.K., Johnston, W.K., Garrett-Engele, P., Lim, L.P., and Bartel D.P. (2005) MicroRNA targeting specificity in mammals: determinants beyond seed pairing. *Mol Cell* **27**, 91–105.
11. Friedman, R.C., Farh, K.K., Burge, C.B., and Bartel, D.P. (2009) Most mammalian mRNAs are conserved targets of microRNAs. *Genome Res* **19**, 92–105.
12. Bartel, D.P. (2009) MicroRNAs: target recognition and regulatory functions. *Cell* **136**, 215–33.
13. Doench, J.G., Petersen, C.P., and Sharp, P.A. (2003) siRNAs can function as miRNAs. *Genes Dev* **17**, 438–42.

Index

Silvia Monticelli (ed.), *MicroRNAs and the Immune System: Methods and Protocols*, Methods in Molecular Biology, vol. 667, DOI 10.1007/978-1-60761-811-9, © Springer Science+Business Media, LLC 2010

N

O

P

Q

R

MIX
Papier aus verantwortungsvollen Quellen
Paper from responsible sources
FSC® C105338

If you have any concerns about our products,
you can contact us on
ProductSafety@springernature.com

In case Publisher is established outside the EU,
the EU authorized representative is:
Springer Nature Customer Service Center GmbH
Europaplatz 3, 69115 Heidelberg, Germany

Printed by Libri Plureos GmbH
in Hamburg, Germany